Parasitology: Echinococcus and Echinococcosis

Parasitology: Echinococcus and Echinococcosis

Editor: Loyd Homewood

AMERICAN
MEDICAL PUBLISHERS
www.americanmedicalpublishers.com

AMERICAN
MEDICAL PUBLISHERS
www.americanmedicalpublishers.com

Cataloging-in-publication Data

Parasitology : echinococcus and echinococcosis / edited by Loyd Homewood.
p. cm.
Includes bibliographical references and index.
ISBN 979-8-88740-361-8
1. Echinococcus. 2. Echinococcosis. 3. Parasitology. I. Homewood, Loyd.
QL391.P7 P37 2023
595.122--dc23

American Medical Publishers,
41 Flatbush Avenue,
1st Floor, New York,
NY 11217, USA

ISBN 979-8-88740-361-8 (Hardback)

Contents

Preface VII

Section 1 Epidemiology 1

Chapter 1 **Molecular and Epidemiology Data on Cystic Echinococcosis in Tunisia** 3
Myriam Oudni-M'rad, Selim M'rad and Hamouda Babba

Chapter 2 **Echinococcosis in Mexico – A Story Worth Sharing** 23
Ana Flisser, Pablo Maravilla, Pilar Mata-Miranda and Fernando Martinez-Hernandez

Chapter 3 **Echinococcosis in Colombia – A Neglected Zoonosis?** 46
Alfonso J. Rodriguez-Morales, Lauren Sofia Calvo-Betancourt, Camila Alarcón-Olave and Adrián Bolívar-Mejía

Chapter 4 **Current Research Advance on Echinococcosis** 74
Shukun Yang, Yumin Zhao, Don Peter McManus and YuRong Yang

Section 2 Biological and Clinical Aspects 89

Chapter 5 **Echinococcosis – Rare Locations and Uncommon Clinical Manifestations** 91
Antonio Di Cataldo, Giuseppe Petrillo, Claudia Trombatore, Stefano Palmucci, Antonella Agodi, Martina Barchitta, Annalisa Quattrocchi, Nunzio Crimi, Silvia Fichera, Stefano Puleo, Amy Giarrizzo, Martina Calabrini, Rosalia Latino and Rosanna Portale

Chapter 6 **Brain Hydatid Cyst** 109
Said Hilmani

Chapter 7 **Radiological Characteristics of Pulmonary Hydatid Cysts** 118
Dilek Emlik, Kemal Ödev, Necdet Poyraz and Hasan Emin Kaya

Chapter 8 ***Echinococcus shiquicus* and *Echinococcus felidis*** 138
Adel Spotin

Chapter 9 **Genitourinary Hydatid Disease** 150
Santosh Kumar and Shivanshu Singh

Section 3 **Treatment and Prevention** 169

Chapter 10 **Hydatidosis and Intervention Strategies** 171
YuRong Yang

Chapter 11 **Immunotherapy Can Enhance Anthelmintic Efficacy in Alveolar Echinococcosis** 187
Emília Dvorožňáková

Chapter 12 **Surgical Management of Hydatid Disease** 222
Angeliki Vidoura, Mariana Parisidou, Christina Chatedaki and Dimitris Zacharoulis

Chapter 13 **Biliary Complications of Hepatic Hydatid Cyst Surgery and Prevention Methods** 229
Can Konca and Deniz Balcı

Permissions

List of Contributors

Index

Preface

This book has been an outcome of determined endeavour from a group of educationists in the field. The primary objective was to involve a broad spectrum of professionals from diverse cultural background involved in the field for developing new researches. The book not only targets students but also scholars pursuing higher research for further enhancement of the theoretical and practical applications of the subject.

Parasitology is a scientific discipline that is concerned with the study of the biology of parasites and parasitic diseases. A parasitic disease caused by infection with tiny tapeworms of the genus Echinococcus is called echinococcosis. It is mainly classified into two categories, namely, cystic echinococcosis and alveolar echinococcosis. The other types include unicystic echinococcosis and polycystic echinococcosis. Unicystic echinococcosis manifests as a slow-growing mass in the body. Alveolar disease generally starts in the liver, but can spread to other parts of the body, such as the lungs or brain. The patient may experience abdominal pain, weight loss, along with yellow-toned skin discoloration due to development of jaundice when the liver is affected. A major cause of the disease includes the consumption of food or water that contains the eggs of the parasite. It can also be caused by coming in close contact with an infected animal. The disease is diagnosed using blood tests and medical imaging tests such as CT scan and MRI. This disease can be prevented by vaccinating the infected animals. This book aims to shed light on some of the unexplored aspects of echinococcosis and the recent researches with respect to this disease. Its aim is to present researches that have transformed the study of this disease. This book will provide comprehensive knowledge to the readers.

It was an honour to edit such a profound book and also a challenging task to compile and examine all the relevant data for accuracy and originality. I wish to acknowledge the efforts of the contributors for submitting such brilliant and diverse chapters in the field and for endlessly working for the completion of the book. Last, but not the least; I thank my family for being a constant source of support in all my research endeavours.

Editor

Section 1

Epidemiology

1

Molecular and Epidemiology Data on Cystic Echinococcosis in Tunisia

Myriam Oudni-M'rad, Selim M'rad and Hamouda Babba

Abstract

Cystic echinococcosis (CE) or hydatidosis is a widespread zoonose in the world. In Tunisia, despite the deployed prevention program, CE remains a serious public health problem. With a human surgical annual incidence averaging 12.6/100000 inhabitants, Tunisia is one of the most endemic areas amongst the Mediterranean countries. Three Echinococcus species have been described: *E. granulosus sensu stricto* (G1 and G3 genotypes), *E. canadensis,* and *E. equinus*. CE, which commonly starts during childhood and described as a young adult disease, may be observed at any age. The liver and the lungs are the most commonly involved organs but the cyst can occur almost anywhere in the body. In production animals, the prevalence of CE is ranged from 16.42% to 40.42% in sheep, 8.56% in cattle, 6% in dromedaries, 2.9% in goats, and 8.48% in donkeys. The elevated number of stray and semi-stray dogs and their frequent contamination by *E. granulosus* infected viscera is the major cause of the CE spread. A high prevalence of *E. granulosus* infection has been reported in Tunisian dogs ranging from 3.75% to 27.1%, depending on the regions. Thus, the sanitary education concerning hydatidosis should be reinforced and efforts should be made to implement a targeted educational program.

Keywords: Cystic echinococcosis, Tunisia, molecular characterization, epidemiology, public health

1. Introduction

Cystic echinococcosis (CE) or hydatidosis, caused by *Echinococcus granulosus*, is a widespread zoonosis in the world, especially in North African countries such as Libya, Algeria, Morocco, and Tunisia [1, 2]. Alveolar echinococcosis (AE), caused by the larval stage of *E. multilocularis* is extremely rare in Maghreb and only three autochthonous cases of human AE were reported in Tunisia and Morocco [3–5]. CE is of veterinary and medical importance because infection with metacestode may cause severe illness and significant socio-economic repercussions. With an annual surgical incidence (SI) averaging 12.6/100000 inhabitants [6] and approximately US$ 10–19 million losses annually in both humans and animals [7], Tunisia is one of the most endemic areas amongst the Mediterranean countries. Neighboring countries such as Italy (SI=1.6), Algeria (SI=3.6–4.6), Morocco (SI=4.6), Libya (SI=4.2), Spain (SI=0.3), and France (SI=0.1) presented lower surgical incidence [1, 8, 9]. In the *E. granulosus* vital cycle the adult tapeworm lives in the intestine of some carnivores (definitive hosts), and the larval stage develops in the herbivores (intermediate hosts) and humans, essentially in the liver and lungs.

2. *Echinococcus granulosus* genotyping

E. granulosus is a complex in which four or five cryptic species are intermixed: *E. granulosus sensu stricto* (genotypes G1 to G3), *E. equinus* (genotype G4), *E. ortleppi* (genotype G5), *E. canadensis* (genotypes G6 to G10), and *Echinococcus felidis* (lion strain) [10–12]. The characterization of the species/genotypes responsible for human and animal hydatidosis is important in order to adapt the measures of control and prevention against this parasitic disease. Indeed, it is known that the genotype influences the life cycle patterns, the host specificity, and the pathology. Four genotypes (G1, G3, G4, and G6) have been described in Tunisia using molecular techniques such as PCR-RFLP analysis of the ribosomal DNA ITS1 fragment and mitochondrial cytochrome C oxidase (Cox1) or elongation factor 1-alpha (ef1a) gene sequencing (Table 1). The G1 genotype was identified in humans, sheep, cattle, and dromedaries [13–16], the G3 genotype in cattle and human isolates [17], the G6 genotype in one human case and in the Southern dromedaries [13, 16], and the G4 genotype in donkeys [16]. Recently, it has been demonstrated that donkeys can be infected by two different species, *E. granulosus s.s* (G1 genotype) and *E equinus*, occurring in sympatry [16].

Origin	No. of cysts	Gene markers	Genotype frequency (%)	Reference
Sheep	102	ITS1 and cox1	G1 (100%)	[13]
	33	12s rRNA	G1 (100%)	[18]
	10	Cox1	G1 (100%)	[17]
	33	Cox1 and ef1a	G1 (100%)	[16]
Cattle	79	ITS1 and cox1	G1 (100%)	[13]
	4	12sRNA	G1 (100%)	[18]

Origin	No. of cysts	Gene markers	Genotype frequency (%)	Reference
	10	Cox1	G1 (90%); G3 (10%)	[17]
	19	Cox1 and ef1a	G1 (100%)	[16]
Human	50	ITS1 and cox1	G1 (100%)	[13]
	10	Cox1	G1 (90%); G3 (10%)	[17]
	241	ITS1 and cox1	G1 (100%)	[15]
	25	Cox1 and ef1a	G1 (100%)	[16]
Dromedary	3	ITS1 and cox1	G6 (100%)	[13]
	13	Cox1	G1 (100%)	[14]
	11	Cox1 and ef1a	G1 (72%); G6 (28%)	[16]
Donkey	37	Cox1 and ef1a	G1 (40%); G4 (60%)	[16]
Goat	14	Cox1 and ef1a	G1 (100%)	[16]

Table 1. Molecular epidemiology of cystic echinococcosis in human and production animals in Tunisia.

The Tunisian situation is grossly the same as other Maghreb countries (Algeria and Libya) where the G1 and the G6 genotypes were reported in livestock and camels [19–22].

In Tunisia, the most frequent genotype associated with CE is the G1 genotype (*E. granulosus sensu stricto*) [13–16]. Currently, at least 43 different haplotypes were described for the Cox1 gene by molecular analysis in humans and different intermediate hosts (Genbank accession numbers: U50464, AY679144, AY679145, AY679146, KM014606-KM014644, Table 2) [13, 16]. The existence of genetic and phenotypic variants inside this genotype has been previously shown by using isoelectric-focusing techniques [23, 24]. Regarding the host origin, it has been demonstrated that there is a slight difference of the G1 genotype in parasite populations between sheep, human, and cattle (Fst values from 0.05 to 0.15) [16, 23]. The cysts originating from human (lung or liver) are intermediary between sheep and cattle origins as considering the genetic variability, whereas cattle and sheep isolates are slightly different [25].

GenBank accession numbers	Mutation	CO1 protein mutation	Host	Cyst localisation	Reference
U50464	C56T	A27V	Human, Sheep , Cattle	Lung and Liver	[13]
AY679144	T123C	None	Sheep	Liver	[13]
AY679145	G312A	None	Human	Lung	[13]
AY679146	T204G	None	Cattle	Lung	[13]
KM014606 to KM014644	-	-	Camels, cattle, goat sheep, human, jackals, donkey, wild boar	-	[16]

Table 2. Molecular epidemiology and G1 genotype genetic diversity observed in Tunisia.

3. Human disease with special focus on pediatric hydatidosis

The *E. granulosus* adult stage infects the Canidae that releases the parasite eggs in the environment through their feces. Humans are a dead-end host that do not play a role in the natural cycle of the parasite. They are contaminated by an accidental consumption of the eggs, resulting from the contact with an infected dog or through the ingestion of contaminated vegetables. Eggs result in the development of one or several unilocular hydatid cysts (Figure 1) that could grow up to 20 cm in diameter [15, 26, 27]. Because of the slow rate of cyst growth, clinical symptoms do not usually arise until several years after infection. The liver and the lungs are the most commonly involved organs but the cyst can occur almost anywhere in the body.

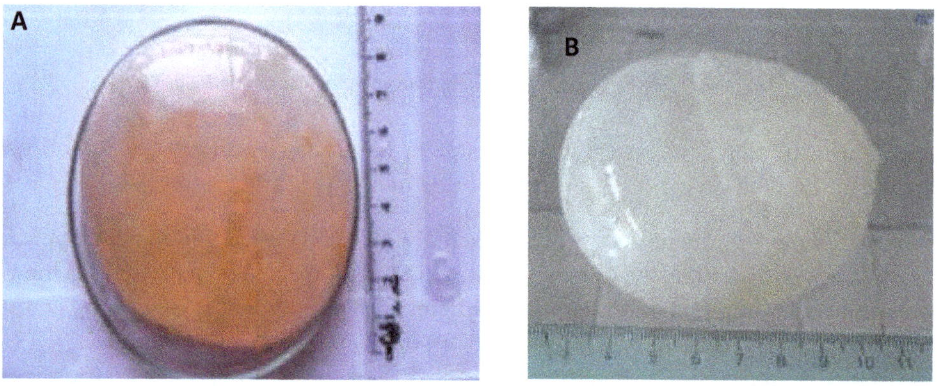

Figure 1. Hydatid cysts from Tunisian children operated at F. Bourguiba Monastir teaching hospital. A: Pulmonary cyst from an eight-year-old child. B: Hepatic cyst from a six-year-old child. Photograph: LP3M: Laboratory of Medical and Molecular Parasitology-Mycology, Faculty of Pharmacy, University of Monastir, Tunisia.

CE remains an important public health problem in Tunisia and despite the deployed prevention program, a slight reduction in the mean annual surgical incidence rate (SI) from 15 to 12.6 cases/100,000 inhabitants was observed during the last 20 years [6, 28]. The endemic status differs from one region to another, based on the SI, and some areas have been defined as hyperendemic (SI>22.6), holoendemic (15 < SI <22.6), mesoendemic (7.5< SI <15), and hypoendemic regions (SI < 7.5) [6]. The geographical repartition of different endemic regions was shown in Figure 2. Hydatidosis is known to be more important in rural areas where the definitive hosts (domestic and wild Canid) and herbivore intermediate hosts are in close contact, but an extension in the urban zones was noted during the past decade.

In Tunisia, several human studies were focusing on pediatric hydatidosis [15, 27, 29–31]. Cystic echinococcosis, which commonly starts during childhood or adolescence and described as a young adult disease, may be observed at any age. Two studies on children hydatid cysts (161 and 241 cysts) were carried out between 1999 and 2009 and assessed that the greatest number of cases was observed in the age groups of 4–9 years [15, 31]. Another retrospective study conducted between 1985 and 2009 and based exclusively on 757 pulmonary cysts of young

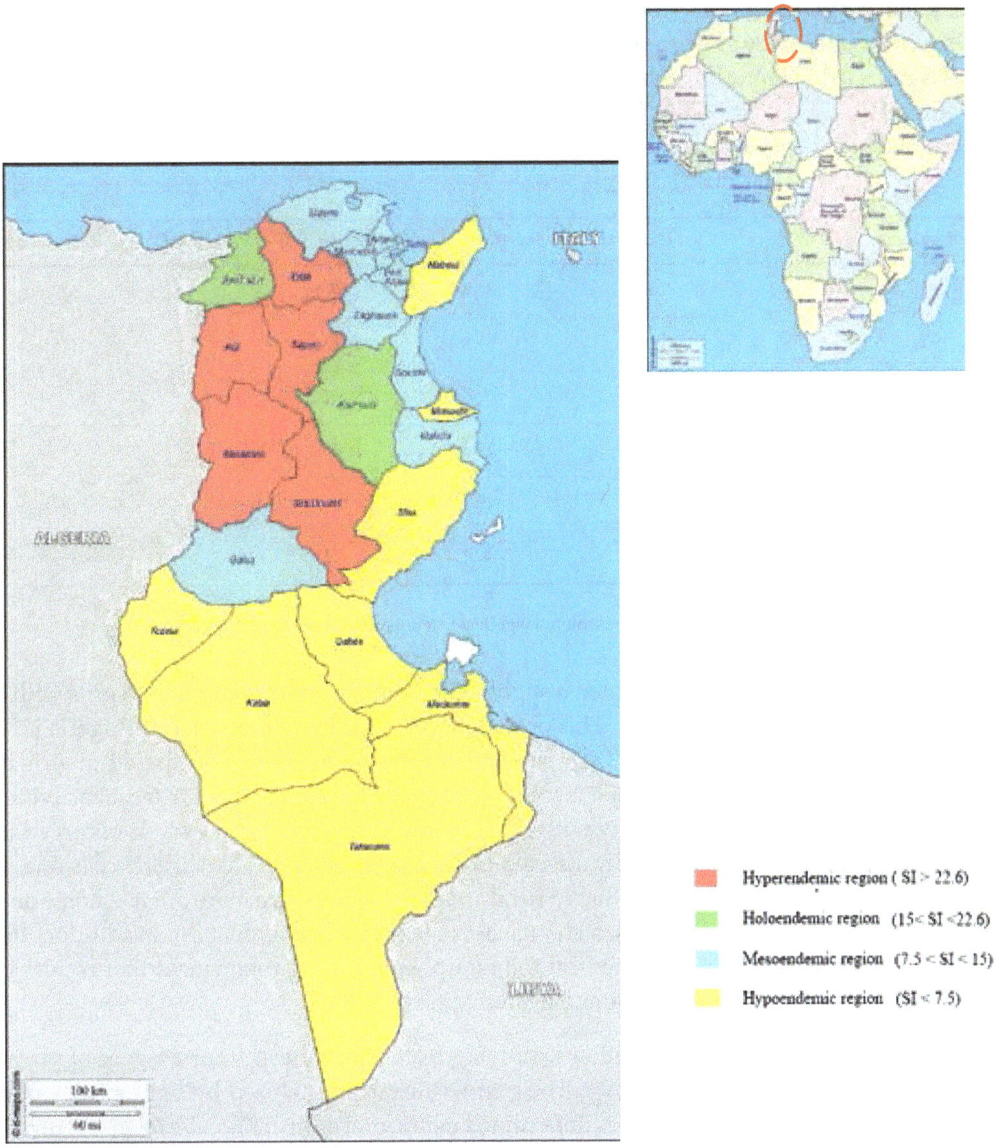

Figure 2. Hydatidosis endemic status based on mean human annual surgical incidence (SI) published by [6]. (The maps of Africa and Tunisia come from http://d-maps.com/).

children (3–7 years) and older children (8–15 years) demonstrated a mean age of 5.7 and 12 years old, respectively [27]. This early infestation has already been described in Turkey [32], Palestine [33], and Jordan [34].

In children, the lungs are the most common sites for hydatid cysts followed by the liver (Table 3) [15, 27, 31]. This could be explained by noisier and earlier symptoms in children where cough, chest pain, and hemoptysis are the most frequently encountered signs [27, 30]. Some exceptional cyst localizations (central nervous system, orbit, spleen, kidney, and heart) were also described [15, 35, 36]. Several organs may be contaminated simultaneously and about 20% of cases reported in literature were involved in multiple cysts with essentially liver associated with lung [15, 27]. The growth of the hydatid is independent of children's age since cysts of high diameter (15 cm) were found in children of 4 years old [15, 31].

No. of patients	No. of cysts	Cyst localization	Frequency (%)	Fertility (%)	Viability (%)	Reference
195	241	Liver	34.8	68.5	77	[15]
		Lung	61.8	83		
		Other	3.4	71		
121	161	Lung	59.5	70	79	[31]
		Liver	36	81.5		
		Other	4.5	71		

Table 3. CE prevalence, cyst fertility, and protoscoleces viability in Tunisian children.

Numerous pediatric studies have noted a slight male predominance compared to girls with a sex ratio of 1.2 to 1.8 [15, 27, 28, 31]. This observation was although reported in Algeria [37], Iran [38], Bulgaria [39], and Jordan [34]. The higher infestation of boys compared to girls in endemic countries is explained by the fact that school-age boys have more external activities than girls, with a greater promiscuity with dogs. In adults, in contrast to what is observed in children, women are more commonly affected than men [28, 40, 41]. This difference is due to their role in the home activities and that in rural areas, the women are more often at home and care very often for dogs and cattle, which increases the risk of contamination. In addition, the adult females have more regular medical follow-up (e.g., during pregnancy) that results in fortuitous cyst discoveries on ultrasound examinations.

The direct examination of the cyst allows studying its fertility (presence or absence of protoscoleces) and the protoscolex viability. The cyst fertility was analyzed by light microscopic observation. Protoscolex viability was determined using vital eosin 0.2% coloration (Figure 3). The fertility of the cyst is independent of its location and its size and no relation with the age of infected children was noticed (Table 3) [15, 27, 42]. The cyst fertility and protoscoleces viability in humans are not involved in the maintenance of the parasite life cycle because human is a dead-end host but they are parameters attesting of the perfect adaptation of the parasite to humans.

As mentioned before in the genotyping section, the most frequent species associated with human hydatidosis is the *E. granulosus sensu stricto* (G1 genotype). Nevertheless, for two children, the *E. granulosus sensu stricto* (G3 genotype) and the *E. canadensis* species were observed. The fact that humans could be infected by different species/genotypes is an epidemiological feature to be taken into account in CE control measures.

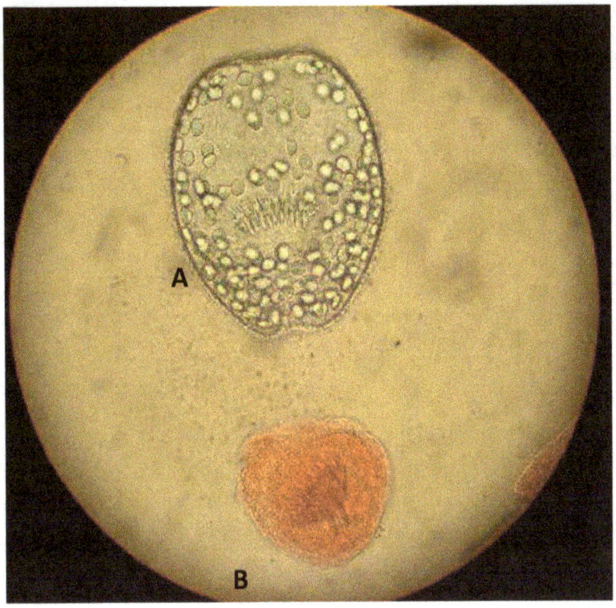

Figure 3. Determination of protoscolex viability by using 0.2% eosin coloration: Alive (A) and dead (B) protoscolex. Photograph: LP3M: Laboratory of Medical and Molecular Parasitology-Mycology, Faculty of Pharmacy, University of Monastir, Tunisia.

4. Cystic echinococcosis in production animals

Livestock echinococcosis leads to economic repercussions because of animal liver and lung condemnations, decrease of the carcass weight, animal fertility, and milk production [43]. In Tunisia, breeding remains mainly traditional and the population practices extensive sheep farming. Livestock are ubiquitous all over Tunisia, especially in rural areas and about 4 million sheep female unit (FU), 700,000 goat FU, 420,000 cattle FU, and 17,000 camel FU are recorded [44]. The CE prevalence in food animals depends on the presence of the intermediate host of the parasite and their close contact with the final host (stray and semi-stray dogs). These intermediate hosts differ from one region to another in function of climatic factors and/or breeding or alimentary practices. Thus, dromedary breeding is essentially located in Southern Tunisia (desertic climate) where camels are most consumed, whereas sheep and cattle breedings are practiced throughout the country. Herbivores acquire the infection through ingestion of *echinococcus* eggs excreted by the dog feces. The breeding of small animals is practiced by farmers, but also commonly practiced by households in rural and urban areas (Figures 4 and 5). The importance of pastoral animal husbandry constitutes a significant risk factor for echinococcosis transmission because of the close contact of production animals with dogs. Thus, the infected livestock that died on the pastures are not buried and dogs or other carnivores are able to access these cadavers and lead to complete the transmission cycle (Figure 6).

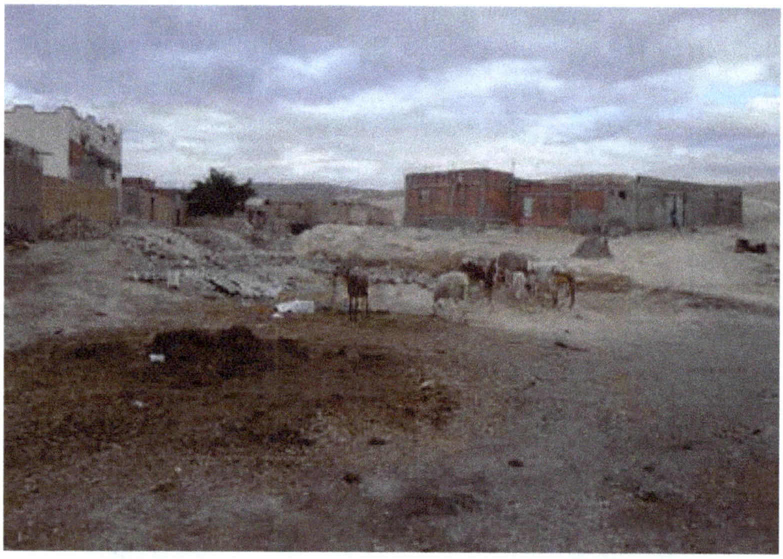

Figure 4. Pastoral sheep breeding in rural areas where sheep are in close contact with dogs. Photograph: LP3M: Laboratory of Medical and Molecular Parasitology-Mycology, Faculty of Pharmacy, University of Monastir, Tunisia.

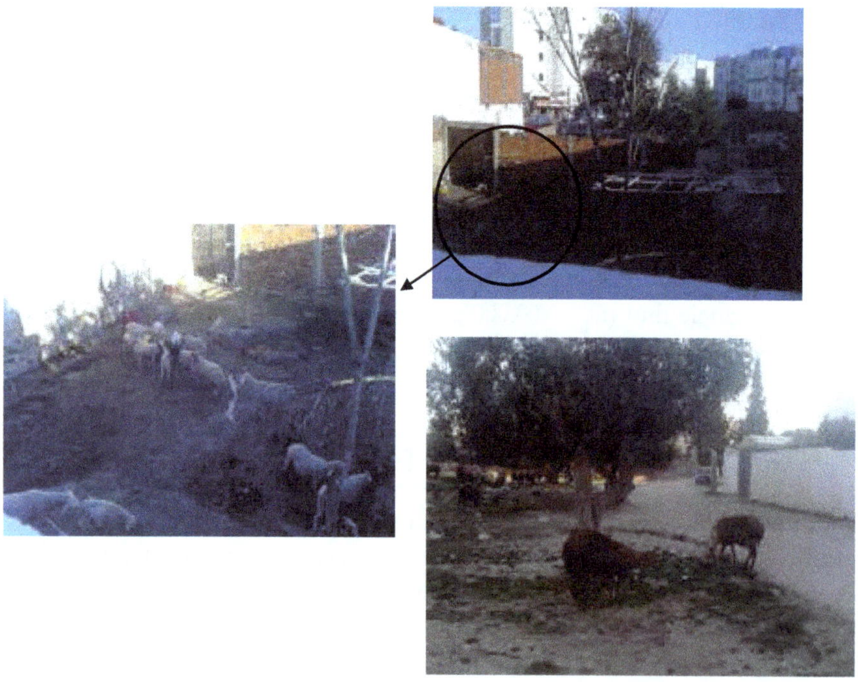

Figure 5. Sheep breeding in urban areas where sheep are in close contact with dogs. Photograph: LP3M: Laboratory of Medical and Molecular Parasitology-Mycology, Faculty of Pharmacy, University of Monastir, Tunisia.

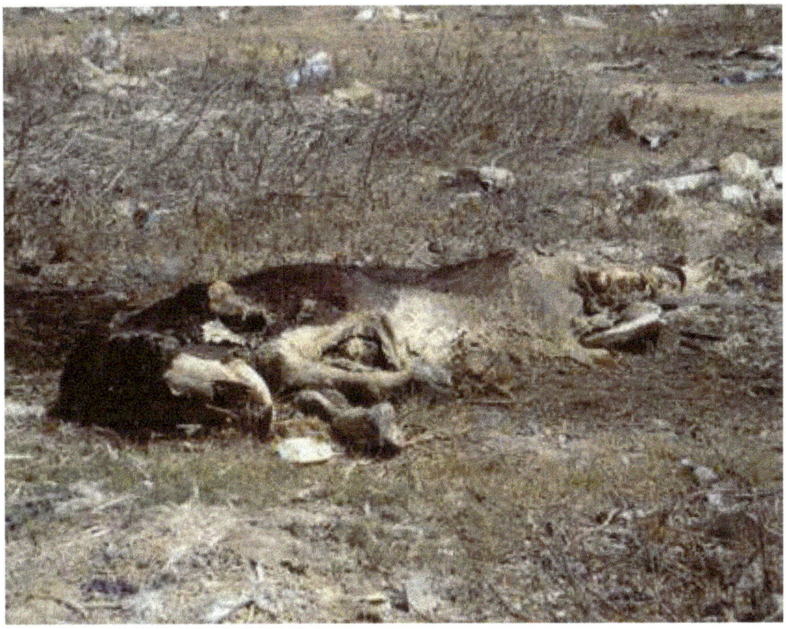

Figure 6. Carcass of dead cattle abandoned on the pasture and accessible to stray dogs. Photograph: LP3M: Laboratory of Medical and Molecular Parasitology-Mycology, Faculty of Pharmacy, University of Monastir, Tunisia.

CE prevalence in production animals was estimated by post-mortem examination of slaughtered animals at abattoirs. A series of studies carried out in Tunisia assessed that the prevalence of *E. granulosus* infection ranged from 16.42% to 40.42% in sheep, 8.56% in cattle, 6% in Dromedaries, 2.9% in goats, and 8.48% in donkeys [14, 45–47] (Table 4). The highest prevalence was observed in sheep, as is the case in Libya (20%) and Italy (11.5%) [21, 48], while the lowest prevalence was noted in goats. In Morocco and Algeria, the cattle (23%) and the camels (25%), respectively, are the most infected animals whereas husbandry and slaughtering practices are grossly the same as in Tunisia [19, 49, 50]. It has been accepted that variations in animal CE prevalence rates can be related to the species/genotype involved in the infection [51]. Nevertheless, in Tunisia, the G1 genotype is predominant in all intermediate hosts with high fertility rates [13] and only some infection cases by others genotypes are reported (see genotyping section). Moreover, a study conducted in Tunisia has demonstrated that the sheep over 8 years old are more often contaminated than sheep of 1-2 years and sheep of 4 years (60% vs. 20% and 40%, respectively) [46]. Consequently, in Tunisia, the difference in prevalence rate is more related to the age of slaughtered herbivores than to the species/genotype implied in the infection. In camels, the prevalence varies largely according to the region because of the difference in camel slaughtering practices. Thus, camels are slaughtered at an older age in South of Tunisia, whereas they are slaughtered at an earlier age (before 3 years) in Center of Tunisia. It has been demonstrated, in opposition to other intermediate hosts, that the camel cysts do not or seldom develop before the age of three [14, 52]. Therefore, it can be assumed that only old camels are implied in the parasite life cycle dog-camel.

Liver and lung are the only organs observed to be infected in production animals. The prevalence of the liver localization of the cyst was higher than that of pulmonary cysts except for the dromadaries where the pulmonary cysts are predominant (Table 4) [14, 45, 46, 53]. The co-infection of both organs in the same host is frequently observed and, contrary to what is usually described in humans, several cysts (up to 50 cysts) may develop in the same organ (Figure 7).

Hosts	No. of animals	Prevalence (%)	Location of cysts	Frequency (%)	Fertility	Protoscolex viability	Period	Reference
Sheep	2722	16.42	Liver	54.97	19.24	74.94	2003-2010	[45]
			Lung	45.02	11.01	66.49	2003-2010	[45]
	1039	40.42	liver	40.42	-	-	2001-2004	[45]
	248	-	Liver	67.33	86	-	2000-2005	[53]
		-	Lung	32.66	63	-	2000-2005	[53]
Cattle	3913	8.56	Liver	62.58	0.55	67.9	2003-2010	[45]
			Lung	37.41	0.40	89	2003-2010	[45]
	203	-	Liver	60.6	76.5	-	2000-2005	[53]
		-	Lung	39.4	27.5	-	2000-2005	[53]
Goat	3779	2.88	Liver	67.82	15.57	25.63	2003-2010	[45]
			Lung	32.14	14.75	14.8	2003-2010	[45]
Dromed-aries	404	5.94	Liver	86.27	22.22	65.86	2003-2010	[45]
			Lung	13.72	22.22	13.72	2003-2010	[45]
	291	6.5	Liver	7.69	-	-	-	[14]
			Lung	92.30	-	-	-	[14]
	8	-	-	-	100	100	2000-2005	[53]
Donkey	2040	8.48	Liver	89.9	3.58	35.80	2006-2007 and 2009	[47]
			Lung	10.09	15.38	32.96	2006-2007 and 2009	[47]

Table 4. CE prevalence and epidemiological data in Tunisian production animals.

However, available CE prevalence in livestock species does not reflect the real endemic situation since it is not considered private or illegal slaughtering. Uncontrolled home slaughtering during religious or local festivities is very common in Tunisia and the infected viscera

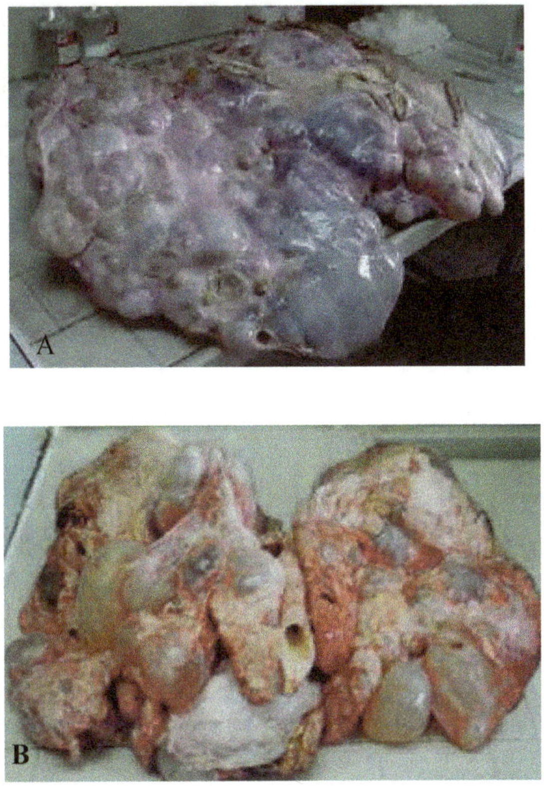

Figure 7. Multiple hydatid cysts in the liver (A) and lungs (B) of a bovine. Photograph: LP3M: Laboratory of Medical and Molecular Parasitology-Mycology, Faculty of Pharmacy, University of Monastir, Tunisia.

unsuitable for consumption are rejected and eaten by dogs. The knowledge of the parasite cycle and its transmission modalities are weak, in spite of a perception of the risk notably in rural areas. For example, a study conducted in 2007 (76 patients, 90 and 100 humans from urban and rural areas, respectively), has demonstrated that 40% of topics interrogated have the false notion that the humans' contamination is consecutive to the consumption of viscera containing hydatic cysts, whereas only 25.8% among them incriminate the dog [54]. The livestock trade in Tunisia is mainly based on weekly markets and exchange of animals all over the country. Thus, the lack of information on the exact geographical origin of livestock makes very difficult the identification of grazing areas at risk and the targeting of prophylactic measures.

Molecular analyses have demonstrated that *E. granulosus* species circulating in Tunisia are *E. granulosus sensu stricto* (G1 and G3 genotypes), *E. canadensis* (G6 genotype), and *E. equinus* (G4 genotype) [13, 16, 17] (see Table 1 in genotyping section). The cyst fertility and the viability of protoscoleces are the main factors that allow the maintenance of the cycle between intermediate and definitive host and leads to the existence of particular life cycles. Cyst fertility varied amongst livestock host populations with average rates of 44.8% (range: 11–86%) in sheep, 15%

in goats, 27.13% (range: 0.4–76.5%) in cattle, 48.5% (range: 22.22–100%) in camels, and 4.77% in donkeys [13, 14, 45, 47, 53] (Table 4). Contrary to what was observed in European countries [48], G1 genotype has a significant fertility rate (46%) in the cattle host in Tunisia [13] and Algeria (from 52% to 70%) [19]. In general, a significant fertility rate, as far as cattle was concerned, was due to the *E. ortleppi* species (G5 genotype) and rarely to *E. granulosus sensu stricto* (G1 genotype) [55, 56]. The findings of fertile hydatid cysts and viable protoscoleces in cattle, suggest that Tunisian and Algerian cattle can act as suitable hosts for the G1 genotype. The perfect adaptation of this genotype to bovine host is a significant parameter risk for human contamination via infected dogs and proved that cattle has more importance in the transmission cycle than previously believed.

5. *Echinococcus* in dogs

The CE is highly endemic in many North African countries and very high infection rates have been reported in dogs (55–58% in Morocco [49], 20–25.8% in Libya [57] and 19–42% in Algeria [58]). In Tunisia, although a sylvatic life cycle involving wild carnivores (golden jackals and red foxes) as definitive hosts was described [59], the *E. granulosus* transmission is typically through a synathropic cycle between dogs and livestock (essentially sheep, cattle, and camels). In Tunisia, the dogs are used primarily to guard livestock and property. The canine population is estimated at 800,000 dogs and composed essentially of feral and semi-feral (free-roaming dogs that are fed by an owner) dogs that rarely receive deworming treatment (Figure 8) [60].

In rural, urban, and semi-urban areas, the canine density is one dog per 3.0 to 5.5 inhabitants, one dog per 16 inhabitants and one dog per 46 inhabitants, respectively. In urban regions, less than 20% of households own a dog, whereas in rural regions there are 7–30 dogs per km^2, and more than 80% of households own at least one dog [61].

The prevalence of *E. granulosus* in dogs is estimated by several techniques including the detection of worms at necropsy, worm antigen in feces (coproantigen), or direct examination of eggs in dog feces. The prevalence of *E. granulosus* infection in Tunisian dogs ranges from 3.75% to 27.1% depending on the regions [59, 62, 63] (Table 5).

No. of dogs	Prevalence (%)	Worm burden (n)	Diagnostic procedure	Period	Reference
60	18.4	848	Necropsy	2007	[59]
375	3.75	-	Purgation	2002-2003	[62]
256	6.9-27.1	2534	Necropsy	1998-1999	[63]

n: mean number of parasites per infected dog

Table 5. Prevalence and molecular epidemiology of *E. granulosus* dog infection in Tunisia.

The study of the vital areas of stray dogs, based on 52 to 285 locations in a semi-urban area of Tunisia, has identified an area ranging between 0.06 and 8.53 km^2 [61]. Thus, considering that

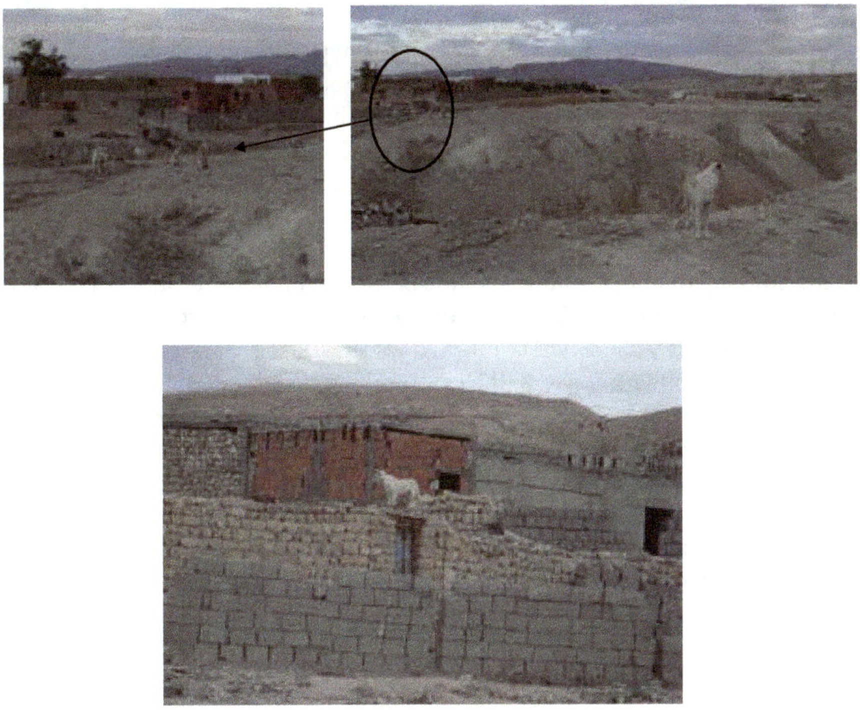

Figure 8. Stray and semi-stray dogs in rural area of Gafsa governorate (South of Tunisia). Photograph: LP3M: Laboratory of Medical and Molecular Parasitology-Mycology, Faculty of Pharmacy, University of Monastir, Tunisia.

the average number of worms per dog is estimated at several thousands [59] and more than 8,000 *Echinococcus* eggs were shed per day [64], dogs cause massive environmental contamination. Using direct examination of dog feces, the overall contamination index of dog feces by *E. granulosus* was estimated to 25.3% and was ranged between 8.3% to 41.3% depending on the regions [65]. Nevertheless, the canine echinococcosis is not necessarily correlated to human CE since transmission of echinococcus is influenced by human activities and behavior [65, 66]. As in many African countries, dog contamination is essentially due to the consumption of uninspected meat during familial or religious slaughtering, improper disposal of offal or carcasses unsuitable for consumption that are eaten by numerous stray and semi-stray dogs, and lack of knowledge about the transmission of the disease [50, 60, 67]. Thus, 38.4% and 44% of butchers and population, respectively, have an inappropriate behavior concerning the management of infected offal. They throw them directly into the trash or bury them superficially leaving them easily accessible to dogs [67].

6. Conclusion

Despite the control programs, essentially based on the systematic condemnation of infected offal in slaughterhouses, cystic echinococcosis remains a major public health in Tunisia. The endemic status differs from one region to another, and some areas have been defined as hyperendemic, holoendemic, mesoendemic, and hypoendemic regions. Hydatidosis is important in rural areas but an extension in the urban zones was noted during the past decade. The characterization of the species responsible for echinococcosis in Tunisia is a significant point that has to be taken into consideration in order to focus and to adapt the control measures. Three *Echinococcus* species (*E. granulosus sensu stricto, E. canadensis* and *E. equinus*) have been described in different intermediate hosts but *E. granulosus sensu stricto* G1 genotype remains predominant. The continuing presence of CE in Tunisia depends on a variety of factors and human behavior plays an important role in the perpetuation of the cystic echinococcosis. The importance of pastoral animal husbandry, the elevated number of unrestrained dogs, and their frequent contamination by *E. granulosus* infected viscera are the major causes of the CE spread. The inadequate deworming treatment, the close contact of untreated dogs with humans, and animals particularly in rural areas, the hygiene level, the poor public awareness about the disease, and the favorable ecological and climatic conditions for the survival of *Echinococcus* eggs in the environment constitute ideal conditions for the transmission of the infection to dogs, humans, and animals. Thus, the sanitary education concerning hydatidosis should be reinforced and efforts should be made to implement a targeted educational program. Awareness should be created for the animal attendants, farmers, customers, slaughterhouse workers, and butchers regarding the CE public health significance.

Acknowledgements

The authors thank Imen Hizem-Attig for her assistance with the linguistic part of this paper.

Author details

Myriam Oudni-M'rad[1*], Selim M'rad[1] and Hamouda Babba[1,2]

*Address all correspondence to: myriam.mrad@gnet.tn

1 LP3M: Laboratory of Medical and Molecular Parasitology-Mycology, LR12ES08, Faculty of Pharmacy, University of Monastir, Monastir, Tunisia

2 Laboratory of Parasitology, teaching hospital F. Bourguiba, Monastir, Tunisia

References

[1] Dakkak A. Echinococcosis/hydatidosis: A severe threat in Mediterranean countries. Veterinary Parasitology 2010;174:2–11.

[2] Sadjjadi SM. Present situation of echinococcosis in the Middle East and Arabic North Africa. Parasitology International 2006;55:197–220.

[3] Robbana M, Ben Rachid MS, Zitouna MM, Heldt N, Hafsia M. Première observation d'échinococcose alvéolaire autochtone en Tunisie. Archives Anatomo–Cytologie Pathologique 1981;29:311–312.

[4] Zitouna MM, Boubaker S, Dallagi K, Ben Safta Z, Hadj Salah H, Robbana M, Ben Rachid MS. Alveolar echinococcosis in Tunisia. A propos of 2 cases. Bulletin de la Société de Pathologie Exotique 1985;78:723–728.

[5] Maliki M, Mansouri F, Bouhamidi B, Nabih N, Bernoussi Z, Mahassini N, Elhachimi A. Hepatic alveolar hydatidosis in Morocco. Médecine tropicale: Revue du corps de santé coloniale 2004;64:379–380.

[6] Chahed MK, Bellali H, Touinsi H, Cherif R, Ben Safta Z, Essoussi M, Kilani T. Distribution of surgical hydatidosis in Tunisia, results of 2001-2005 study and trends between 1977 and 2005. Archives de l'Institut Pasteur deTunis 2010;87(1-2):43–52.

[7] Majorowski M, Carabin H, Kilani M, Ben Salah A. Echinococcosis in Tunisia: A cost analysis. Transactions of the Royal Society of Tropical Medicine and Hygiene 2005;99:268–278.

[8] WHO Regional Office for Europe, Copenhagen, Denmark. Centralized Information System for Infectious Diseases, Communicable Diseases, Surveillance and Response. http://data.euro.who.int/cisid (accessed 2014).

[9] Brundu D, Piseddu T, Stegel G, Masu G, Ledda S, Masala G. Retrospective study of human cystic echinococcosis in Italy based on the analysis of hospital discharge records between 2001 and 2012. Acta Tropica 2014;140:91–96.

[10] Hüttner M, Nakao M, Torsten W, Siefert L, Boomker JDF, Dinkel A, Sako Y, Mackenstedt U, Romig T, Ito A. Genetic characterization and Phylogenetic position of *Echinococcus felidis* (Cestoda : Taeniidae) from the African lion. International Journal for Parasitology 2008;8:861–868.

[11] Nakao M, McManus DP, Schantz PM, Craig PS, Ito A. A molecular phylogeny of the genus *Echinococcus* inferred from complete mitochondrial genomes. Parasitology 2007;134:713–722.

[12] Nakao M, Yanagida T, Okamoto M, Knapp J, Nkouawa A, Sako Y, Ito A. State-of-the-art *Echinococcus* and Taenia: Phylogenetic taxonomy of human-pathogenic tapeworms and its application to molecular diagnosis. Infection Genetic and Evolution 2010;10(4):444–452.

[13] M'rad S, Filisetti D, Oudni M, Mekki M, Belguith M, Nouri A, Sayadi T, Lahmar S, Candolfi E, Azaiez R, Mezhoud H, Babba H. Molecular evidence of ovine (G1) and camel (G6) strains of *Echinococcus granulosus* in Tunisia and putative role of cattle in human contamination. Veterinary Parasitolology 2005;129:267-272.

[14] Lahmar S, Debbek H, Zhang LH, McManus DP, Souissi A, Chelly S, Torgerson PR. Transmission dynamics of the *Echinococcus granulosus* sheep–dog strain (G1 genotype) in camels in Tunisia. Veterinary Parasitolology 2004;121:151–156.

[15] M'rad S, Oudni-M'rad M, Boubaker G, Bouazzi L, Gorcii M, Nouri A, Mezhoud H, Babba H. Etude rétrospective de la distribution et de la fertilité des kystes hydatiques chez l'enfant en Tunisie. Pathologie Biologie 2012;60:166-169.

[16] Boufana B, Lahmar S, Rebaï W, Ben Safta Z, Jebabli L, Ammar A, Kachti M, Aouadi S, Craig PS. Genetic variability and haplotypes of *Echinococcus* isolates from Tunisia. Transactions of the Royal Society of Tropical Medicine and Hygiene 2014;108(11): 706-714.

[17] M'rad S, Oudni-M'rad M, Filisetti D, Mekki M, Nouri A, Sayadi T, Candolfi E, Azaiez R, Mezhoud H, Babba H. Molecular Identification of *Echinococcus granulosus* in Tunisia: First Record of the Buffalo Strain (G3) in Human and Bovine in the Country. The Open Veterinary Science Journal 2010;4:27–30.

[18] Farjallah S, Busi M, Mahjoub MO, Slimane BB, Said K, D'Amelio S. Molecular characterization of *Echinococcus granulosus* in Tunisia and Mauritania by mitochondrial rrnS gene sequencing. Parassitologia 2007;49:239–246.

[19] Bardonnet K, Benchikh-Elfegoun MC, Bart JM, Harraga S, Hannache N, Haddad S, Dumon H, Vuitton DA, Piarroux R. Cystic echinococcosis in Algeria: Cattle act as reservoirs of sheep strain and may contribute to human contamination. Veterinary Parasitology 2003;116:35–44.

[20] Maillard S, Benchikh-Elfegoun MC, Knapp J, Bart JM, Koskei P, Gottstein B, Piarroux R. Taxonomic position and geographicaldistribution of the common sheep G1 and camel G6 strains of *Echinococcus granulosus* in three African countries. Parasitology Research 2007;100:495–503.

[21] Tashani OA, Zhang LH, Boufana B, Jegi A, McManus DP. Epidemiology and strain characteristics of *Echinococcus granulosus* in the Benghazi area of eastern Libya. Annals of Tropical Medicine and Parasitology 2002;96:369–381.

[22] Abushhewa MH, Abushhiwa MHS, Nolan MJ, Jex AR, Campbell BE, Jabbar A, Gasser RB. Genetic classification of *Echinococcus granulosus* cysts from humans, cattle and camels in Libya using mutation scanning-based analysis of mitochondrial loci. Molecular and Cellular Probes 2010;24:346–351.

[23] Oudni-M'rad M, M'rad S, Mekki M, Belguith M, Cabaret J, Pratlong F, Sayadi T, Nouri A, Mezhoud H, Babba H, Azaiez R. Genetic relationships between sheep, cattle and human *Echinococcus* infection in Tunisia. Veterinary Parasitology 2004;121:95–103.

[24] Oudni-M'rad M, Cabaret J, M'rad S, Bouzid W, Mekki M, Belguith M, Sayadi T, Nouri A, Lahmar S, Azaiez R, Mezhoud H, Babba H. Genetic difference between Tu-

nisian camel and sheep strains of the cestode *Echinococcus granulosus* revealed by SSCP. Parasite 2006;13:131–136.

[25] Oudni-M'rad M, Cabaret J, M'rad S, Mekki M, Belguith M, Sayadi T, Nouri A, Mezhoud H, Babba H. P-33. *Echinococcus granulosus* G1 genotype in three hosts (sheep, cattle and man) in Tunisia: Same or several? Proceedings of the International Symposium, Innovation for the Management of Echinococcosis, March 27–29, 2014, Besançon, France. Parasite 2014,;21:28.

[26] Ghedira-Besbes L, Haddad S, Ben Meriem C, Hammami S, Nouri A, Gueddiche MN. Giant hydatid lung cysts: About two paediatric cases. Respiratory Medicine 2010;3:174–178.

[27] Marghli A, Zairi S, Ammar J, Mohamed J, Ouerghi S, Boudaya MS, Smati B, Hamzaoui A, Kilani T. Pulmonary hydatidosis: A single-center study comparing older and small children. Journal de pédiatrie et de puériculture 2012;25:81–90.

[28] Ministère de la Santé Publique. Incidence chirurgicale de l'hydatidose en Tunisie: 1988-1992. Rapport interne de la D.S.S.B: Direction des soins de santé de base 1993.

[29] Chaouachi B, Nouri A, Ben Salah S, Lakhoua R, Saied H. Les kystes hydatiques du poumon chez l'enfant. À propos de 643 cas. Pédiatrie 1988;43:769–773.

[30] Chaouachi B, Ben Salah S, Lakhoua R, Hammou A, Gharbi HA, Saied H. Les kystes hydatiques chez l'enfant. Aspects diagnostiques et thérapeutiques. A propos de 1195 cas. Annales de pédiatrie 1989;36:441–449.

[31] Oudni-M'rad M, M'rad S, Gorcii M, Mekki M, Belguith M, Harrabi I, Nouri A, Azaiez R, Mezhoud H, Babba H. L'échinococcose hydatique de l'enfant en Tunisie: Fertilité et localisation des kystes. Bulletin de la Société de Pathologie Exotique 2007;100:10–13.

[32] Anadol D, Göçmen A, Kiper N, Ôzçelik U. Hydatid disease in childhood: A retrospective analysis of 376 cases. Pediatric Pulmonology 1998;6:190–196.

[33] Abu-Hassan N, Daragmeh M, Adwan K, Al-Qaoud K, Abdel-Hafez SK. Human cystic echinococcosis in the West Bank of Palestine: surgical incidence and seroepidemiological study. Parasitology Research 2002;88:107–112.

[34] Al-Qaoud KM, Craig PS, Abdel-Hafez SK. Retrospective surgical incidence and case distribution of cystic echinococcosis in Jordan between 1994 and 2000. Acta Tropica 2003;87:207–214.

[35] Limaiem F, Bellil S, Bellil K, Chelly I, Mekni A, Khaldi M, Haouet S, Zitouna M, Kchir N. Primary hydatidosis of the central nervous system: A retrospective study of 39 Tunisian cases. Clinical Neurology and Neurosurgery 2010;112:23–28.

[36] Jeblaoui Y, Bouguila J, Yacoub K, Bouguila H, Ben Neji N, Besbes G. Orbital hydatid cyst. Revue de Stomatologie et de Chirurgie Maxillo-faciale 2008;109:117–119.

[37] Zait H, Achir I, Guerchani MK, Hamrioui B. Profil épidémiologique de 290 cas d'échinococcose kystique humaine diagnostiqués au CHU Mustapha d'Alger (2006 à 2011). Pathologie Biologie 2013;61:193–198.

[38] Mamishi S, Sagheb S, Pourakbari B. Hydatid disease in Iranian children. Journal of Microbiology, Immunology and Infection 2007;40:428–431.

[39] Todorov T, Boeva V. Echinococcosis in children and adolescents in Bulgaria: a comparative study. Annals of Tropical Medicine and Parasitology 2000;94:134–144.

[40] Lahmar S, Rebaï W, Boufana BS, Craig PS, Ksantini R, Daghfous A, Chebbi F, Fteriche F, Bedioui H, Jouini M, Dhibi M, Makni A, Ayad MS, Ammous A, Kacem MJ, Ben Safta Z. Cystic echinococcosis in Tunisia: Analysis of hydatid cysts that have been surgically removed from patient. Annals of Tropical Medicine and Parasitology 2009;103:593–604.

[41] Bellil S, Limaiem F, Bellil K, Chelli I, Mekni A, Haouet S, Kchir N, Zitouna M. Profil épidémiologique des kystes hydatiques extra pulmonaires: A propos d'une série tunisienne de 265 cas. Tunisie Médicale 2009;87:123–126.

[42] M'rad S, Oudni-M'rad M, Chaabane-Bennaoues R, Hizem A, Bannour-Ben Abdeljelil A, Ksia A, Lamiri R, Mekki M, Nouri A, Mezhoud H, Babba H. P-32. Identification of *Echinococcus granulosus* species and case distribution of hydatid cysts in children in Tunisia: Proceedings of the International Symposium, Innovation for the Management of Echinococcosis, March 27–29, 2014, Besançon, France. Parasite 2014;21:28.

[43] Torgerson PR. Economics effects of echinococcosis. Acta Tropica 2003;85:113–118.

[44] Ministère de l'agriculture, Direction de la production agricole. Ressources génétiques et animales en Tunisie. Presentation presented at: A symposium; 2013 Avril 14-15; Abidjan, Côte d'Ivoire. http://www.au-ibar.org/events/au-ibar/237-the-9th-conference-of-ministers-responsible-for-livestock-in-africa?showall=&start=1.

[45] Lahmar S, Trifi M, Ben Naceur S, Bouchhima T, Lahouar N, Lamouchi I, Maamouri N, Selmi R, Dhibi M, Torgerson PR. Cystic echinococcosis in slaughtered domestic ruminants from Tunisia. Journal of Helminthology 2013;87(3):318–325.

[46] Lahmar S, Ben Chéhida F, Petavy AF, Hammou A, Lahmar J, Ghannay A, Gharbi HA, Sarciron ME. Ultrasonographic screening for cystic echinococcosis in sheep in Tunisia. Veterinary Parasitology 2007;143:42–49.

[47] Lahmar S, Boufana B, Jebabli L, Craig PS, Ayari H, Basti T, Dhibi M, Torgerson PR. Modelling the transmission dynamics of cystic echinococcosis in donkeys of different ages from Tunisia. Veterinary Parasitology 2014;20:119–124.

[48] Cardona GA, Carmena D. A review of the global prevalence, molecular epidemiology and economics of cystic echinococcosis in production animals. Veterinary Parasitology 2013;192:10–32.

[49] Azlaf R, Dakkak A, Chentoufi A, El Berrahmani M. Modelling the transmission of *Echinococcus granulosus* in dogs in the northwest and in the southwest of Morocco. Veterinary Parasitology 2007;145:297–303.

[50] Seimenis A. Overview of the epidemiological situation on echinococcosis in the Mediterranean region. Acta Tropica 2003;85:191–195.

[51] McManus DP. Molecular discrimination of taeniid cestodes. Parasitology International 2006;55:31–37.

[52] Ibrahem MM, Craig PS. Prevalence of cystic echinococcosis in camels (*Camelus dromedarius*) in Libya. Journal of Helminthology 1998;72:27–31.

[53] M'rad S. Etude par les techniques PCR-RFLP et séquençage du polymorphisme génétique d'*Echinococcus granulosus* isolé chez l'homme et l'animal en Tunisie. [PhD Thesis]. Sfax, University of Sfax; 2006.

[54] Benabid M, Chahed MK, Nouira R, Galai Y, Bouratbine A, Aoun K. Knowledge, behaviour and implications on hydatidosis. Revue Tunisienne d'Infectiologie 2007;1(4): 22–28.

[55] Thompson RC, McManus DP. Towards a taxonomic revision of the genus *Echinococcus*. Trends in Parasitology 2002;18:452–457.

[56] Thompson RCA, Kumaratilake LM, Eckert J. Observation on *Echinococcus granulosus* of cattle origin in Switzerland. International Journal for Parasitology 1984;14(3):283–291.

[57] Buishi IE, Njoroge EM, Bouamra O, Craig PS. Canine echinococcosis in northwest Libya: Assessment of coproantigen ELISA, and a survey of infection with analysis of risk factors. *Veterinary Parasitology 2005;130(3-4):223–232.*

[58] Bentounsi B, Meradi S, Ayachi A, Cabaret J. Cestodes of Untreated Large Stray Dog Populations in Algeria: A Reservoir for Herbivore and Human Parasitic Diseases. The Open Veterinary Science Journal 2009;3:64–67.

[59] Lahmar S, Boufana B, Lahmar S, Inoubli S, Guadraoui M, Dhibi MH, Bradsha W, Craig PS. *Echinococcus* in the wild carnivores and stray dogs of northern Tunisia: The results of a pilot survey. Annals of Tropical Medicine and Parasitology 2009;103(4): 323–331.

[60] Aoun K, Bouratbine A. Epidemiological data concerning hydatidosis in Tunisia, Médecine et Maladies Infectieuses 2007;37:40–42.

[61] Food and Agriculture Organization of the United Nations. Renforcement de la surveillance et des systèmes d'alerte pour la fièvre catarrhale ovine, la fièvre du Nil occidental et la rage au Maroc, en Algérie et en Tunisie. 2009. 17p. Projet GCP/RAB/002/ FRA.

[62] Lahmar S, Sarciron ME, Rouiss M, Hammouda A, Youssfi M, Mensi M. *Echinococcus granulosus* and other intestinal helminths in semi-stray dogs in tunisia : infection and re-infection rates. La Tunisie médicale 2008;86(3):279–286.

[63] Lahmar S, Kilani M, Torgerson PR. Frequency distribution of *Echinococcus granulosus* and other helminths in stray dogs in Tunisia. Annals of Tropical Medicine and Parasitology 2001;95(1):69–76.

[64] Gemmell MA, Lawson JR, Roberts MG. Population dynamics in echinococcosis and cysticercosis: Evaluation of the biological parameters of Taenia hydatigena and T. ovis and comparison with those of Echinococcus granulosus. Parasitology 1987;94(1): 161–180.

[65] Chaabane-Banaoues R, Oudni-M'rad M, Cabaret J, M'rad S, Mezhoud H, Babba H. Infection of dogs with *Echinococcus granulosus*: causes and consequences in an hyperendemic area. Parasites & Vectors 2015;8(1):231.

[66] Jenkins EJ, Schurer JM, Gesy KM. Old problems on a new playing field: Helminth zoonoses transmitted among dogs, wildlife, and people in a changing northern climate. Veterinary Parasitology 2011;182:54–69.

[67] Besbes M, Sellami H, Cheikhrouhou F, Makni F, Ayadi A. L'abattage clandestin en Tunisie: Enquête sur les connaissances et les pratiques des bouchers face à l'hydatidose. Bulletin de la Société de Pathologie Exotique 2003;96(4):320–322.

2

Echinococcosis in Mexico — A Story Worth Sharing

Ana Flisser, Pablo Maravilla, Pilar Mata-Miranda and Fernando Martinez-Hernandez

Abstract

At the beginning of the XXI millennium, while working at a general hospital in Mexico City, a young lady arrived with a previous diagnosis of liver amebiasis given six years earlier. Different treatments in various clinical settings were provided. In the hospital, the first approach was an ultrasound study and unexpectedly an *Echinococcus granulosus* cyst was clearly identified. The patient received adequate treatment and accepted to participate as the index case in an epidemiological survey performed in her community. Inhabitants, dogs, cattle, pigs, and sheep were studied; cysts in humans, pigs, and sheep were searched by ultrasound and dogs by coproantigens, livestock, and dogs were negative for larval or adult stages respectively. The use of ultrasound allowed the detection of two cases (overall prevalence 0.95). DNA of the patient's cyst recovered by surgery was purified, amplified, sequenced, and multiple alignments were performed and analyzed, identifying to *Echinococcus ortleppi*. Subsequently, in a population genetics study focused to evaluate the presence and genetic variability of the intestinal tapeworm in dogs and of cystic echinococcosis in livestock in central areas from Mexico, *Echinococcus canadensis* G7 was identified and was found only in pigs. Based on a genetic network analysis, the following deductions were made: 1) *E. canadensis* G7 in Mexico is very diverse and was probably introduced from abroad several times from different sources and from different countries; 2) G7 haplotypes grouped in the North American wildlife cluster are placed far from Mexican isolates, thus they might be ruled out as sources of introduction to Mexico; and 3) the species status for G7, formally named *E. canadensis*, is still controversial, because biologically different strains (G6 to G10) are currently unified, though ecological and genetic data appear to indicate otherwise.

Keywords: Cystic echinococcosis, *Echinococcus canadensis*, *Echinococcus granulosus*, hydatid cyst, Mexico

1. Introduction

Echinococcosis, a well-known helminthic disease [1, 2] is practically absent in Mexico since there were only 10 clinical cases of this disease reported in PubMed since 1962. Between 1990 and 1998, only 33 hospitalized cases with postoperative diagnosis of echinococcosis were reported in the yearbook statistics of the Mexican Ministry of Health. Except for two, all cases were in adult men: 10 were reported in 1993 and 21 in 1996. Furthermore, cases might have been in immigrants or travelers but there is no information available [3].

On the other hand, taxonomy of the genus *Echinococcus* has been a matter of controversy and some confusion, particularly for *E. canadensis,* since ecological and geographical strains have been unified into a single species [4-8]. In Mexico, the pig-dog cycle is mainly present and maintains the pig strain of *E. granulosus* sensu lato (s.l.) or genotype (G)7. Some epidemiological studies performed from northern Mexico indicate the presence of the larval stage or cystic echinococcosis (CE) in livestock [9-11]. In addition, *E. oligarthra* has been recorded in a wildcat (*Lynx rufus texensis*) [12], *E. granulosus* sensu stricto (s.s.) in a rural pig [13], and *E. ortleppi* (*E. granulosus* s.l., G5) in a patient [14]. However, there is no evidence that these species are being maintained in Mexico, because only isolated cases have been documented [15, 16]. Here we review and discuss those studies conducted on *Echinococcus granulosus* s.l. in Mexico.

2. The clinical case

In the year 2000, a 38-year-old female from a community in the State of Mexico, two hours NW from Mexico City, attended the General Hospital "Dr. Manuel Gea Gonzalez". She had never lived or visited outside her community. She was treated six years before for cholecystectomy; the surgical finding was a normal bile vesicle, as commented by the patient. Her main complaint was pain in the right hypochondrium without migration that started two months before admission to the hospital, fever, malaise, fatigue, moderate pain with spontaneous exacerbation, and partial remission. Her family history had no importance for the present disease. Previous medical treatment included various antibiotics and metronidazole for the treatment of a hepatic amebic abscess. These drugs were provided simultaneously with painkillers, thus the patient partially improved. A private clinician performed an ultrasonography study (US) and found an undefined cyst with an internal calcification and referred her to the General Hospital "Dr. Manuel Gea Gonzalez".

One of the hospital clinicians undertook physical examination. No cardiopulmonary abnormalities were seen and peristalsis was normal. On palpation, muscular resistance in the right hypochondria, hepatomegaly, and no signs of acute abdomen were found. Laboratory tests were normal. US showed a solitary cyst that measured around 6 cm and contained undulating hyperechogenic membranes floating inside the cyst fluid (Figure 1a). Computed tomography (CT) image showed a similar pattern (Figure 1b). Since both images resembled a hydatid cyst, an intradermal Casoni test was performed. A thickening of 4 cm at 15 minutes and at 24 hours was detected. Since this test cross-reacts with other helminthes [17], coproparasitological tests were performed for larva and eggs and the results were negative. Albendazole at 800 mg daily was given for two weeks.

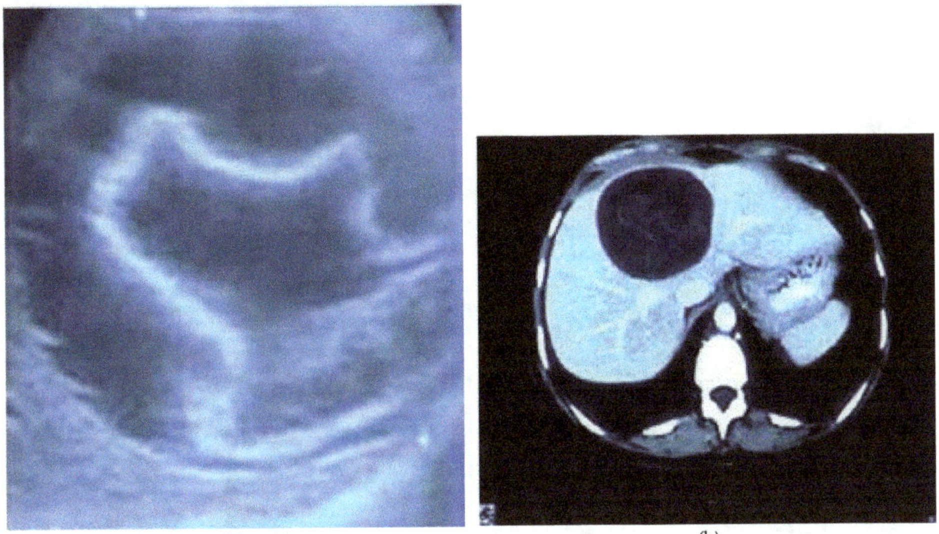

(a) (b)

Figure 1. Hepatic hydatid cyst of the patient; the ultrasonographic image shows a solitary cyst that measured around 6 cm and contained undulating hyper-echogenic membranes floating inside the cyst fluid (a); the CT shows a similar hiperdense pattern (b).

A colangic-pancreatographic retrograde endoscopy (CPRE) was performed to eliminate the possibility of communicating biliary ducts. The result of this procedure was negative but the patient developed severe post-CPRE pancreatitis, thus enteral feeding was started and albendazole was stopped after one week. Laparoscopic surgery was performed two weeks later by the surgical team of the hospital, using percutaneous aspiration-instillation-reaspiration (PAIR) [18-21]. The cyst was punctured to extract the intracystic fluid (Figure 2a) and instill 100 cc of hypertonic saline solution (17.7% NaCl) as a scolicidal agent (Figure 2b) that was left for 10 minutes. The upper part of the cyst was also irrigated and opened; exploration within the cyst clearly showed the germinal membrane (Figure 2c) that was totally extracted (Figure 2d). No complications arose during the surgical procedure. Seven days later, the patient was sent home without any symptoms. A CT performed 60 days after surgery showed a fluid filled cavity with 50% size reduction. In spite of our lack of experience in the treatment of liver cystic echinococcosis, the decision to perform laparoscopy was taken since the cyst was free in the right liver lobule and the patient could have a surgical procedure of minimal invasion as a definitive treatment for the parasitic disease, which came out successful, without complications or recurrence according to the TC performed 14 and 60 days later.

At the Center for Disease Control and Prevention in Atlanta (CDC), USA, ELISA and western blot were done with the serum samples taken before, 2, 3, and 11 weeks after surgery. All were positive to echinococcosis, and the western blot showed the 8 kDa diagnostic band [22]. At

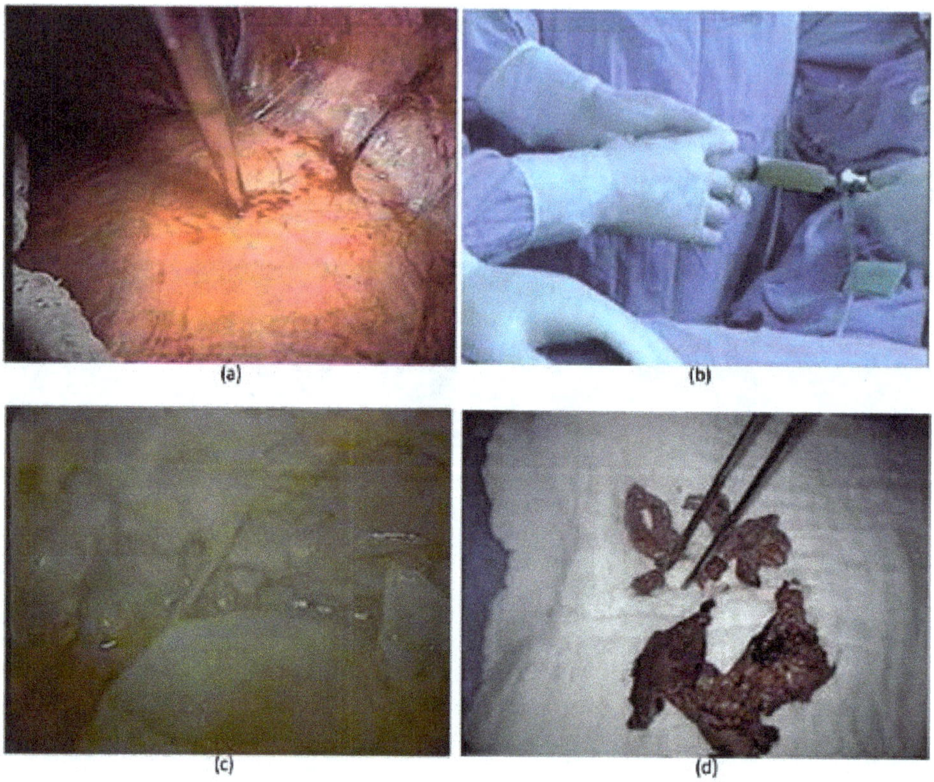

Figure 2. The hydatid cyst was punctured to extract the cyst fluid (a) and instill hypertonic saline solution (b); the germinal membrane could be seen from the inner surface of the cyst capsule, in the lower part of the figure the parasite's membrane is smooth, while the host's capsule, seen in the upper side of the figure (c) is rough, probably due to the inflammatory reaction; the germinal membrane was fully extracted (d).

laparoscopy, 90 ml hydatid fluid was collected, immediately low-speed centrifuged, and the pellet was analyzed. Light microscopy showed many protoscolices, mostly damaged (Figure 3a), while the sample obtained after PAIR treatment contained only debris (Figure 3b). These images are probably due to the effect of albendazole and the hypertonic solution, respectively. We tried to confirm and pursue the infection by orally introducing around 500 protoscolices into a young dog, but coproparasitoscopic studies were negative after two months and no parasites were detected at necropsy. Worthwhile mentioning is that for several years the patient received treatments without definitive diagnosis, since bacterial infections, amebic liver abscess, and vesicular problems were presumed. CE is a well-known parasitic disease, its diagnosis, medical treatment, and epidemiology have been exhaustively published [1, 2], imaging techniques are available, and cysts are specific. Nevertheless, differential diagnosis of CE in gastrointestinal malaise is not considered in Mexico [23, 24].

DNA from the germinal layer of the cyst obtained during laparoscopic surgery was obtained and analyzed by RAPD, 18s rRNA PCR-RFLP, and *coI* PCR-sequencing techniques. Banding profiles and sequence analysis matched 100% to *Echinococcus ortleppi* (*E. granulosus* s.l. G5,

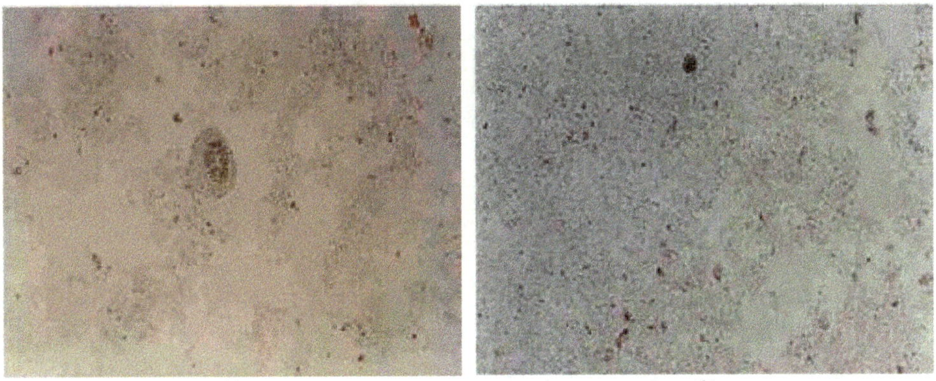

(a) (b)

Figure 3. Micrograph of the pellet obtained after centrifugation of the cyst fluid before instilling the hypertonic solution (a) and after this process (b). An *Echinococcus* protoscolex can be seen in (a) but only detritus in (b).

cattle strain). Interestingly, there are few human cases documented for CE in humans by *E. ortleppi* in the world. DNA analysis of partly calcified cyst recovered from an infected Dutch boy suggested that this *Echinococcus* species can be infective to humans [25] since in regions such as the Netherlands and Switzerland where the cattle strain occurs, cattle may act as a source of human infection. In addition, a first case of cattle strain (G5) in humans in South America was also reported in a rural community of Argentina [26].

3. Epidemiologic study

Between September and November 2002, a cross-sectional study was undertaken in the area of the index case, Santa Cruz, Tepozotlan, State of Mexico [3]. The objective of this work was to determine the prevalence and distribution of human echinococcosis and its probable risk factors. This US-based study was a pilot to search for autochthonous human echinococcosis in Mexico. Initially, authorization to perform the study was obtained from the jurisdiction, local authorities, and the clinician in charge of the Health Center. Ethics and Research Commissions of the Hospital General "Dr. Manuel Gea González" approved the research protocol. Household census was used to randomly select houses, visits were done in order to obtain cartography from the community and to identify street names and house numbers. Demographic, household characteristics, and animals were registered. The community, Santa Cruz, is located in the municipality of Tepozotlan, State of Mexico at 19°42′50″ N and 99°13′24″ W at 2300 masl. The municipality belongs to a warm zone bordered by 4 mountain ranges: Sierra Madre Occidental, Eje Neovolcanico, Sierra Madre Oriental y Sierra Madre del Sur (Figure 4a).

An initial field exercise was performed in the community Cañadas de Cisneros, close to Santa Cruz, in order to train the field workers, to evaluate if the content of the family questionnaire was clearly understood and to register the average time that each worker needed to fill one family questionnaire. One hundred people were interviewed during the exercise and the

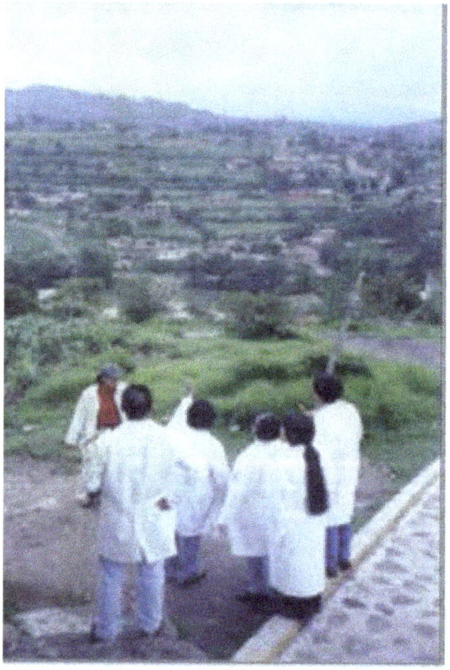

(a)

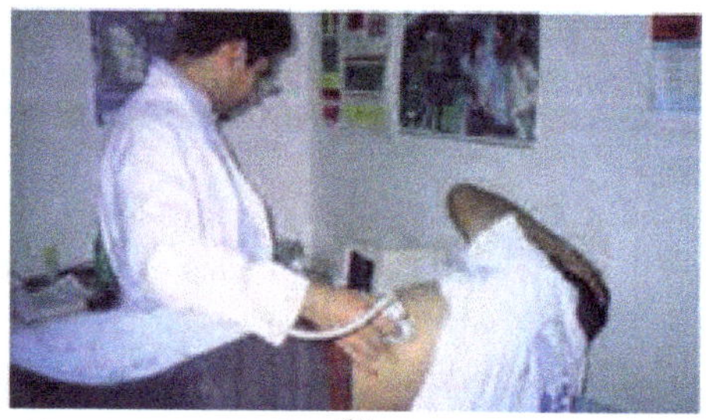

(b)

Figure 4. Scenery of the community of Santa Cruz (a), an ultrasound participant of the community (b).

average time for answering one questionnaire was 10 minutes. Most questions were clearly understood, except when asked if inhabitants had animals, 60% answered no but many had dogs, so another question specific on having dogs was added. This questionnaire was used for the investigation of risk factors in a larger population.

Santa Cruz had then 405 houses (11 were uninhabited), 98% of the streets were paved, electric power, telephone, and drinking water were available, the latter by a chlorine facility. There was no drainage thus latrines were used. Of the 375 houses that were submitted to a census 1,911 inhabitants were found, with an average of 5 (from 1 to 17) per house. Women constituted 63%, average age was 27; 20% of men and women were between 3 and 24 years and 30% were between 25 and 44 years; 48% were single, 41% married, the remaining were widows, couples separated or living together; 39% studied primary school, 24% middle school, 17% high school, 5% kindergarten, 3% bachelor, and 7% illiterate. Male workers made almost half of the population; students (30%) and house workers (23%) constituted the other half. Most houses were built of brick, sand, and had latrines, although 3% used the field. Drinking water was available in 86% of the houses, half of which boil the water before drinking, those lacking drink water from a well. Dogs were present in 83% of houses, 79% were vaccinated for rabies, most slept outside, although half of the dogs were kept tied. Of the 426 dogs in the community, feces were collected from 414 to examine for cestode eggs. After treatment and purge, 3 dogs had *Taenia pisiformis* but none had *Echinococcus*. Also, 83% of people had livestock, 77% were kept close to the house.

Sample size was defined for prevalence, each house was considered a unit; 94 houses were randomly selected and the index case and her family were also included. Families were visited to inform them about the study and invite them to participate; a written informed consent was requested. All members of the selected families were also invited to attend the Health Center for a free US; those units that did not accept, the house to the right replaced them. Cysts were searched in liver, spleen, and kidneys and cyst characteristics were recorded. Blood was drawn from people with images suggestive of CE, serum samples were sent to CDC for diagnosis confirmation, and an in-depth questionnaire was applied to them.

Only 331 people out of the 543 that were invited to have a US attended (Figure 4b). To avoid bias, families that attended and those that did not attend were compared for differences in demographic data. A high proportion of students and house workers were observed; the opposite was found with male workers who were less in the group that undertook a US; this was to be expected because workers could not lose a working day. Regarding knowledge of the disease, 8% of participants older than 18 years said they heard of hydatid cysts or "sand (arenilla)" and 15% referred having seen cysts in livestock viscera. Concerning interaction with dogs, 37% said dogs were guardians, 34% said they were friends or pets, 20% were companions or toys, and 9% said that dogs transmit diseases. How do people show kindness to dogs? 32% pet them, 25% talk to them, and 9% hug and kiss their dogs. While 26% of dogs lick their owners, 22% play or jump, 15% touch their legs, 12% bark, and 25% did not answer. Out of 331 US performed, 2 people had images suggestive of hydatid cysts; added to the index case give a prevalence of 0.9%. Cases were distributed in the same sector of the community (Figure 5). The close distribution of cases suggests the same exposure source.

The index case has been described at the beginning of this chapter in all clinical aspects. Epidemiologic data showed that the husband was a veterinarian. They lived with 12 other family members; all were submitted to diagnostic assays; Casoni test was positive in 3 people at 15 minutes but negative at 48 hours, all 12 were negative in ELISA, and in coproparasitoscopic studies. The house had a cement floor and walls, they had a small farm with 4 sheep, 3 cows, 2 horses, and 1 pig; they also grew vegetables and had 4 dogs that are fed with fresh viscera from livestock slaughtered in the backyard. Dogs were held in the same place for 3 days in order to collect feces to look for the adult parasite, and the results were negative.

The second case detected during the US survey was an 89-year-old married male, without digestive or abdominal symptomatology. The US showed one irregular 76 x 72 mm lesion with a defined wall in the right hepatic lobule, having two densities, one anechoic and internal echoes like snowflakes (Figure 6a). The serum sample was negative. He lived with 6 people in a brick house with a cement floor; he grew vegetables, fresh water was kept in a cistern, drinking water in flasks and had a latrine. He had 2 dogs that were held at the entrance of the house, slept outside, and were fed with leftovers, never with fresh viscera.

The third case, also detected during the US screening survey, was a 46-year-old married female. The US showed one 55 x 48 mm lesion in the left hepatic lobule with a wall slightly limited by a hyperechoic round ring (Figure 6b). The serum sample was negative. There were 4 households, she finished primary school, lived in a brick house with a cement floor, had a latrine,

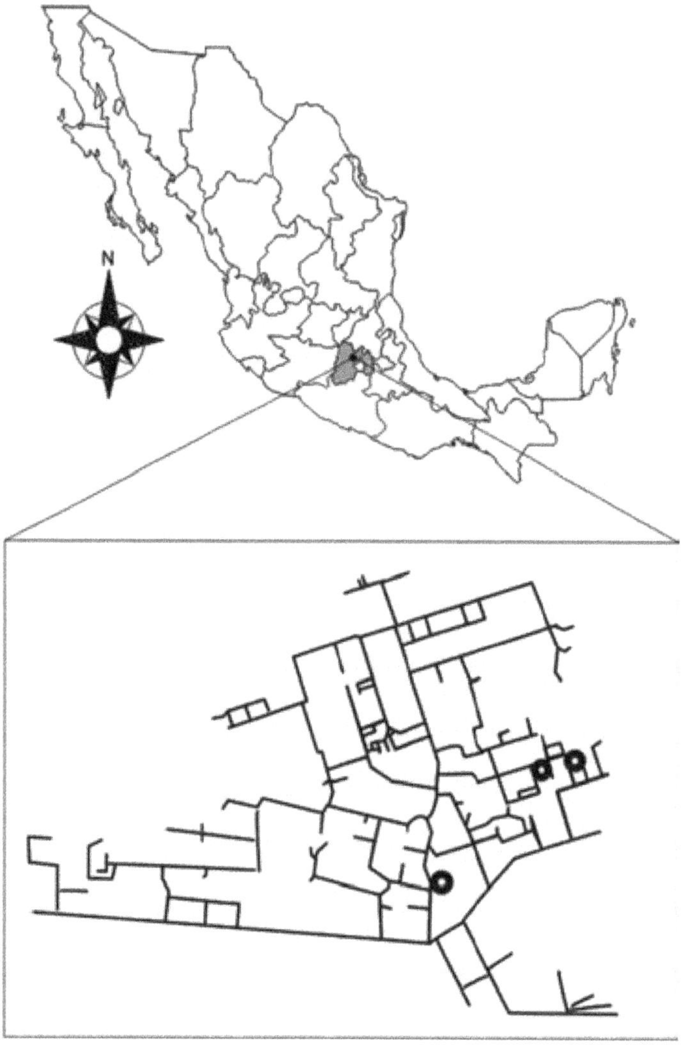

Figure 5. Location of the community of Santa Cruz in Mexico and of the cases in the community. Kindly reproduced with permission of the American Society of Tropical Medicine.

fresh water was kept in a small cistern, they boiled drinking water and kept it in flasks. They did not grow vegetables and did not have dogs.

These 2 cases were not confirmed by molecular techniques since, being asymptomatic, they were not offered any treatment at that time. Nevertheless, interestingly, in addition to the fact that the cases lived more or less close by, is the finding that the hydatid cysts of both cases detected in the community had similar sizes (between 5 cm and 7 cm). It is known that hydatid cysts grow approximately 1 cm per year [1, 2], suggesting that exposure occurred around 6 years earlier, and also that possibly one dog harboring *E. granulosus* s.l. adult parasites, living at that time in close contact with their houses, could have infected both patients.

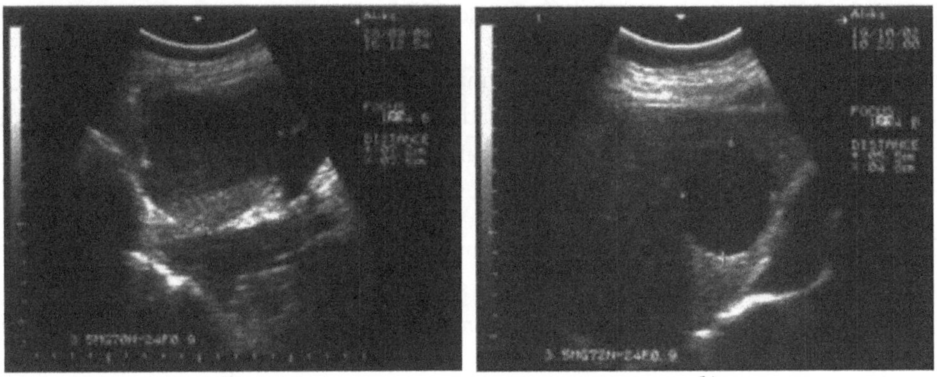

(a) (b)

Figure 6. US of the second (a) and third probable (b) cases. Kindly reproduced with permission of the American Society of Tropical Medicine.

4. Population genetics study for *Echinococcus*

Due to scarce source of genetic information and as an attempt to clarify the status of *Echinococcus granulosus* s.l. and genetic variability in Mexico, the presence of the intestinal tapeworms in dogs and of CE in livestock of north and central areas from Mexico with informal reports of this parasite was conducted [16].

5. CE in slaughterhouses

Several sanitary inspections to the municipal slaughterhouse of Calera, Zacatecas took place between December 2005 and June 2006 to identify CE in visceral organs, as well as to obtain data regarding the infected animals, place of origin, owner information, and number and size of cysts. In this slaughterhouse, formal farm and backyard livestock animals are accepted, coming from Zacatecas and nearby states (Aguascalientes, Morelos, and San Luis Potosi), thus offal from 387 pigs, 243 bovines, and 32 sheep were inspected for the larval stage of *Echinococcus*. Of the more than 660 animal viscera inspected in the Calera slaughterhouse, 18 pigs showed CE (7 males and 11 females, $P<0.05$), with a mean of 8 hepatic cysts per animal with average size of 3.7±1.7 cm. Interestingly, a similar tendency about gender in infected animals was observed in the experimental model of CE in mice, where female have a higher number of cysts in liver than male [27]. The global frequency of 5% of CE in pigs seen in the municipal slaughterhouse of Calera and the community studied are similar to previous data of Mexico [9, 13], but lower than those from other Latin American countries that can be as high as 12% for livestock [28]. Samples of fluid cysts from 9 pigs (6 from Zacatecas, 2 from Aguascalientes, and 1 from Morelos) were recovered and stored in 70% ethanol and processed for molecular analysis. PCR for amplifying a partial sequence of mitochondrial cytochrome oxidase I (*coI)* of size ≈450 bp [29], were performed to fluid cysts and amplicons were purified, sequenced, and compared with several *coI* sequences from the GenBank.

5.1. Epidemiological study for CE in livestock

Based on the presence of the parasite in the municipal slaughterhouse of Calera, Zacatecas, a rural community, was selected to identify the adult and larval stages. The community is located in the northern state of Zacatecas, in the central area at 22°55′N, 102°48′W; it has a semi-arid-dry weather, mild temperature (mean 15.4°C), with average rainfall of 448 mm H_2O.

In 2006, an initial census showed that the community was organized in 39 blocks with 155 houses, 140 were inhabited with 526 peoples, showing a mean of 4±2 people/house, a range from 1 to 11 and a mode of 2. Also, 266 were women and 260 were men, 174 (33%) were younger than 18 years old. On the other hand, 26% were economically active population (136/526) and 74% of households derive their income from a single person; the main activity was agriculture (83%) followed by crafts (10%) and trade (7%). The community had electricity, chlorinated drinking water, and telephone services; 45% of the streets are paved. Of the 140 housing, 49 (35%) had 60 dogs, while in 79 (56%) several livestock were recorded, such as sheep (586 animals/18 houses), cattle (441 animals/58 houses), pigs (124 animals/44 houses), and horses (31 animals/ 24 houses).

5.2. Identification of Echinococcus and treatment of dogs

With the owners' verbal consent, feces obtained by rectal spoon of all 60 dogs in the community were recovered and analyzed by Faust technique [3, 30] and by Coproantigen ELISA (CpAg ELISA) [31, 32]. Coprological study showed that 5 dogs were infected with *Toxocara canis* (8.3%), 2 with teniids (3.4%) and 1 with *Ancylostoma caninum* (1.6%), while 11 samples positive for *E. granulosus* antigens (18.3%) were detected. Fecal samples were obtained after treatment and used for egg and antigen detection; none was positive.

For Copro-PCR, only in those 11 positive samples by CpAg ELISA were analyzed; JB3 and JB4 primers [29] only 3 samples yielded one amplicon of ≈450 bp and those were purified and sequenced, showing a high identity with *E. canadensis* G7 genotype.

Positive dogs for taeniid eggs or coproantigens were purged and treated; for this they were isolated in cages with fecal collection facilities, which were maintained in the backyards of their homes, and were treated orally with praziquantel and with arecoline bromide. Dogs were kept in the cage and after collection of feces the dogs were released. However, no tapeworms were recovered after treatment, probably because it was administered 3 months after diagnosis, since arecoline bromide is rarely available in Mexico. Fecal samples were obtained after treatment and used for egg and antigen detection; none was positive.

In addition, a questionnaire was applied to search for possible risk factors in the population, and showed that having fed pig and/or sheep raw offal to dogs was significantly associated with *Echinococcus* antigen positivity (odds ratio=5.9, 95% confidence interval=1.11-31.3, P=0.023).

5.3. Identification of CE in pigs and sheep

From July 2006 to January 2007, 586 sheep and 55 adult pigs were examined using US for hydatid cysts in the community. For this, standing sheep were immobilized and US was performed with a transductor between the 4th and the 7th intercostal ribs of the shaved right side, no sedation was required for the sheep. Pigs were intramuscularly sedated and positioned for the transducing process. All sheep in the community were submitted to US, except: piglets, pregnant or nursing females, as well as stallions or pigs destined for early human consumption. In the community, sheep and pigs are confined in small flocks inside semi-closed backyard areas where they had access to open feeding, and that were accessible to dogs, cats, and other small wilds animals.

Three local abattoirs in the community were identified; regular visits were undertaken, mainly during pig and sheep sacrifice in order to recover potential infected viscera. Before sacrifice, animals were submitted to US and afterwards, during viscera inspection, spleen, liver, and lungs were meticulously checked. Only 3 female pigs had CE during necropsy, but only in 1 case was the diagnosis previously established using US. However, it was not possible to recover any fluid cysts for DNA analysis.

5.4. Phylogenetic and population genetics analyses

All sequences obtained of 9 hydatid cysts and 3 by Copro-PCR, were subjected to BLAST search in the GenBank database; multiple alignments were performed with the CLUSTAL W [33] and MUSCLE [34] programs, with manual adjusted in MEGA program v5 [35]. The multiple alignments were used to determine the appropriate model of molecular evolution in the Modeltest 3.7 program [36]. The *coI* sequences for *E. granulosus* s.l. were analyzed with the General Time Reverse model, using gamma distribution (GTR+G). The phylogenetic reconstruction using Bayesian inference was performed with Mr Bayes 3.2.1 program [37-39]. Analysis was executed for 10 million generations; trees were sampled every 100 generations. Trees with scores lower than those at the stationary phase were discarded from the analysis, while those that reached the stationary phase were collected and used to build consensus trees. In addition, unrooted haplotype networks were created using NETWORK 4.611 software. These networks were nested according to the rules in Median-Joining networks [40], in which interior/tip status was considered a clade/haplotype and the ancestral haplotype had priority over missing haplotypes. An analysis of genetic diversity within and between populations was performed using DnaSPv4 [41] and included nucleotide diversity (π), haplotype polymorphism (θ), expected heterozygosity (H_S), genetic differentiation index (F_{ST}), and Tajima's D test.

Up to 335 sequences for *coI* of *E. granulosus, E. canadensis, E. equinus, E. ortleppi, E. shiquicus* and *E. multilocularis* were analyzed, 68 haplotypes were found. GenBank has many more sequences of *E. granulosus* (232) than of other species, H_S and π values were lower than *E. canadensis* (Table 1). Also, θ values were very small (~0.3 for *E. granulosus* and *E. canadensis* and <0.01 for other species), whilst Tajima's D test exhibited negative values. When we matched different *Echinococcus* species, the F_{ST} value was close to 1, suggesting a very high differentiation between species and corroborating the taxonomic status among these species (Table 2).

Species	N[1]	Haplotypes	π^2	θ^3	Tajima's D
E. granulosus s.s.	232	31	0.0085	0.0423	-2.3523
E. canadensis	70	18	0.0118	0.0336	-2.1235
E. shiquicus	16	9	0.0054	0.0076	-1.0886
E. equines	10	6	0.0061	0.0075	-0.7831
E. ortleppi	3	2	0.0023	0.0022	ND[4]
E. multilocularis	4	2	0.0019	0.0015	ND

[1]N, number of sequences analyzed

[2]π, nucleotide diversity

[3]θ, haplotype polymorphism

[4]ND, not determined

Table 1. Genetic polymorphism indexes among *Echinococcus* species obtained with the use of *coI* GenBank sequences.

Population A (Species A)	Population B (Species B)	F_{ST}
E. canadensis	*E. equinus*	0.8498
E. canadensis	*E. granulosus* s.s.	0.8243
E. canadensis	*E. ortleppi*	0.7023
E. canadensis	*E. shiquicus*	0.8578
E. canadensis	*E. multilocularis*	0.8840
E. equinus	*E. granulosus* s.s.	0.9156
E. equinus	*E. ortleppi*	0.9390
E. equinus	*E. shiquicus*	0.9198
E. equinus	*E. multilocularis*	0.9517
E. granulosus s.s.	*E. ortleppi*	0.9068
E. granulosus s.s.	*E. shiquicus*	0.9269
E. granulosus s.s.	*E. multilocularis*	0.9429
E. ortleppi	*E. shiquicus*	0.9455
E. ortleppi	*E. multilocularis*	0.9540
E. shiquicus	*E. multilocularis*	0.9557

F_{ST}, genetic differentiation index

Table 2. Genetic differentiation index values between different paired sequences of *Echinococcus* species.

Sequences for *coI* of *E. canadensis* from Africa, Asia, Europe, and Latin and North America deposited in the GenBank databases (58), as well as our 12 sequences were analyzed (from KF734649 to KF734660, GenBank accession numbers). High identity (>98%) between Mexican, Peruvian, and Polish pig sequences was found. Globally, G6 was compared to G7 and to G8 and showed lower value of H_S (~0.26) and the pair between G6 and G7 exhibited the lowest value of F_{ST} (~0.10); the other genotypes had F_{ST} ≥0.6. When G6 and G7 were separated by geographic area, the main pairs had F_{ST} ≤0.1, except Europe vs. Africa. We did not find available sequences of G7 in humans, however, there are some sequences for G6 in humans from Africa (Mauritania) and Asia (China, Iran, Mongolia) that presented similar H_S and F_{ST} values as those sequences for G6 and G7 obtained from livestock (Table 3).

Population A	Population B	H_S [1]	F_{ST} [2]
G6	G7	0.2712	0.1018
G6	G8	0.2618	0.9169
G6	G10	0.3836	0.6339
G7	G8	0.5306	0.9198
G7	G10	0.5981	0.6484
G8	G10	0.6447	0.9030
Mexico (G7)	Europe[3] (G7)	0.8017	0.0988
Latin America[4] (G7)	Europe (G7)	0.7815	0.0938
Latin America (G7)	Africa[5] (G6)	0.5993	0.0773
Latin America (G7)	Asia[6] (G6)	0.6393	0.0773
Latin America (G7)	Africa-Asia[7] (G6)	0.8146	0.0542
Europe (G7)	Africa (G6)	0.2370	0.2
Europe (G7)	Asia (G6)	0.2666	0.2
Europe (G7)	Africa-Asia (G6)	0.5222	0.1142

[1]H_S, expected heterozygosity within each population

[2]F_{ST}, genetic differentiation index

[3]include sequences from Italy, Poland, and Rumania

[4]include sequences from Mexico and Peru

[5]include sequences from Algeria, Ethiopia, Mauritania, and Sudan

[6]include sequences from Iran and Kazakhstan

[7]include sequences of patients from China, Iran, Mauritania, Mongolia, and Russia

Table 3. Expected heterozygosity and genetic differentiation indexes between different paired sequences of *Echinococcus canadensis* genotypes obtained from animals.

Regarding the phylogenetic analyses, a Bayesian tree showed that all Mexican sequences obtained were grouped in the *E. canadensis* cluster with a value of 0.80 of posterior probability (Figure 7a), while a second Bayesian inference performed with only *E. canadensis* grouped to Mexican sequences with a G6 and G7 cluster from different reservoirs and different countries (Figure 7b).

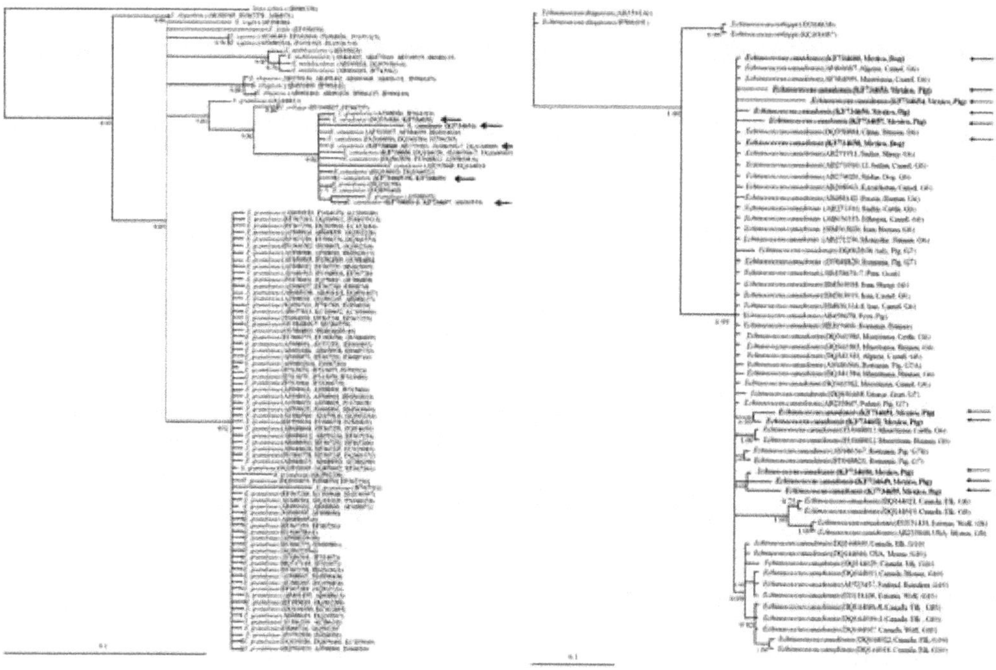

(a) (b)

Figure 7. Bayesian phylogenetic trees of *Echinococcus* species (a) and *Echinococcus canadiensis* (b) using *coI* sequences; Bayesian analysis with the *coI* data; Values at nodes indicate the posterior percentage probabilities using 10 million generations. The Mexican sequences are identified by arrows.

The haplotype network inferences showed consistent results with the values of genetic differentiation previously obtained (Figure 8); some sequences of *E. granulosus* were placed in the *E. canadensis* clade, probably because at the time they were submitted to GenBank, their taxonomic status had not been fully established. However, clearly 6 clades can be identified that correspond to *E. granulosuss.s.*, *E. multilocularis, E. canadensis, E. equinus, E. oligarthra,* and *E. shiquicus*. Other network trees, which were built only with sequences of *E. canadensis*, exhibited a similar distribution profile according to their host (Figure 9a) and origin country (Figure 9b). Thus, 3 clusters were identified: one for Canada, USA, Finland, Estonia, Mongolia, Kazakhstan with elk, wolf, and moose; the 2nd, for African, Asian, Latin-American, and European countries with camel, cattle, sheep, dog, pig, goat, and human and interestingly, the Mexican G7 haplotypes were placed around core dispersion center; finally, the 3rd cluster grouped other haplotypes G7 from Romania, Mauritania, and Peru and identified in pigs, humans, camels, and cattle.

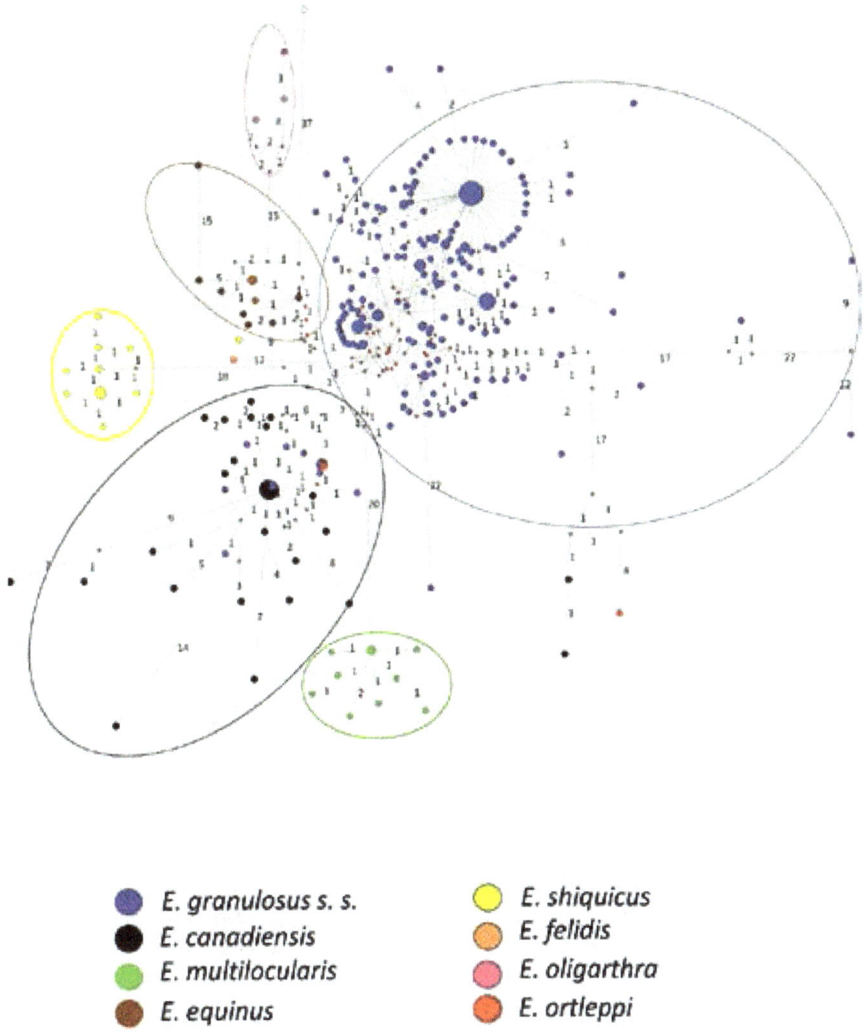

Figure 8. Median joining network of *Echinococcus* species using *coI* sequences. Bigger sizes of circles represent higher frequency of each haplotype in each species. Numbers in branches refer to mutational changes.

5.5. What can we interpret about the population genetics study about Echinococcus in Mexico?

Current revisions accept 9 *Echinococcus* species based on clinical, molecular, epidemiological, and biological data, as well as characteristics of their host-parasite relationship: *E. granulosus* s.s. , *E. felidis, E. multilocularis, E. shiquicus, E. equinus, E. oligarthra, E. vogeli, E. ortleppi* and *E. canadensis* [5-7, 10]. Field and laboratory findings have revealed a significant phenotypic and genetic variability among isolates of *Echinococcus,* mainly for *E. granulosus* s.l. from different intermediate hosts. Recent phylogenetic studies based on both mitochondrial and nuclear DNA genes have showed that *E. granulosus* s.l. consists of 10 strains or genotypes (G1 to G10)

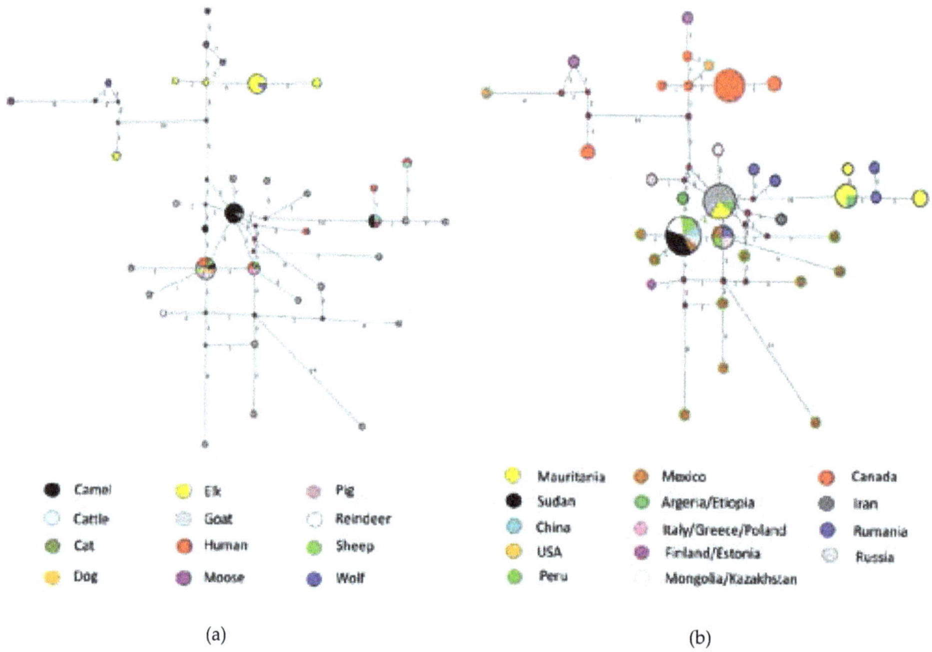

Figure 9. Median joining network trees of *Echinococcus canadensis* from different reservoirs (a) and countries (b), built using *coI* sequences. Numbers in branches refer to mutational changes; sizes of circles are proportional to haplotype frequencies, thus, bigger circles represent ancestral haplotypes, small red circles represent missing haplotypes.

with at least 4 valid species: *E. granulosus* s.s. (G1-G3; sheep strains [G1 and G2] and buffalo strain [G3]), *Echinococcus equinus* (G4; horse strain), *Echinococcus ortleppi* (G5; cattle strain), and *Echinococcus canadensis* (G6-G10: camel strain [G6], pig strain [G7], cervid strains [G8 and G10] and human strain [G9, under a controversial status]) [4, 5, 42, 43]. Nonetheless, the species status of *E. canadensis* is still controversial [4-8, 11, 44], because few biological differences have been identified among all strains (from G6 to G10) proposing them as a single species. However, ecological and geographical differences between camel and pig strains to cervid strains show clear differences, suggesting a diversification process. In this way, some authors have suggested that G6 and G7 should be treated as a single species designated as *E. intermedius* [4, 8, 11], and even G8 as *E. borealis* and G10 as *E. canadensis* have also been proposed [8]. In contrast, Nakao et al. [6, 7, 45], advise that G6 to G10 should be retained by the specific name *E. canadensis*, pending further population genetic studies, using particularly nuclear DNA markers to clarify the status of the taxon.

A contrasting phenomenon is observed for CE by *E. canadensis* (G7) in humans, because the pig strain is the main genotype identified in patients from Eastern and Southeastern European countries [46, 47]. There are few human cases of CE reported in Mexican patients, although none by G7 has been identified by molecular techniques. There are only 2 genetic studies performed in samples of CE from Mexico; Cruz-Reyes et al. [11] documented that G7 parasites of Mexican and Polish pig isolates showed similar patterns by RFLP of rDNA ITS1 and RAPD techniques, although PCR-sequencing analysis of mitochondrial *coI* gen fragment was performed, no polymorphism data were reported. Saarma et al. [48] identified 2 variants (A, B) inside of G6/G7 group consisting of samples from Mexico and Argentina, using 5 nuclear markers (elongation factor 1 alpha, transforming growth factor beta receptor kinase, thioredoxin peroxidase, calreticulin, and ezrin-radixin-moesin-like protein).

In general, the genetic population parameters reported by Rodriguez-Prado et al. [16] were similar to those reported by Haag et al.[49], who using mitochondrial (*nad*) and nuclear (*ActII, Hbx2, AgB*) sequences of *Echinococcus*, found π=0.0005 for *E. multilocularis*, and π=0.0090 for *E. granulosus*. In addition, a study focused in the genetic diversity of *Echinococcus granulosus* s.s. hydatid cysts from 4 European countries (Bulgaria, Hungary, Romania, and Italy) evaluated by DNA sequence analysis of the *coI*, showed F_{ST} values that ranged from 0.018 to 0.187 with higher negative values for Tajima's D that ranged from -0.515 to -1.066 [50]. Analyzing Mexican and other sequences, it was observed that among *E. canadensis* populations, they have a moderate differentiation (F_{ST} ~0.1), while the other genotypes of *E. canadensis* exhibited a high differentiation among them (F_{ST} >0.6). When G6 and G7 were divided in geographic areas, similar genetic differentiation was observed with F_{ST} <0.1, except when Europe (G7) was matched with Africa or Asia (F_{ST}=0.2). However, in both cases, this phenomenon could be interpreted as a moderate genetic differentiation within these populations. Also, we found negative values for Tajima's D, similarly to Casulli et al. [50] data, indicating that a size expansion due to a bottleneck event might have occurred in the past.

Based in the network analyses and according to Rodriguez-Prado et al. [16], the following inferences can be done: 1) *E. canadensis* in Mexico is very diverse and has probably been introduced from abroad several times from different sources because 6 Mexican isolates have from 4 to 14 mutational changes between the isolate and the main haplotype; 2) haplotypes grouped in the North American wildlife cluster (G10) are closer within them, with 1 or 2 mutational changes and they are placed far of the Mexican isolates, thus they might be ruled out as sources of introduction to Mexico; 3) differentiation between G6 and G7 would not make any sense based on the differentiation of genetic indexes found for both genotypes (F_{ST} close to 0.1), besides one of the main ancestral dispersion centers in the network analysis, clustered identical haplotypes of G6 and G7 from China, Mexico, Peru, Sudan, and Russia.

6. Final remarks

The first human CE case identified by molecular techniques was reported in 2006 in the United Kingdom (UK) in a male with clinical and CT scan images consistent with CE that was surgically treated for the removal of a hydatid cyst, which was subsequently confirmed as *E. granulosus* G1 [51]. This case was similar to the Mexican one: it was unexpected and wrongly diagnosed for a long time. Also in the UK, recent *Echinococcus* isolates from intermediate and definitive animal hosts, as well as from human CE cases were analyzed to determine species and genotypes within these hosts. *E. equinus* was identified from horse hydatid isolates, while *E. granulosus* s.s. was identified from hydatid cysts of sheep and cattle, as well as in DNA extracted from a farm dog, foxhound fecal samples, and from human cystic echinococcosis isolates. Low genetic variability for *E. equinus* using *coI* sequences (π=0.000666±0.000620) indicates the presence of a dominant haplotype; in contrast, greater haplotypic variation was observed for *E. granulosus* s.s. (π=0.000955±0.000790). Furthermore, a haplotype phylogenetic inference showed a star-shaped network with a centrally placed main haplotype that was reported from other world regions [52].

Four new cases of CE in Mexican patients were reported since 2009, a 38-year-old female from the State of Mexico, who was submitted to surgery to remove a liver cyst [53]; 2 cases referred to a tertiary-care oncology hospital with an initial diagnosis of liver and lung cancer, respectively. The liver cyst case was resolved with percutaneous drainage and administration of albendazole for 2 months, while the lung cyst was resolved solely with 2 months of albendazole [54]. The last case was a 16-year-old female from the state of Puebla, Mexico with a liver cyst that was surgically removed [55]. Unfortunately, in all cases, molecular assays were not performed so identification of *Echinococcus* strains was not possible.

7. Conclusion

We wish to finalize this chapter by pointing out that the correct diagnosis and adequate management of the initial case, the subsequent epidemiological follow-up of human echinococcosis at a community level in Mexico and the in-depth genetic study of the parasite, integrate a comprehensive and unique study of *Echinococcus granulosus,* s.l. and support the very low frequency of this disease in Mexico.

Although no data on cystic echinococcosis caused by *E. canadensis* G7 have previously been documented in Mexican patients, the high number of infected patients in central Europe by the G7 genotype, points to the potential public health importance of this strain or species, as well as the necessity to perform molecular and epidemiological studies focused to clarify this contrasting situation and the controversial taxonomic status of *E. canadensis* species.

Author details

Ana Flisser[1*], Pablo Maravilla[2], Pilar Mata-Miranda[3] and Fernando Martinez-Hernandez[2]

*Address all correspondence to: flisser@unam.mx

1 Departamento de Microbiologia y Parasitologia, Facultad de Medicina, Universidad Nacional Autonoma de Mexico, DF, Mexico

2 Departamento de Ecologia de Agentes Patogenos, Hospital General "Dr. Manuel Gea Gonzalez", Secretaria de Salud, DF, Mexico

3 Coordinación Auxiliar de Investigación en Salud, Delegación Veracruz Norte, Xalapa, Veracruz, Mexico

References

[1] Eckert J, Gemmell MA, Meslin FX, Pawlowski ZS, editors. WHO/OIE Manual on echinococcosis in humans and animals: A public health problem of global concern. World Organization for Animal Health and World Health Organization. Paris, France. 2001;265.

[2] Flisser A, Craig PS. Larval cestodes. In: Cox FEG, Wakelin D, Gillespie SH, Despommier DD, editors. Topley & Wilson's microbiology and microbial infections.10th ed. Arnold, London. 2005;5:677-712.

[3] Mata-Miranda P, Osnaya-Palma I, Rodríguez-Prado U, Gutiérrez-Marín A, Tawil M, Hernández-González S, Solano-Ceh M, Villalvaso L, Martínez-Maya JJ, Maravilla P, García-de-la-Torre, G, Flisser A. Epidemiologic and ultrasonographic study of echinococcosis in a community in the State of Mexico. Am J Trop Med Hyg. 2007;77:500-555.

[4] Thompson RC. The taxonomy, phylogeny and transmission of *Echinococcus*. Exp Parasitol. 2008;119:439-446.

[5] McManus DP. Current status of the genetics and molecular taxonomy of *Echinococcus* species. Parasitology. 2013;11:1-7.

[6] Nakao M, Yanagida T, Konyaev S, Lavikainen A, Odnokurtsev VA, et al. Mitochondrial phylogeny of the genus *Echinococcus* (Cestoda: Taeniidae) with emphasis on relationships among *Echinococcus canadensis* genotypes. Parasitology. 2013;140:1595-1601.

[7] Nakao M, Lavikainen A, Yanagida T, Ito A. Phylogenetic systematics of the genus *Echinococcus* (Cestoda: Taeniidae). Int J Parasitol. 2013;43:1017-1029.

[8] Lymbery AJ, Jenkins EJ, Schurer JM, Thompson RC. *Echinococcus canadensis, E. borealis,* and *E. intermedius*. What's in a name?. Trends Parasitol. 2015;31:23-29.

[9] Martínez-Maya JJ, Zuñiga A, Jaramillo A, Cardenas L, Navarro F. Caracterizacion epidemiologica de la equinococosis/hidatidosis en Zacatecas, Mexico. Vet Mex. 1994;25:231-237.

[10] Schantz PM, Chai J, Craig PS, Eckert J, Jenkins DJ, et al. Epidemiology and control of hydatid disease. In: Thompson RCA, Lymbery AJ editors. *Echinococcus* and hydatid disease. Wallingford, Oxon, UK: CAB International. 1995:233-331.

[11] Cruz-Reyes A, Constantine CC, Boxell AC, Hobbs RP, Thompson RC. *Echinococcus granulosus* from Mexican pigs is the same strain as that in Polish pigs. J Helminthol. 2007;81:287-292.

[12] Salinas-Lopez N, Jimenez-Guzman F, Cruz-Reyes A: Presence of *Echinococcus oligarthrus* (Diesing, 1863) Lühe, 1910 in *Lynx rufus texensis* Allen, 1895 from San Fernando, Tamaulipas state, in North-east Mexico. Int J Parasitol. 1996;26:793-796.

[13] Villalobos N, González LM, Morales J, de Aluja AS, Jiménez MI, et al. Molecular identification of *Echinococcus granulosus* genotypes (G1 and G7) isolated from pigs in Mexico. Vet Parasitol. 2007;147:185-189.

[14] Maravilla P, Thompson RCA, Palacios-Ruiz JA, Estcourt A, Ramirez-Solis E, et al. *Echinococcus granulosus* cattle strain identification in an autochthonous case of cystic echinococcosis in central Mexico. Acta Trop. 2004;92:231-236.

[15] Rodriguez-Prado U, Gutiérrez-Marín A, Martínez-Ocaña J, Romero-Valdovinos M, Olivo-Díaz A, Hernández-Castro R, Flisser A, Maravilla P, Martínez-Maya JJ. Estudio coprológico y ultrasonogáfico en perros y borregos de una comunidad suburbana en el Estado de México para la búsqueda de *Echinococcus spp.* Vet Mex. 2014;Supp:53-58.

[16] Rodriguez-Prado U, Jimenez-Gonzalez DE, Avila G, Gonzalez AE, Martinez-Flores WA, Mondragon de la Peña C, Hernandez-Castro R, Romero-Valdovinos M, Flisser A, Martinez-Hernandez F, Maravilla P, Martinez-Maya JJ: Genetic variation of *Echinococcus canadensis* (G7) in Mexico. Am J Trop Med Hyg. 2014;91:1149-1153. doi: 10.4269/ajtmh.14-0317.

[17] Ceruzzi O, Osimani JJ, Botto C, Rodríguez N, Cabrera R. Algunos factores a considerar en la evaluación de la intradermorreacción de Casoni para hidatidosis. Bol Chile Parasitol. 1976;31:50.

[18] Alper A, Emre A, Hazar H, Özden I, Bilge O, Acarli K, Ariogul O. Laparoscopic surgery of hepatic hydatid disease: Initial results and early follow-up of 16 patients. World J Surg 1995;19:725.

[19] Khoury G, Jabbour-Khoury S, Bikhazi K. Results of laparoscopic treatment of hydatid cyst of the liver. Surg Endosc. 1996;10:57.

[20] Saglam A. Laparoscopic treatment of liver hydatid cysts. Surg Laparosc Endosc. 1996;6:16.

[21] Sayek I, Onat D. Diagnosis and treatment of uncomplicated hydatid cyst of the liver. World J Surg. 2001;25:21.

[22] Maddison SE, Slemenda SB, Schantz PM, Fried JA, Wilson M, Tsang VCW. A specific diagnostic antigen of *Echinococcus granulosus* with an apparent molecular weight of 8 KDa. Am J Trp Med Hyg. 1989;40:377-383.

[23] Palacios JA, Ramírez-Solis ME, Cárdenas-Mejia A, Maravilla P, Flisser A. Hypertonic saline in hydatid disease. World J Surg. 2002;26:1398.

[24] Palacios-Ruíz JA, Ramírez-Solís E, Moreno-Moller M, Cárdenas-Mejía A, Mata-Miranda P, Maravilla P, Flisser A. Identificación y manejo integral de un caso autóctono de hidatidosis en México. Rev Mex Gastroenterol. 2003;68:41-45.

[25] Bowles J, Van Knapen F, McManus DP. Cattle strain of *Echinococcus granulosus* and human infection. Lancet.1992;39:1358.

[26] Scott, JC, McManus, DP. The random amplification of polymorphic DNA can discriminate species and strains of *Echinococcus*. Trop. Med. Parasitol. 1994;45.

[27] Blancas Mosqueda M, Herrera Esparza R, Rodríguez Padilla C, Tavizón García JP, Mercado Reyes M, et al. Gender as a factor of susceptibility to infection in experimental hydatidosis.Rev Latinoam Microbiol. 2007;49:31-37.

[28] Moro P, Schantz PM. Echinococcosis: A review. Int J Infect Dis. 2009;13:125-133.

[29] Bowles J, McManus DP. Genetic characterization of the Asian *Taenia*, a newly described taeniid cestode of humans. Am J Trop Med Hyg. 1994;50:33-44.

[30] Faust EC, Sawitz W, Tobie J, Odom V, Peres C, Lincicome DR. Comparative efficiency of various techniques for the diagnosis of protozoa and helminth in feces. J Parasitol. 1939;25:241-261.

[31] Allan JC, Craig PS, Garcia Noval J, Mencos F, Liu D, et al. Coproantigen detection for immunodiagnosis of echinococcosis and taeniasis in dogs and humans. Parasitology. 1992;104:347-356.

[32] Moro PL, Lopera L, Bonifacio N, Gonzales A, Gilman RH, et al. Risk factors for canine echinococcosis in an endemic area of Peru. Vet Parasitol. 2005;130:99-104.

[33] Thompson JD, Higgins DG, Gibson TJ, Clustal W. Improving the sensitivity and progressive multiple sequence alignment through sequence weighting, positions-specific gap penalties and weight matrix choice. Nucleic Acids Res. 1994;22:4673-4680.

[34] Edgar RC. MUSCLE: multiple sequence alignment with high accuracy and high throughput. Nucleic Acids Res. 2004;32:1792-1797.

[35] Tamura K, Peterson D, Peterson N, Stecher G, Nei M, et al. MEGA5: Molecular Evolutionary Genetics Analysis using maximum likelihood, evolutionary distance, and maximum parsimony methods. Mol Biol Evol. 2011;28:2731-2739.

[36] Posada D, Crandall KA. Modeltest: testing the model of DNA substitution. Bioinformatics.1998;14:817-818.

[37] Huelsenbeck JP, Ronquist F, Nielsen R, Bollback JP. Bayesian inference of phylogeny and its impact on evolutionary biology. Science. 2001;14:2310-2314.

[38] Holder M, Lewis PO. Phylogeny estimation: traditional and Bayesian approaches. Nat Rev Genet. 2003;4:275-284.

[39] Ronquis F, Huelsenbeck JP. MrBayes 3: Bayesian phylogenetic inference under mixed models. Bioinformatics. 2003;19:1572-1574.

[40] Bandelt HJ, Forster P, Röhl A. Median-joining networks for inferring intraspecific phylogenies. Mol Biol Evol. 1999;16:37-48.

[41] Rozas J, Sanchez-Del Barrio JC, Messeguer X, Rozas R. DNA sequence Polymorphism (DNAsp) ver. 4.10.9. Departamento de Genetica, Universidad de Barcelona. 2006.

[42] Thompson RC, McManus DP. Towards a taxonomic revision of the genus *Echinococcus.* Trends Parasitol. 2002;18:452-457.

[43] Alvarez Rojas CA, Romig T, Lightowlers MW. *Echinococcus granulosus* sensu lato genotypes infecting humans—Review of current knowledge. Int J Parasitol. 2014;44:9-18.

[44] Yanagida T, Mohammadzadeh T, Kamhawi S, Nakao M, Sadjjadi SM, et al. Genetic polymorphisms of *Echinococcus granulosus* sensu stricto in the Middle East. Parasitol Int. 2012;61:599-603.

[45] Nakao M, McManus DP, Schantz PM, Craig PS, Ito A. A molecular phylogeny of the genus *Echinococcus* inferred from complete mitochondrial genomes. Parasitology. 2007;134(Pt 5):713-722.

[46] Schneider R, Gollackner B, Schindl M, Tucek G, Auer H. *Echinococcus canadensis* G7 (pig strain): An underestimated cause of cystic echinococcosis in Austria. Am J Trop Med Hyg. 2010;82:871-874.

[47] Dybicz M, Gierczak A, Dąbrowska J, Rdzanek Ł, Michałowicz B. Molecular diagnosis of cystic echinococcosis in humans from central Poland. Parasitol Int. 2013;62:364-367.

[48] Saarma U, Jõgisalu I, Moks E, Varcasia A, Lavikainen A, Oksanen A, Simsek S, Andresiuk V, Denegri G, González LM, Ferrer E, Gárate T, Rinaldi L, Maravilla P. A novel phylogeny for the genus *Echinococcus,* based on nuclear data, challenges relationships based on mitochondrial evidence. Parasitology. 2009;136:317-28.

[49] Haag KL, Zaha A, Araújo AM, Gottstein B. Reduced genetic variability within coding and non-coding regions of the *Echinococcus multilocularis* genome. Parasitology. 1997;115:521-529.

[50] Casulli A, Interisano M, Sreter T, Chitimia L, Kirkova Z, La Rosa G, Pozio E. Genetic variability of *Echinococcus granulosus* sensu stricto in Europe inferred by mitochondrial DNA sequences. Infect Genet Evol. 2012;12:377-383.

[51] Craig PS, Woods ML, Boufana B, O´Loughlin B, Gimpel J, San Lett W, Mcmanus DP. Cystic echinococcosis in a fox-hound hunt worker, UK. Pathogens and Global Health. 2012;106:373-375.

[52] Boufana B, Lett WS, Lahmar S, Buishi I, Bodell AJ, Varcasia A, Casulli A, Beeching NJ, Campbell F, Terlizzo M, McManus DP, Craig PS. *Echinococcus equinus* and *Echino-*

coccus granulosus sensu stricto from the United Kingdom: Genetic diversity and haplotypic variation. Int J Parasitol. 2015;45:161-6. doi: 10.1016/j.ijpara.2014.10.005.

[53] Steta J, Torre A. Mexican-native human echinococcosis: Case report of an underestimated disease. Ann Hepatol. 2009;8:251-254.

[54] Cornejo-Juárez P, Espinosa-Altamirano A, Ibarra-del-Río M, Pacheco-Bravo I, Volkow-Fernández P. Cystic echinococcosis: A disease mimicking cancer in a non-endemic country report of two cases. West Indian Med J. 2013;62:266-269.

[55] Orea-Martínez JG, Pérez-Corro MA, Contreras-Vera RA, Bretón-Márquez JH. A case of hydatid cyst caused by *Echinococcus granulosus* in Puebla, Mexico, that resulted in successful surgical treatment. Rev Gastroenterol Mex. 2013;78:116-119. doi: 10.1016/j.rgmx.2012.10.007.

3

Echinococcosis in Colombia — A Neglected Zoonosis?

Alfonso J. Rodriguez-Morales,
Lauren Sofia Calvo-Betancourt,
Camila Alarcón-Olave and Adrián Bolívar-Mejía

Abstract

Echinococcosis or hydatid disease is a near-cosmopolitan parasitic zoonosis caused by the larval stages of cestodes of the genus *Echinococcus*, whose spectrum of clinical manifestations can vary from asymptomatic infection to death, the liver being the most frequently affected organ. In the absence of an adequate treatment, case fatality rate of affected patients may reach 100%, so clinical suspicion should always be accompanied by a complete workup and a prompt treatment. Like other zoonotic parasitic diseases, echinococcosis is associated with low socioeconomic and cultural levels, especially affecting rural areas of developing countries, not only by the morbidity and mortality it produces, but also by the economic impact associated to health care costs and productivity losses. Despite this, in Colombia and in other South American countries, epidemiological studies of this disease are limited, so it is not known with certainty the incidence, the prevalence, and the burden of the disease. The objective of this chapter is to summarize and describe epidemiological and clinical updated aspects of the disease, focusing on evidences and published research articles on echinococcosis in Colombia, finally questioning if this cestode zoonotic disease has been largely neglected.

Keywords: Echinococcosis, *Echinococcus*, Colombia, neglected diseases, zoonotic infectious diseases

1. Introduction

Echinococcosis or hydatid disease is a near-cosmopolitan parasitic zoonosis caused by the larval stages (paratenic for humans) of cestodes of the genus *Echinococcus* (Figure 1) [1, 2]. This helminthiasis causes an important economic loss over agricultural and pastoral regions of limited resources, particularly in developing countries [3]. In addition, it is also important to notice that this is one of the important infectious disease groups caused by larval stages of cestodes, which also include cysticercosis (caused by larval stages of *Taenia solium*), coenuriasis (caused by larval stages of *Taenia multiceps gaigeri*), and sparganosis (caused by larval stages of *Spirometra*), among others.

Biologically and taxonomically, although in the past it was considered as part of the genus *Taenia*, *Echinococcus* genus belongs to the family *Taeniidae* (order Cyclophyllidea, subclass Eucestoda, class Cestoda, phylum Platyhelminthes). Family *Taeniidae* also includes the genus *Taenia*. Order Cyclophyllidea has two important families that infect humans: *Hymenolepididae* (*Hymenolepis*) and *Dipylidiidae* (*Dipylidium*). Subclass Eucestoda includes the order Diphyllobothriidea that belongs to family *Diphyllobothriidae* and genus *Diphyllobothrium*.

Although, 12 species have been recognized, only four are of public health concern and produce human pathology: *Echinococcus granulosus* (cystic echinococcosis), *E. multilocularis* (alveolar echinococcosis), *E. vogeli*, and *E. oligarthrus* (both causing polycystic echinococcosis). The first two species are etiological agents of life-threatening diseases, having high fatality rate and poor prognosis if careful clinical management is not given [2]. *E. vogeli* and *E. oligarthrus* are responsible for polycystic echinococcosis in Central and South America [2]. Majority of the cases reported in these regions, till 2008, have corresponded to *E. vogeli* (54 of 172; 31.4%) and *E.* cf. *vogeli* (*confer, species affinis*) (114 of 172; 66.3%) [3]. Only three cases (1.7%) have been identified that have corresponded to *E. oligarthrus* and one has corresponded to *E. granulosus* (0.6%) [3]. In the past, it was believed that *E. multilocularis* was not present in Central and South America.

Living or having lived in rural areas where farming and animal husbandry are common is an important risk factor for this disease, in some areas particularly where people frequently come in contact with dogs that accompany paca hunters as well as where wild animal hunting for food is common practice (e.g., hunters and aboriginal people) [4]. In addition, new population migration patterns over the past four decades have caused a change in the profile of this disease, allowing its worldwide distribution [4]. In addition, in general, now it is considered that there is a risk of getting echinococcosis infection, as well other cestodiasis, while traveling to endemic zones.

This disease is related with extensive livestock or poor health infrastructures; usually associated with a low socioeconomic level and lack of education. Its public health importance is related not only to the high fatality rate in humans but also with reduced work performance, costs of hospitalization, interventions, and disabilities [5].

Although echinococcosis has been recognized for centuries (at the 17th century, Francesco Redi illustrated that the hydatid cysts of echinococcosis were of "animal" origin), in some countries of the neotropic region, such as Colombia, this disease was discovered during 20th century). Studies in this context in this country, as well as in other countries of South America, are still limited. Therefore, the objective of this chapter is to summarize and describe epidemiological and clinical updated aspects of this disease, focusing on evidences and published research articles on echinococcosis in Colombia, finally questioning if this cestode zoonotic disease has been largely neglected [1-84].

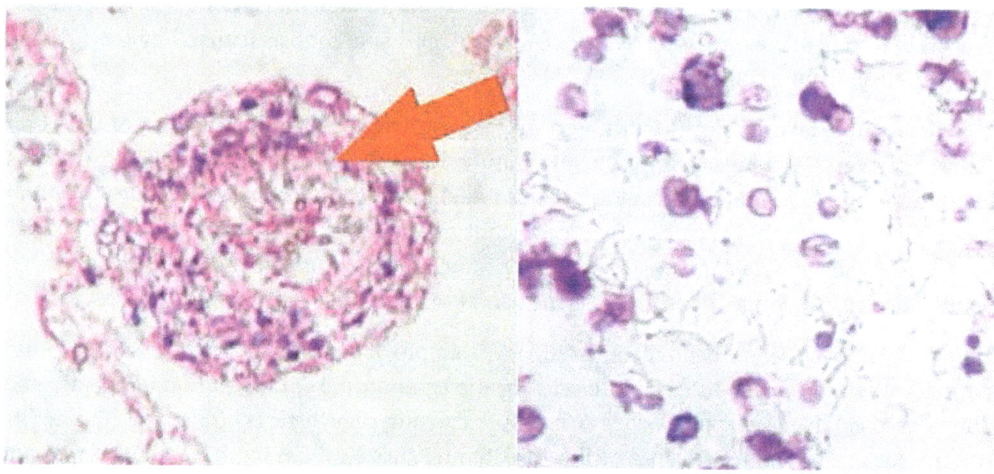

Figure 1. Scolex and hooks of *Echinococcus granulosus* (pictures by A. J. Rodriguez-Morales).

2. Organisms causing human disease

2.1. *Echinococcus granulosus*

(Cystic echinococcosis)

E. granulosus is a cestode whose life cycle involves dogs (*Canis lupus familiaris*) and other canids (coyote, dingo, red fox, among others) as definitive hosts for the intestinal tapeworm, which are infected by ingestion of food containing hydatid cysts with viable protoscoleces, and domestic and wild ungulates as intermediate hosts for the tissue invading metacestode (larval) stage (Figure 1) [1]. The metacestode (or hydatid cyst) consists of two parasite-derived layers: an inner nucleated germinal layer, and an outer acellular laminated layer surrounded by a host-derived fibrous capsule [2]. Intermediate host species depends on the infecting strain of *E. granulosus*, regional or local differences in the availability of the various intermediate host species, and other factors [2], but would include primarily ungulates, also marsupials [which for the case of Colombia would make think the possibility of occurrence in the country given the wide presence of them, such as *Didelphis marsupialis* (locally called "chucha")]. Ten strains of *E. granulosus* have been identified so far (G1–G10) with different host affinities: G1–G2 being sheep strains, G3 and G5 bovid strains, G4 a horse strain, G6 a camelid strain, G7 a pig strain,

G8 a cervid strain, G9 has been described in swine in Poland, and G10 in reindeer in Eurasia [1, 81]. The sheep strain (G1) is most commonly associated with human infections [1]. The presence of diverse strains of *E. granulosus* has important implications for public health. The shortened maturation time of the adult form of the parasite in the intestine of dogs suggests that the interval period for administering anti-parasite drugs to infected dogs will have to be shortened in those areas where the G2, G5, and G6 strains are found [1]. The adult *E. granulosus* is 2.0 to 7.0 mm in length. It has three proglottids (range 4–6). It is supposed that *E. granulosus* is found worldwide; however, in many countries (including Colombia and other countries in South America), its presence has not been confirmed both in humans and in animals. Hydatid cysts are predominantly found in liver and lungs (Figure 1).

2.2. *Echinococcus multilocularis*

(Alveolar echinococcosis)

E. multilocularis is the etiological agent of the alveolar echinococcosis, its infection is perpetuated in a sylvatic cycle, with wild carnivores—mainly red (*Vulpes vulpes*) and arctic (*Alopex lagopis*) foxes—regarded as the most important definitive hosts. Domestic dogs and cats may be involved in a synanthropic cycle, and also raccoon dog and coyotes [2]. Small mammals (usually microtine and arvicolid rodents) act as intermediate hosts. The metacestode of *E. multilocularis* is a tumor-like, infiltrating structure consisting of many small vesicles embedded in stroma of connective tissue. The metacestode mass usually contains a semisolid matrix rather than fluid. The adult tapeworm is different in size than adult *E. granulosus* (1.2–4.5 mm) and its eggs are indistinguishable by light microscopy. The hydatid cysts do not form hyaline membrane and the scolices, which are abundant in rodents but absent in humans. People become exposed to *E. multilocularis* by handling of infected hosts, or by ingestion of food contaminated with eggs of the parasite [2].

It is endemic in North America, Alaska, Europe, Central Russia, China, Turkey, Japan, Uruguay, and Argentina. In humans, the most frequently affected organs are the liver (80%), lungs (10%), brain (5%), and other organs such as kidney and pancreas (5%) [6]. *E. multilocularis* has five proglottids (range 2–6). Hydatid cysts are primarily hepatic, with metastases in lungs, brain, and bones among other organs.

2.3. *Echinococcus oligarthrus*

(Polycystic echinococcosis)

E. oligarthrus is the smallest species of the genus, it only measures, in its adult form, 2.2 to 2.9 mm. Definitive hosts are different species of wild felidae (pampas cats, Geoffrey's cat, ocelot, jaguar, cougar, jaguarandi, puma, boat cats) and intermediate hosts are rodents like rats (spiny rat), agoutis, and pacas (both, very highly distributed in the whole territory of Colombia and in most of the tropical areas of South America, including Brazil, Paraguay, Bolivia, Peru, Ecuador, Venezuela, Guyana, Suriname, and French Guyana) [6]. Hydatid cysts are located in an extrahepatic location, mostly in the intermuscular tissue, pleural, and peritoneal cavity [6].

E. oligarthrus has three proglottids. Larval parasite of this species can be also located in eye and heart.

2.4. *Echinococcus vogeli*

(Polycystic echinococcosis)

E. vogeli also causes polycystic echinococcosis and has been reported only in Central and South America. However, not every country in this region has reported cases of *E. vogeli*. Brazil (98 cases) and Colombia (30 cases) have been the countries with the highest number of reported cases, till 2010 (including *E.* cf. *vogeli*) [6]. The adult tapeworm measures 5.6 mm. The eggs are similar to that of the *Taenia* genus. Definitive hosts are domestic and wild dogs (bush dog and domestic dog). The bush dog, *Speothos venaticus*, is widely distributed in South America, particularly not only in Brazil (>80% of the territory) but also in most parts of Venezuela, Guyana, Suriname, and French Guyana, as well as in some areas of Colombia, Panama, Ecuador, Peru, Paraguay, Argentina, and Uruguay. Intermediate hosts are rodents, but mainly the agoutis and pacas. In this species, the hydatid cyst is of endogenous proliferation and it forms bags or folds inside the primary bladder [6]. While in rodent the larvae is limited, in humans it disseminates, due to exogenous vesiculation and due to the amount of scolice inside the cyst, which can cause reinfection when it breaks spontaneously or by medical manipulation [6]. The adult *E. vogeli* is 3.9 to 5.6 mm in length. *E. vogeli* has three proglottids.

The results of a survey (carried out to detect *Echinococcus* infections) involving more than 4,000 Colombian mammals showed interesting findings regarding *E. vogeli* and *E. oligarthrus*. Adult worms were found in 5 of 121 carnivores: *E. oligarthrus* in 1 of 11 ocelots, 2 of 9 jaguarundi cats, and single puma; and *E. vogeli* in 1 of 15 domestic dogs. Although bush dogs were present, none could be examined. Polycystic larvae were found in 96 of 325 pacas (29.5%) and in 6 of 1,168 (0.5%) spiny rats, *Proechimys spp*. None of the 118 agouti showed hydatid cysts but an infected heart was provided by hunters. The paca's infection rate increased with age but was not related to gender or geographic region. In 73 of 96 pacas, the infection was due to *E. vogeli*, and the cysts were located in the liver. In three cases, it was due to *E. oligarthrus* and the hydatid cysts were extrahepatic, mainly attached to muscles. In the remaining 20, the species involved could not be determined. The parasites in two of the spiny rats, and in the agouti heart were *E. oligarthrus* [48]. Although most of the infected animals were collected in the eastern plains, other records and verbal information indicate that, at least in Colombia where man has not exterminated pacas, agoutis, wild canids, and felids, one still can find enzootic neotropical *Echinococcus* infection. The cycle of *E. vogeli* involves the bush dog and paca as hosts, and that of *E. oligarthrus*, the paca, agouti, spiny rat, and several species of wild felids [48].

Other species in the genus *Echinococcus* have also been discovered and identified. Currently, there are 12 species, including those four causing human pathology, six identified in animals: *E. canadensis* (main intermediate host: cervids; known definite hosts: wolves, dog), *E. equinus* (main intermediate host: horses; known definite host: dogs), *E. felidis* (main intermediate host: warthogs; known definite host: lions), *E. intermedius* (main intermediate hosts: camels, pigs, sheep; known definite hosts lions), *E. ortleppi* (main intermediate host: cattle; known definite hosts dogs), and *E. shiquicus* (main intermediate host: pika; known definite host: Tibetan fox);

and two to be assigned to name species (*Echinococcus sp.* GL-2010 and *Echinococcus sp.* GL-2012) (http://www.ncbi.nlm.nih.gov/Taxonomy/Browser/wwwtax.cgi?id=6209) [46].

Some authors have recently exposed that all these species would be infectious for humans, probably with the exception of *E. equinus*, *E. felidis*, and *E. shiquicus*, and also the two to be assigned to name species [46]. Probably, with more studies in molecular epidemiology in the future, their role will become clear.. However, it is interesting to note that at the GenBank (http://www.ncbi.nlm.nih.gov/gene/?term=echinococcus), there are 271 genes identified from different species of *Echinococcus*: *E. oligarthrus* (36 genes), *E. vogeli* (36 genes), *E. shiquicus* (36 genes), *E. canadensis* (36 genes), *E. equinus* (36 genes), *E. felidis* (36 genes), *E. ortleppi* (14 genes), *E. multilocularis* (12 genes), and *E. granulosus* (12 genes). At GenBank, there are also 43,971 sequences of proteins of the genus *Echinococcus* (http://www.ncbi.nlm.nih.gov/protein/?term=echinococcus): *E. granulosus* (24,310 sequences), *E. multilocularis* (18,670 sequences), *E. canadensis* (476 sequences), *E. shiquicus* (111 sequences), *E. equinus* (77 sequences), *E. ortleppi* (66 sequences), *E. vogeli* (51 sequences), *E. oligarthrus* (47 sequences), and *E. felidis* (34 sequences).

More importantly, a draft genomic sequence for *E. granulosus* comprising 151.6 Mb encoding 11,325 genes has been achieved [47], including the evaluation of the regulation of genes in the adult, oncosphere, hydatid cyst, and protoscoleces, which would be of great significance for further studies in diagnostic as well in the immunology and vaccine development, among other things.

3. Life cycle

The adult *E. granulosus* lives in the small intestine of the definitive hosts (dogs or other canids) (Figure 2). Gravid proglottids release eggs that are passed in the feces of these animals (which would come in close contact with humans). After ingestion by a suitable intermediate host (sheep, goat, swine, cattle, horses, camel, under usual natural conditions), embryonated eggs are hatched in the small intestine of the intermediate host and release the oncosphere which penetrates the intestinal wall and migrates through the circulatory system into various organs, especially the liver and lungs (Figure 2).

In these organs, the oncosphere develops into a cyst that enlarges gradually, producing protoscolices and daughter cysts that fill the cyst interior (Figure 2). The definitive host becomes infected by ingesting the cyst-containing organs of the infected intermediate host (Figure 2). After ingestion, the protoscolices evaginate, attach to the intestinal mucosa, and develop into adult stages in approximately 32 to 80 days (Figure 2). Humans can also get infected by ingesting eggs from feces of definitive hosts infected, then resulting with the release of oncospheres in the intestine and the development of cysts in different organs (mainly liver and lungs) (Figure 2).

The same life cycle occurs with *E. multilocularis*, *E. vogeli*, and *E. oligarthrus*, with the differences in the definitive or main hosts and the intermediate hosts involved for these species (Figure 2).

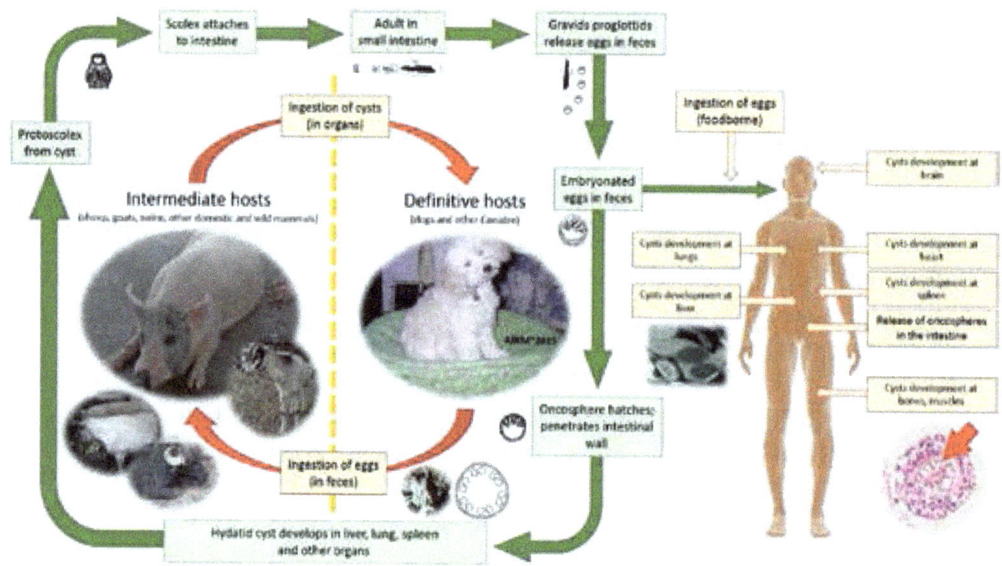

Figure 2. Life cycle of echinococcosis (pictures by A. J. Rodriguez-Morales).

4. Geographical distribution

Cystic echinococcosis or cystic hydatidosis (caused by *E. granulosus*) is an important public health problem in South America, the Middle East and Eastern Mediterranean, some sub-Saharan African countries, China, the former Soviet Union, Russia, and the new related countries (Figure 3) [7, 8]. The overall prevalence of echinococcal infection is underestimated in many countries because systematic population surveys are not performed in all endemic areas, and this disease is not under surveillance neither in humans nor in animals in most of these countries [9]. Even more, in some countries, such as Colombia, there are reports from animal health authorities claiming that echinococcosis as a disease has "never" been registered in the country [49]. In endemic areas, its incidence has been estimated to be around 50 cases per 100,000 population per year [10].

In South America, although there is underreporting, it has been estimated that each year there would be occurring 2,000 cases [3], but these are not the exact figures. Uruguay has reported 9.2 cases per 100,000 population in 1995, and Chile has reported between 6.6 and 8.4 new cases per 100,000 population per year. Besides this, echinococcosis is also a health problem in Argentina, Bolivia, Brazil, and Peru [10, 82]. In the Peruvian Andes, observed prevalence rates in one study among humans, canines, and sheep were 9%, 46%, and 32%, respectively [9].

World Health Organization (WHO) had developed a global map of the distribution of *E. granulosus* and cystic echinococcosis (hydatidosis, 2009); however, there is no recent official WHO map for distribution of other *Echinococcus* species (Figure 3) [50]. However, in 2001, WHO and World Organization for Animal Health also developed a map of the approxi-

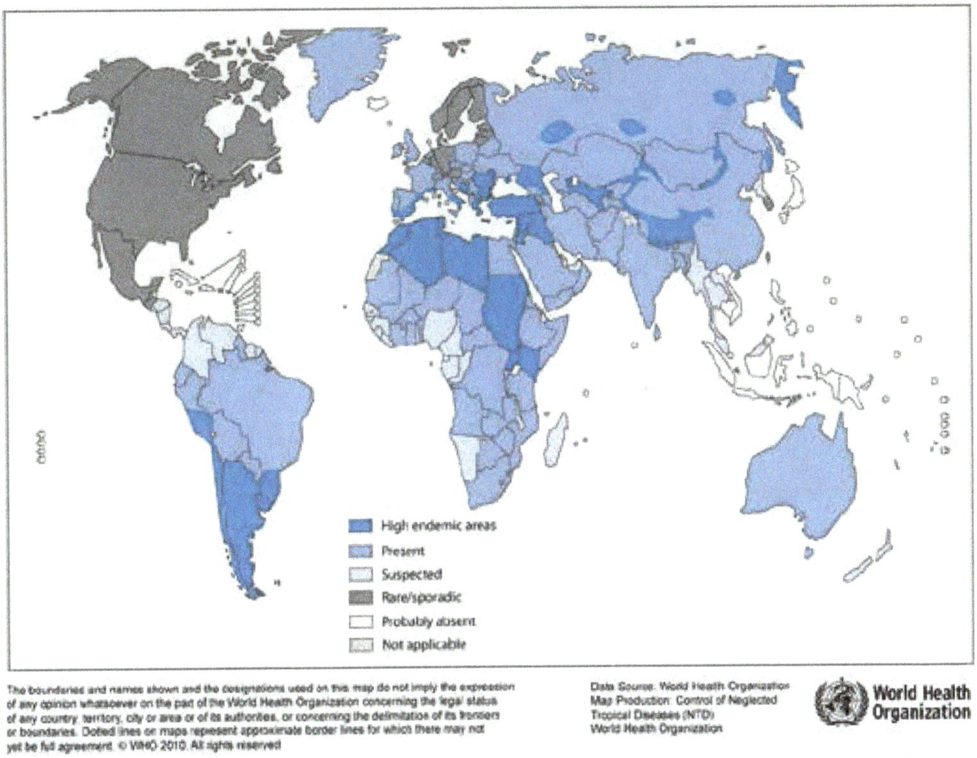

Figure 3. Distribution of *Echinococcus granulosus* and cystic echinococcosis (hydatidosis), 2009 (2010) [50].

mate geographical distribution of *E. multilocularis* and alveolar echinococcosis (1999) (Figure 4) [51, 52].

E. multilocularis is limited to the northern hemisphere (Figure 4). It occurs in Central and Eastern Europe, the former Soviet Union (now Russia), Turkey, Iraq, northern India, central China, some Japanese islands, some provinces of Canada, Alaska, and some north central states of the United States [9] (Figure 4).

Distribution of *E. oligarthrus* and *E. vogeli* is limited to South and Central America, but there is no precise map regarding their presence in the countries of these regions.

Since definitive host of *E. vogeli* exists only from Panama to the North of Argentina, cases of polycystic hydatidosis outside of this region of the world are probably imported by *E. oligarthrus* [9]. However, there are no precise estimations of *E. oligarthrus*. An attempt to map the distribution of *E. vogeli* was presented in 2005 by Colombian authors (Figure 5).

Normally, infections from species of the genus *Echinococcus* involve wild and rural hosts; however, due to human actions (temporary by recreation and work, but also definitive) which have permanently used dogs in work grazing and fed them with viscera of sacrificed animals, this cycle has been altered [6]. Since all types of echinococcosis or hydatidosis are acquired by ingestion of water or food contaminated with the eggs in the feces shed by the carnivores, it

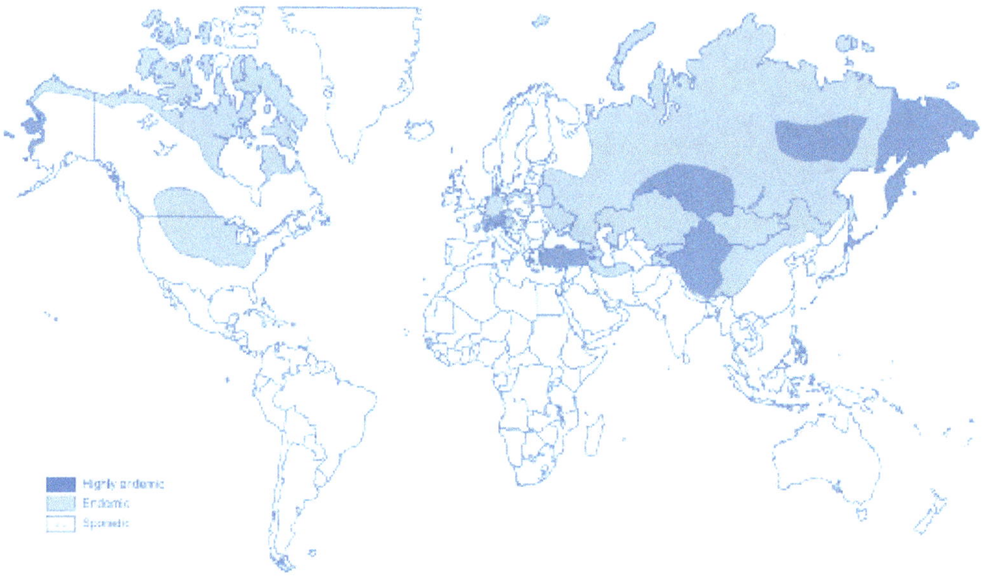

Figure 4. Approximate geographical distribution of *Echinococcus multilocularis* and alveolar echinococcosis (1999) [51, 52].

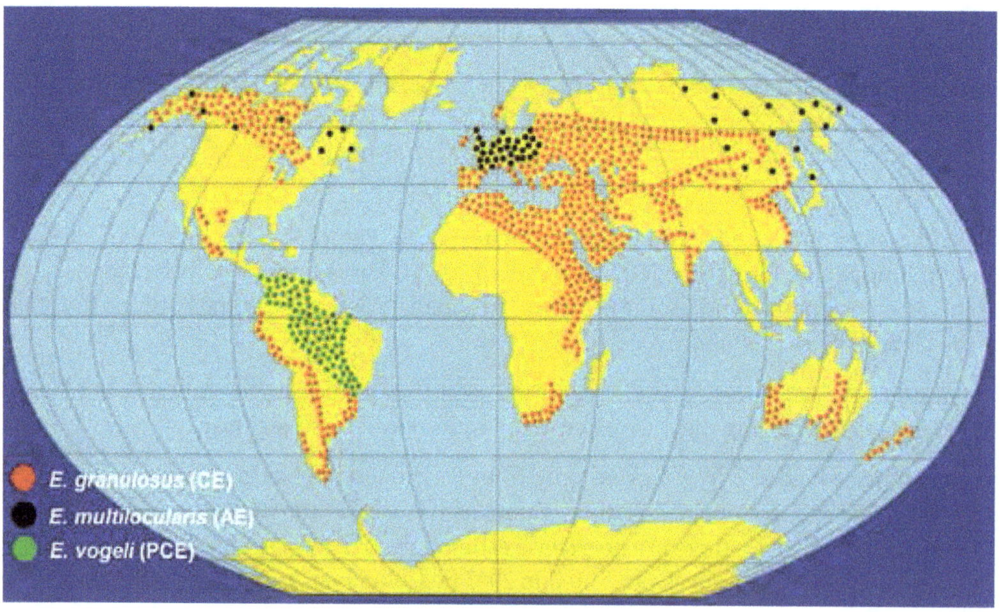

Figure 5. Drawing illustrates the geographic distribution of hydatid disease from *Echinococcus granulosus* (red dots), *E. multilocularis* (black dots), and *E. vogeli* (green dots). *E. granulosus* is the most common of the *Echinococcus* species (1999) [53]. This is not precise and requires more specific information from the countries regarding the distribution of cases by the territories included in the map.

is advisable to take special care with the feces of these animals, especially when considering that these eggs resist partial desiccation for several months [6].

5. Echinococcosis studies in Colombia

In Colombia, echinococcosis does not seem to be a major problem if we base such assumptions from human and animal health authorities [49]. But, as has been evidenced, cases of infection with the larval forms of *E. granulosus* have been reported [11]. However, prevalence and incidence of this entity have not been determined. Echinococcosis is not under surveillance and there is no obligation to report cases related to this infection to health authorities in the country; then known cases have been just those reported in national and international biomedical literature (Figure 6).

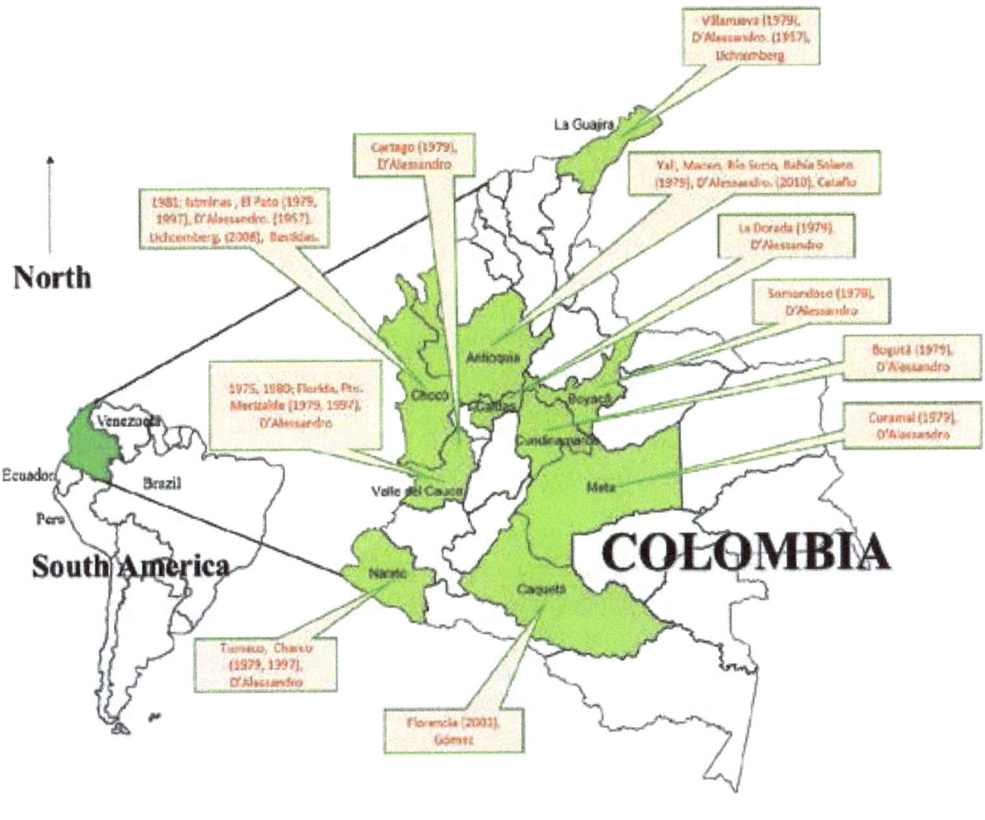

Figure 6. Departments of Colombia where cases of echinococcosis have been reported. (First date reported is the year of the case, then the location, year of publication in parenthesis, and main author.)

The first case was reported in 1941 [12], but since 1957, more cases had been reported [54] (Figure 6). Two decades later, D'Alessandro began studies in the country. This author found more than a dozen of human cases of polycystic echinococcosis produced by the larval stage of *E. vogeli* whose definitive hosts were wild and domestic dogs and intermediate host was paca ("guagua," *Cuniculus paca*) [3, 55], after suspecting the presence of disease due to four cases of calcified hydatid cysts [55].

Most of the infected people were native from Colombia who acquired the disease by ingesting food or water contaminated with dog feces and by eating raw viscera of "guagua." Botero et al. describe three more unpublished cases: two from the coast of the Pacific Ocean and one from Santa Marta [13, 14]. D'Alessandro's studies demonstrated that in Colombia, the guagua is the main intermediate host and the wild dogs known as gouache fox is the definitive host. The guatin, which is also an edible animal for Colombian indigenous tribes, is a more specific host for *E. oligarthrus* [6].

Till 2008, the country in South America with the highest number of cases reported was Brazil, with 99 cases, followed by Colombia with 29 (Figure 6) [3, 50-60]. In Colombia, some authors believe that there are more cases not reported, in fact due to the lack of records. This also probes that occurrence of echinococcosis is more evidently reported, when people in the rural and jungle areas receive health services and physicians are more aware of the disease [60].

Two years later, in 2010, another and the last case till March 2015, has been reported [61]. A case of cardiac echinococcosis, detected in echocardiographic finding in an 18-year-old woman diagnosed in Medellin, Antioquia [61]. Fortunately in this case, physicians suspected of this cestode infection; however, more awareness among physicians regarding the compromise of cardiovascular system in many parasitic diseases is still necessary, particularly in endemic areas [63-67].

Based on this review of cases, including information from the departments of the country where this disease has been reported, a map for Colombia has been proposed (Figure 6). This map shows the departments of the country (including locations of origin of one or more cases), where echinococcosis have been reported (Figure 6). At least 10 departments (out of 32 in total) have reported cases of echinococcosis (Figure 6) [14, 54, 59-61, 72].

Beyond this, with an increasing number of published reports concerning this disease, medical personnel in tropical areas, as in Colombia and more recently in Brazil, have been keenly interested in undertaking epidemiological surveys [3, 68, 69]. Even more, there is a significant zoonotic potential, given the fact that the investigations in Colombia demonstrated a large enzootic areas of transmission in the oriental plains of that country [3, 58], where multiple species and a high number of animals have been found positive in the evaluations for *Echinococcus*, particularly *E. oligarthrus*.

As in other zoonotic diseases, parasitic and of other etiologies, there is a clear need of more studies, as well as more interaction between physicians and veterinarians. More research is necessary; currently, there are just 10 reports available in Medline for Colombia (using the terms "Colombia" AND "Echinococc*" [means *Echinococcus* and/or echinococcosis]) [53, 55-60, 62, 70, 71]. There is no significantly different information available at Scopus. At SciELO, there is one additional case, a patient with hepatic hydatidosis who appeared as an eosinophilic pleural effusion serologically confirmed, treated with combined therapy with albendazole and the percutaneous aspiration-injection-reaspiration drainage technique [72].

Finally, an undergoing research of our group is analyzing a new source of information for communicable diseases, which are not under surveillance and require compulsory notification. In Colombia, there is a service, which is now available for analyses, the so-called personal health records (*Registro Individual de Prestación de Servicios*, RIPS), where diagnoses are classified according to WHO cause groups International Classification of Diseases version 10 (ICD-10). At this system, we retrieved the cases of echinococcosis between years 2009 and 2013, finding 303 cases (Figure 7).

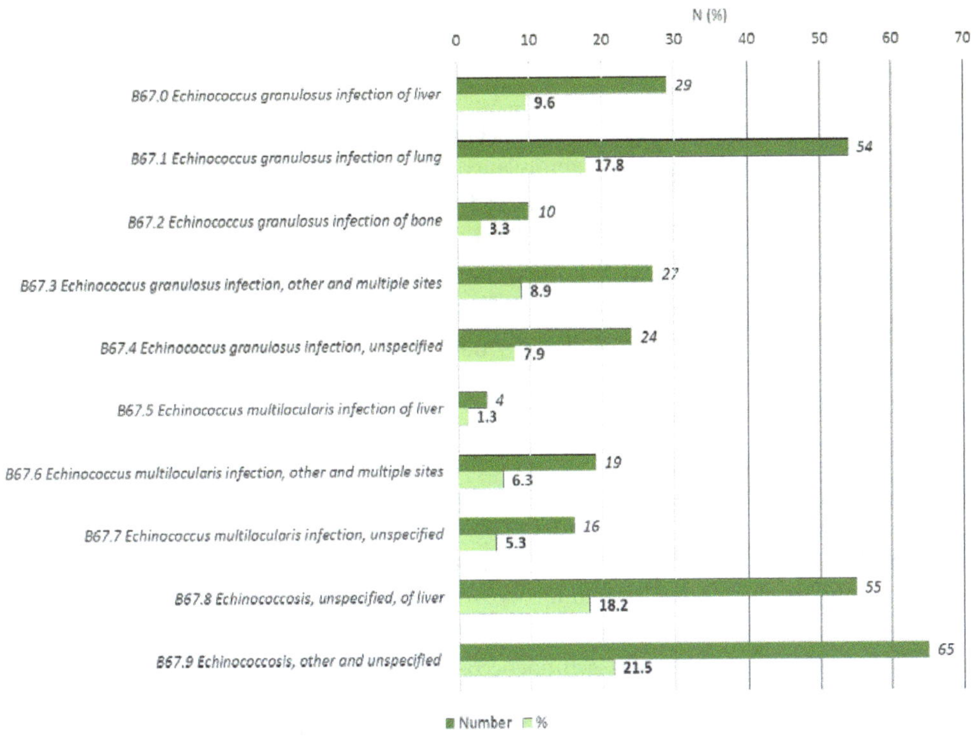

Figure 7. Cases of echinococcosis (ICD-10 codes B67.0 to B67.9) reported to the personal health records of Colombia (RIPS) during 2009–2013.

Although these cases corresponded in 18.2% to "Echinococcosis, unspecified, of liver" (B67.8) and 21.5% to "Echinococcosis, other and unspecified" (B67.9), there are 60.4% (n = 183) of them classified as infection due to *E. granulosus* (47.5%) and *E. multilocularis* (12.9%) in different organs (Figure 7), mainly lung for *E. granulosus* (17.8%) (Figure 7). Although there are limitations to this source, there is useful information that should be further analyzed. Epidemiological factors (geographic distribution, age groups, gender) involved in these cases would be of high interest in describing the situation of echinococcosis in the country.

In these cases, looked retrospectively, the limitation in the approach is that there is no information regarding the diagnostic techniques implemented in each case, and how these cases were therapeutically managed. Then, based on this information, cross-sectional and prospective studies should be implemented in the countries, and there should also be an increase in the awareness about the existence and occurrence of such diseases in different areas of the country, and particularly in those that had previously reported case reports and case series since early decades (Figure 6).

6. Economic burden of echinococcosis

According to the World Bank, economic losses due to this disease stand at the fourth position after other diseases and trauma [3].

Echinococcosis also affects the economy of the endemic regions. In humans, losses are due to costs of hospitalization, treatment, disability, etc. However, in livestock, losses are due to lost productivity, losses in quality of the wool and meat, and decreased milk production and fertility [15]. Estimated annual economic losses in Peru are $ 178,705 [10]. In Colombia, estimation of the economic burden of this disease has not been reported, but given the increase in the number of economic evaluations of infectious diseases in the country and in the region [73, 74], there would be more clear details once the number of cases reported would be defined.

7. Clinical manifestations

Regardless of the etiology, a new concept of organ compromise was proposed in 2014, when two or more organs are affected by echinococcosis at the same time in a patient. This has been defined as multivisceral echinococcosis, simultaneous localization of hydatid cysts in more than one organ [83]. Multivisceral echinococcosis should be differentiated from multiple echinococcosis [83]. The latter is the localization of multiple cysts in one organ [83]. Even in paired organs (lungs, kidneys) if both are compromised, it will be a case of multivisceral echinococcosis, given the implications not just in diagnosis, but particularly in surgical management.

7.1. *Echinococcus granulosus*

Echinococcosis is a larval infection caused in humans by *Echinococcus* species, a metacestode with the ability to create a large spectrum of clinical manifestations, including the asymptomatic infection, and a severe and fatal disease. There are four species of echinococcosis that have been recognized that cause various forms of the disease, specifically the *E. granulosus* species which is responsible for cystic echinococcosis [16].

7.1.1. Cystic echinococcosis

As a general rule, the phase of primary infection is always asymptomatic because the cysts are located in different organs, characterized by their small size, which is less than 5 cm and are encapsulated. This first phase is not been associated with major pathology and might remain asymptomatic for a long period or permanently [16, 17]. The incubation period is undefined but it could be in around months or even years, before the infection becomes symptomatic. There have been reported cases of spontaneous cure due to cyst calcification and collapse and on the other hand, there are cases of early symptomatology because of cyst rupture [16, 18].

7.1.2. Patient characteristics

Cystic echinococcosis is seen in all ages, including patients aged below 1 year and above 75 years, with a majority between 6 and 15 years, 21 and 30, and 30 and 40 years. The most risky profession involves farm labors [16].

7.1.3. Symptoms

There is a huge spectrum of clinical manifestations that are variable among the patients and none of these are considered as pathognomonic of echinococcosis [16]. All the symptoms might depend on different characteristics such as the host-parasite interaction, the different organs involved, cyst size, and the presence of different complications such as cyst rupture or trauma [16, 18]. The most commonly compromised organs are the liver, followed by lung, kidney, spleen, and less common organs like muscles, skin, abdominal cavity, and pelvic cavity. The symptoms may vary in accordance with the organ involved [16-18].

Liver infections include symptoms such as hepatomegaly, cholecystitis, jaundice, liver abscess, or secondary biliary cirrhosis. Lung infections include symptoms like chest pain, expectoration, hemoptysis, and dyspnea [19]. Other severe manifestations include cyst getting rupture into biliary tree causing biliary colic, jaundice and can be confused with pancreatitis or cholangitis [16, 19].

7.1.4. Liver involvement

The liver is the most commonly involved organ, representing around two-thirds of the cases. The right lobe is compromised in the majority of the cases (60% to 80%) but it frequently does not produce symptoms and when these once occur, it is estimated that the cyst size is around 10 cm [20, 21]. Once a cyst develops a larger size, hepatomegaly might occur and other symptoms like right upper quadrant pain, nausea, and vomiting can also result. Due to the mass defect of the cyst compression of the portal and hepatic veins, it can result in Budd-Chiari syndrome [19, 20].

7.1.5. Lung involvement

The most common symptom of lung infection is the presence of cough in around 53% to 62% of the patients, followed by chest pain, dyspnea, and hemoptysis. But generally, most of the patients with lung infection are asymptomatic [21, 22].

7.1.6. Other organs

Heart infection might generate rupture with pericardial tamponade, cardiac insufficiency, embolism or pericardial effusion [23-25, 60, 64, 66]. The central nervous system can lead to seizures or symptoms due to an increase in the intracranial pressure [26]. Kidney disease can cause hematuria, and even glomerulonephritis and nephrotic syndrome have been described. Bones are mostly asymptomatic and only develop manifestations when a pathological fracture occurs [23].

7.1.7. Outcome

Surgeries are performed in around 15% of the patients after the initial diagnosis. And in patients without surgery, majority would remain asymptomatic through many years [18].

7.2. *Echinococcus multilocularis*

The most common presenting complaints include malaise, weight loss, and right upper quadrant discomfort due to hepatomegaly. Cholestatic jaundice, cholangitis, portal hypertension, and the Budd-Chiari syndrome can also occur. The clinical presentation may mimic that of hepatocellular carcinoma [18].

Extrahepatic primary disease is very rare (1% of cases). Multiorgan disease was described in 13% of cases in one series in which metacestodes involved the lungs, spleen, or brain in addition to the liver [2]. If left untreated, more than 90% of patients will die within 10 years of the onset of clinical symptoms, and virtually 100% will die by 15 years [18].

7.3. *Echinococcus oligarthus* and *Echinococcus vogeli*

These species cause polycystic echinococcosis, but they represent a very rare cause of echinococcosis disease, found in muscles and skin but it has been only described in a few cases in Brazil, Venezuela, and Surinam [16, 18, 28, 29].

8. Diagnosis

For an optimal diagnosis, both imaging and serological tests are required.

8.1. Imaging

The cysts may be visualized by ultrasonography, computed tomography (CT), or magnetic resonance imaging (MRI). However ultrasonography is the most commonly employed technique due to its easy performance and low cost. The sensitivity of ultrasonography for the evaluation of echinococcosis is 90% to 95% and the appearance of a cyst in the ultrasound is as an anechoic and smooth cyst. Another important aspect of the ultrasonography is that it helps in the classification of the disease, according to the WHO echinococcosis classification based on their ultrasound appearance. CT has an overall sensitivity of 95% to 100% and is the preferred imaging test to describe the size, location, and number of cysts. MRI has the same sensitivity as that of CT and has no major advantages over CT, but it is better for the determination of intra- and extra-hepatic changes; however, it is not usually a routine examination technique in the patients [18, 27].

8.2. Serological tests

They are used in the diagnosis and follow-up of the patients. Some of the laboratory tests include complement fixation, latex agglutination, and indirect immunofluorescence [27, 84]. However, there are two important antigens of the *E. granulosus* disease [18]:

- Antigen 5 which is a parasite antigen; however, the studies have shown low specificity of its extensive use in the diagnosis [18].
- Antigen B is a lipoprotein and is related with a superior specificity in comparison with the antigen 5 [18].

8.3. Other laboratory tests for diagnosis

Nonspecific leukopenia or thrombocytopenia, mild eosinophilia, and nonspecific liver function may be detected but are not diagnostic. Hypergammaglobulinemia and elevated serum IgE levels are present in more than 50% of cases.

Imaging: On ultrasonography or CT, the lesions usually have an irregular contour with no well-defined wall, central necrosis, and irregular intralesional and wall calcifications.

8.4. Comparing serologies

Serologic tests are more reliable for diagnosis of *E. multilocularis* infection than for *E. granulosus* infection; sensitivity and specificity rates are 95% to 100%. A specific *E. multilocularis* antigen such as the affinity purified Em2 antigen from alveolar echinococcosis metacestodes is often used; the Em2-ELISA can discriminate between *E. granulosus* and *E. multilocularis* in 95% of cases. Serology usually remains positive indefinitely; following complete surgical resection, serology may normalize within a few years [18].

Cyst aspiration or biopsy: In the absence of a positive serologic test, percutaneous aspiration or biopsy may be required to confirm the diagnosis by demonstrating the presence of protoscolices, hooklets, or hydatid membranes.

Polymerase chain reaction: Polymerase chain reaction techniques are limited to research settings but may play a diagnostic role in the future. DNA probes using Southern hybridization tests are also being developed.

9. Treatment

Echinococcosis treatment includes a multidisciplinary conduct and a general overview of the patient condition in order to provide the best management that includes surgical treatment, pharmacological treatment, the "watch and wait," and both of them, depending on the specific characteristics of the disease and most importantly the type of Echinococcosis that the patient develops. The overall approach depends on the different species that infect humans, particularly two of them: *E. granulosus* and *E. multilocularis*, causing cystic echinococcosis (CE) and alveolar echinococcosis (AE), respectively [85].

9.1. Cystic echinococcosis

As mentioned earlier, the treatment is complex, and even these days there are no clinical trials and studies that compare the different modalities to say which one is superior to the other. However, it is accepted that the surgical treatment can potentially remove all the *E. granulosus* cysts for complete cure [30]. The different treatment strategies include surgery, percutaneous management, pharmacological management, and observation [31].

Overall, the diagnosis approach depends on the WHO diagnostic classification, performed in 2003, when the Informal Working Group on echinococcosis established a standardized ultrasound classification based on the status of the cyst by its ultrasound appearance. This classification has the intention to promote uniform standards of diagnosis and treatment, and has important implications for the clinical decision.

There are three different stages, including CE1 and CE2 that are cyst-containing protoscolices. The CE3 stage is divided in CE3a, a detached endocyst, and CE3b, a solid cyst with daughter cysts [32]. Recommendations indicate that CE1 and CE3a stages, in which the cyst size is less than 5 cm, should be treated with albendazole only. Stages CE1 and CE3a with cyst size more than 5 cm may be treated with albendazole in combination with percutaneous treatment via PAIR (puncture, aspiration, injection, and reaspiration). The CE2 and CE3b stages are characterized by multiple cyst compartments that require individual puncture, and these patients usually require PAIR. However, the optimal choice among the different approaches (PAIR, surgery, or drug therapy) is uncertain. Finally, stages CE4 and CE5 involve inactive cysts that only require observation [33, 34].

9.2. Treatment options

9.2.1. Surgery

It is the first treatment option in cases of complicated cysts, including a cyst rupture or infection and hemorrhage. It is also an alternative treatment option for those cysts with many daughter vesicles that are not suitable for percutaneous treatment. Another indications are large liver cysts, cyst diameter more than 10cm, extrahepatic disease (lung, bone, or brain), cysts situated superficially with high risk of rupture, and cysts affecting the biliary tree [31, 35]. Contraindications are relative to each patient; for example, old-aged people, people suffering from concomitant diseases, pregnant women, or patients with small cysts [7]. As far as the complications are concerned, secondary infection, intra-abdominal abscess, fistula, or sclerosing cholangitis have been reported. Recurrent echinococcosis may occur in e 2% to 25% of the cases, depending basically on the surgeon's experience [35].

Before choosing the surgical technique, it's important to administrate drug therapy to minimize the surgical risk of secondary echinococcosis from seeding of protoscolices in the abdominal cavity. Usually, albendazole is administered a week before surgery, and continued at least four weeks after the surgery. Praziquantel is another option, but there is no specific evidence regarding its efficacy [31, 36].

Surgical approach must be individualized, depending on each patient disease and its characteristics. There are two options; the first one is to remove the intact cyst, and another option is to open the cyst with protoscolicidal agents, such as hypertonic saline, followed by the evacuation of the cyst contents and removal of the cyst [31]. Other protoscolicidal used includes 70% to 95% ethanol and 0.5% cetrimide solution. The protoscolicidal agent must be in contact with the germinal layer for at least 15 minutes to make its effect. Albendazole, ivermectin, and praziquantel have been also used as protoscolicidal agents, but their efficacy and safety need more studies. Protoscolicidal agents should not be used in the presence of biliary communication, because of the risk of sclerosing cholangitis or pancreatitis [31, 35].

There is also the possibility of laparoscopic surgery for the treatment of echinococcosis; however, there are no randomized trials done yet comparing the efficacy of laparoscopy with open procedures. Possible indications for laparoscopic treatment are the presence of anteriorly located hepatic cysts, although this procedure is related with associated risk of spillage because of the elevation of intra-abdominal pressures due to the pneumoperitoneum. Contraindications include deep intraparenchymal cysts, the presence of calcified walls cyst, and cysts located next to the vena cava [31].

In a review article published in 2014 with the aim to study the world literature of the laparoscopic treatment of liver hydatid cyst, a total of 914 patients were identified to evaluate the mortality, morbidity, and clinical outcomes of the laparoscopic treatment. It was found that the most common procedure was cystectomy in 60.39% of patients, followed by partial pericystectomy with 14.77% of patients, and finally pericystectomy with 8.21% of patients, and the rest of them were treated via segmentectomy. They also reported that conversion of laparoscopy to open laparotomy occurred in the 4.92% of the cases, due to anatomical limitations and inaccessible locations. Mortality was reported in 0.22% of the patients and morbidity was reported in 15.07% of the patients. There was no intraoperative deaths reported and the most reported complication was bile leakage. In general terms, they concluded that the laparoscopic procedure is safe, with acceptable ranges of mortality and morbidity and clinical outcomes comparable to open surgery [37].

9.2.2. Percutaneous management

There are two percutaneous techniques. The first one called PAIR (puncture, aspiration, injection of a protoscolicidal agent, and reaspiration) is usually effective in the treatment of cysts without daughter cysts. And the second one, that involves the evacuation of the cyst with a large bore catheter. This technique helps in cases in which the drain becomes difficult or tends to relapse after PAIR, like in the case of WHO stages CE2 and CE3b cysts [31, 38].

Percutaneous treatment is associated with anaphylaxis, happening according to a review in the 1.6% of the patients [39]. And as in surgery, albendazole must be administered for at least one month after the percutaneous treatment [31].

9.2.3. PAIR procedure

It was first introduced in the mid-1980s and includes the realization of percutaneous puncture of the cyst by ultrasonic guidance, aspiration of the cyst fluid, injection of a protoscolicidal substance, and finally reaspiration of the cyst fluid. PAIR has the advantages of being less invasive than surgery and can be a diagnostic and therapeutic procedure and it has a success rate of more than 95%. This procedure may be used in cases of echinococcosis of WHO stages CE1 and CE3a as primary treatment and for the relapse after medical therapy in stages CE1 and CE3a, and in case of relapse after surgery. PAIR also showed to be successful in the management of liver cysts and in those cysts located in other abdominal parts such as kidney, spleen, and in the abdominal cavity. There are controversies in the use of PAIR in pregnant women and in children, although the application of PAIR is indicated in symptomatic pregnant women [16, 31, 38].

The procedure is performed by ultrasound or by CT guidance. Then the cyst is punctured and the fluid aspiration is realized and a histopathological study must be done to evaluate the presence of protoscolices. After the administration of protoscolicidal agent, the reaspiration must be done for at least 10 to 15 minutes. Four hours before PAIR, adjunctive drug therapy with albendazole or mebendazole should be administrated. Recommendations indicate that albendazole should be continued after a month of the procedure and mebendazole should be continued for three months. The most important contraindications of the PAIR are the following: the presence of cysts without drainable solid material, superficial cyst with risk of rupture in the abdominal cavity, calcified cysts, and cyst with biliary communication [31, 40].

9.2.4. Drug therapy

In most of the cases, it is useful as an adjunctive therapy to surgery and percutaneous treatment. The use of pharmacological approach as definitive management is indicated in few cases. The recommendations indicate that in cases of small cysts of WHO stages CE1 and CE3a with cyst size less than 5 cm, the initial management with only drug therapy is appropriate, with optimal duration of treatment depending on the clinical factors, but usually estimated in around one to six months. The effectiveness of pharmacological therapy decreases with the presence of a cyst size more than 5 cm, with multiple compartments of cysts [16, 31, 39].

As an adjunctive treatment, albendazole is used as perioperative drug therapy in surgery or in percutaneous treatment. It reduces the risk of recurrent disease by the inactivation of the protoscolices. There is no general consensus of the duration of the treatment, but generally it is initiated four days before surgery and continued at least one month after the surgery in case of albendazole and for three months in case of mebendazole [16, 31, 40, 42].

Albendazole is the first drug option and the primary antiparasitic agent for treatment of *E. granulosus*, and in cases of absence of albendazole, mebendazole may be used as an alternative, but it is less absorbed than albendazole. The primary action of albendazole is that it inhibits microtubules assembly, causing a glycogen depletion, followed by the degeneration of the mitochondria and the endoplasmic reticulum, finally causing the cell death. It is reported that albendazole helps cyst resolution in 30% of the patients, cyst size reduction in 30% to 50% patients, and in 20% to 40% of the patients, there are no changes in the cysts. However, the outcome of the treatment with albendazole depends on multiple factors like the clinical characteristic of the patient, the cyst size, and its location [31, 43].

However, albendazole has more advantages than mebendazole. For example, albendazole is well tolerated by patients and it takes a shorter duration of therapy. Dose of albendazole is usually 10 to 15 mg/kg per day divided in two doses and mebendazole dose is 40 to 50 mg/kg per day divided in three doses. Adverse effects include hepatotoxicity in 1% to 5% of the patients, cytopenia, and alopecia in less than 1% of the patients. Due to hepatotoxicity, there might be an increase in aminotransferase enzymes. Other rare side effect like agranulocytosis has also been reported. Contraindications of using albendazole include patients with liver disease or bone marrow suppression [31, 44]. Patients with pharmacological therapy must be monitored every two to three weeks for first three months and then monthly [31]. Praziquantel has protoscolicidal activity, but its efficacy in clinical studies is variable, but is considered as an alternative when the albendazole treatment cannot be administrated [44, 45].

Observation: Also known as the "watch and wait," indicated in the WHO stages CE4 and CE5, in patients with absence of complications or inactive liver cysts [40].

9.3. Alverolar echinococcosis

Unfortunately, the treatment of alveolar echinococcosis is less effective than the treatment of cystic echinococcosis. The general approach to the treatment is based on surgery. The main idea is to remove all the infected tissue and sometimes it is necessary to also remove part of the host tissue. Management with albendazole is recommended after surgery with an uncertain optimal duration. The benefit of preoperative albendazole administration has not been reported [31].

10. Conclusions

Echinococcosis has always been neglected worldwide and especially in Colombia. Particularly in this country, research was done and published only between 1950s and 1990s. There is no subsequent interest in the occurrence of this disease and all its implications.

Due to the impact of echinococcosis, the burden it creates, and the consequences in the patients, it becomes important to create strategies in order to improve and have a better control on this disease in our country. This probably should begin at medical schools, where more emphasis on teaching about this parasitic disease, would increase awareness about it. As has been mentioned earlier, there should be regular interaction among physicians, biologists and veterinarians to better understand the implications of this zoonotic disease, which at least from an enzootic point of view is clearly extended. As an additional reflection in the middle of the process and discussion about peace in Colombia, there are chances that once this would be reached, after the La Habana discussions, more people, not only missionary, health, and military corps, would be allowed to enter in the guerrillas-controlled areas, which are precisely located where enzootic evidences of echinococcosis have been reported, increasing the exposure to species of *Echinococcus* and probably making more visible the occurrence of this disease in the country [78].

Even more, it's not clear yet, if Colombia would be considered properly a risky area for travelers visiting the country in the view of acquisition of echinococcosis. But certainly in other highly endemic countries, echinococcosis is included in the list of infectious diseases that can be acquired during travel, and cases of echinococcosis, as well from other cestodiasis, have been reported increasingly during the last few years [75-78].

Therefore, it becomes crucial to create a clear and easy consensus to help and guide the physicians to make a better approach towards helping the patients in finding the opportune diagnosis and the best treatment option. The creation of a normative and the global vision of echinococcosis as a public health problem might help improve the control of this disease.

Echinococcosis, and other zoonotic diseases, can re-emerge just when they are considered to be under control or eliminated. They can go into hiding in the animal reservoirs, so there is no possibility for complacency [78]. Epidemiology of zoonoses such as echinococcosis is complex and dynamic, being influenced by varying parameters that can roughly be categorized as human-related, pathogen-related, and climate/environment-related [79, 80]. But certainly for echinococcosis, there is still much to understand.

Acknowledgements

Authors would like to thank the critical comments of anonymous reviewers. Also, Dr. Rodriguez-Morales would like to thank Dr. Juliana Buitrago-Jaramillo, Dean, Faculty of Health Sciences, Universidad Tecnológica de Pereira, Pereira, Risaralda, Colombia, for her support to his research group during the activities in year 2014, including presentation and conferences at major international meetings (mainly in Peru, Mexico, and Cuba), and also in 2015 (Ecuador). The authors would also like to thank the Asociación Colombiana de Infectología and International Society for Chemotherapy, for supporting the research and presentations of studies in zoonoses since 2011 (Italy, Japan, Brazil, Ecuador, Mexico, Peru, Cuba). Finally, the authors would like to thank the Ministry of Health of Colombia, for the access to SIVIGILA and RIPS databases through the system Cubo de datos del SISPRO.

Author details

Alfonso J. Rodriguez-Morales[1,2,3*], Lauren Sofia Calvo-Betancourt[4], Camila Alarcón-Olave[5] and Adrián Bolívar-Mejía[6]

*Address all correspondence to: arodriguezm@utp.edu.co

1 Public Health and Infection Research Group, School of Medicine and School of Veterinary Medicine and Zootechnics, Faculty of Health Sciences, Universidad Tecnológica de Pereira, Pereira, Risaralda, Colombia

2 Committee on Zoonoses and Haemorrhagic Fevers, Asociación Colombiana de Infectología, Bogotá, DC, Colombia

3 Working Group on Zoonoses, International Society for Chemotherapy, Aberdeen, United Kingdom

4 Fundación Cardiovascular de Colombia, Floridablanca, Santander, Colombia

5 Universidad Autónoma de Bucaramanga, Bucaramanga, Santander, Colombia

6 Clínica FOSCAL Internacional, Floridablanca, Santander, Colombia

References

[1] Moro P, Schantz P. Echinococcosis: A review. Int J Infect Dis. 2009;13: 125-133.

[2] McManus D, Zhang W, Li J, Bartley P. Echinococcosis. Lancet. 2003;362:1295-1304.

[3] D'Alessandro A, Rausch RL. New aspects of neotropical polycystic (Echinococcus vogeli) and unicystic (Echinococcus oligarthrus) echinococcosis. Clin Microbiol Rev. 2008;21(2):380-401.

[4] Khanfar N. Hydatid disease: A review and update. Curr Anaesth & Crit Care. 2004;15:173-183.

[5] Soledad S, Rodríguez V, Candia M, Bonastre P. Hidatidosis Pulmonar. Revista de Posgrado de la VIa Cátedra de Medicina. 2005;152:16-18.

[6] Bonilla C. Hidatidosis: Una zoonosis de múltiples Presentaciones clínicas. Revista Investigación y Desarrollo Social. Universidad Militar Nueva Granada. 2001;24:89-106.

[7] Jenkins DJ, Romig T, Thompson RC. Emergence/re-emergence of Echinococcus spp. A global update. Int J Parasitol. 2005;35:1205-1219.

[8] Romig T, Dinkel A, Mackenstedt U. The present situation of echinococcosis in Europe. Parasitol Int. 2006;55:S187-S191.

[9] Moro P. Epidemiology and control of echinococcosis. UpToDate. Last updated October 15, 2014.

[10] Salgado, DS, Suárez-Ognio, L & Cabrera, R. Características clínicas y epidemiológicas de la equinococosis quística registrados en un área endémica en los andes centrales del Perú. Neotrop Helminthol. 2007;1(2):69-83.

[11] Moro P, Schantz P. Cystic echinococcosis in the Americas. Parasitol Int. 2006;55:S181-S186.

[12] Perez V. Origen, desarrollo y extensión de la hidatidosis en América. Boletín de la oficina sanitaria panamericana. February 1949; 124-156.

[13] Botero D. Parasitosis intestinales, cisticercosis e hidatidosis. Iatreia. 1990;3(3):165-171.

[14] Alessandro A. Polycystic echinococcosis in tropical America: Echinococcus vogeli and E. oligarthrus. Acta Trop. 1997;67:43-65.

[15] Torgerson, PR. Economic effects of echinococcosis. Acta Trop. 2003;85:113-118.

[16] WHO Informal Working Group. International classification of ultrasound images in cystic echinococcosis for application in clinical and field epidemiological settings. Acta Trop. 2003;85(2):253-261.

[17] Gottstein B, Wang J, Blagosklonov O, et al. Echinococcus metacestode: In search of viability markers. Parasite. 2014;21:63. Epub; November 28, 2014.

[18] Moro P. Clinical manifestations and diagnosis of echinococcosis. UpToDate. Last updated October 21, 2014.

[19] Touma D, Sersté T, Ntounda R, et al. The liver involvement of the hydatid disease: A systematic review designed for the hepato-gastroenterologist. Acta Gastroenterol Belg. 2013;76(2): 210-218.

[20] Stojkovic M, Junghanss T. Cystic and alveolar echinococcosis. Handb Clin Neurol. 2013;114:327-334.

[21] Santivanez S, Garcia HH. Pulmonary cystic echinococcosis. Curr Opin Pulm Med. 2010;16:25.

[22] Arinc S, Kosif A, Ertugrul M, et al. Evaluation of pulmonary hydatid cyst cases. Int J Surg. 2009;7:192.

[23] Dziri C, Haouet K, Fingerhut A, Zaouche A. Management of cystic echinococcosis complications and dissemination: where is the evidence? World J Surg. 2009;33:1266.

[24] Turgut AT, Altinok T, Topçu S, Koşar U. Local complications of hydatid disease involving thoracic cavity: Imaging findings. Eur J Radiol. 2009;70:49.

[25] Díaz-Menéndez M, Pérez-Molina JA, Norman FF, et al. Management and outcome of cardiac and endovascular cystic echinococcosis. PLoS Negl Trop Dis. 2012;6:e1437.

[26] Nourbakhsh A, Vannemreddy P, Minagar A, et al. Hydatid disease of the central nervous system: A review of literature with an emphasis on Latin American countries. Neurol Res. 2010;32:245.

[27] Wuestenberg J, Gruener B, Oeztuerk S, at al. Diagnostics in cystic echinococcosis: Serology versus ultrasonography. Turk J Gastroenterol. 2014;25(4):398-404.

[28] Soares Mdo C, Rodrigues AL, Moreira Silva CA, et al. Anatomo-clinical and molecular description of liver neotropical echinococcosis caused by Echinococcus oligarthrus in human host. Acta Trop. 2013;125(1):110-114.

[29] Zimmerman DM, Douglass M, Reavill DR, Greiner EC. Echinococcus oligarthrus cystic hydatidosis in Brazilian agouti (Dasyprocta leporina). J Zoo Wildl Med. 2009;40(3):551-558.

[30] Brunetti E, Kern P, Vuitton DA. Expert consensus for the diagnosis and treatment of cystic and alveolar echinococcosis in humans. Acta Trop. 2010;114(1):1-16.

[31] Moro P. Treatment of echinococcosis. UpToDate. Last updated March 06, 2013.

[32] Brunetti E, Filice C. Echinococcosis Hydatid Cyst Workup. Medscape. Last updated October 19, 2011.

[33] Rinaldi F, Brunetti E, Neumayr A, et al. Cystic echinococcosis of the liver: A primer for hepatologists. World J Hepatol. 2014;6(5):293-305.

[34] Stojkovic M, Rosenberger K, Kauczor HU, Junghanss T, Hosch W. Diagnosing and staging of cystic echinococcosis: How do CT and MRI perform in comparison to ultrasound? PLoS Negl Trop Dis. 2012;6(10):e1880.

[35] McNanus D, Gray DJ, Zhang W, Yang Y. Diagnosis, treatment, and management of Echinococcosis. BMJ. 2012;344:e3866.

[36] Bygott JM, Chiodini PL. Praziquantel: Neglected drug? Ineffective treatment? Or therapeutic choice in cystic hydatid disease? Acta Trop. 2009;111:95.

[37] Tuxun T, Zhang JH, Zhao JM, et al. World review of laparoscopic treatment of liver cystic echinococcosis—914 patients. Int J Infect Dis. 2014;24:43-50.

[38] Ormeci N. PAIR vs Örmeci technique for the treatment of hydatid cyst. Turk J Gastroenterol. 2014;25(4):358-364.

[39] Neumayr A, Troia G, de Bernardis C, et al. Justified concern or exaggerated fear: the risk of anaphylaxis in percutaneous treatment of cystic echinococcosis-a systematic literature review. PLoS Negl Trop Dis. 2011;5:e1154.

[40] Rinaldi F, De Silvestri A, Tamarozzi F, at al. Medical treatment versus "Watch and Wait" in the clinical management of CE3b echinococcal cysts of the liver. BMC Infect Dis. 2014;14:492.

[41] Neumayr A, Tamarozzi F, Goblirsch S, Blum J, Brunetti E. Spinal cystic echinococcosis—a systematic analysis and review of the literature: Part 2. Treatment, follow-up and outcome. PLoS Negl Trop Dis. 2013;7(9):e2458.

[42] Popa GL, Tanase I, Popa CA, et al. Medical and surgical management of a rare and complicated case of multivisceral hydatidosis: 18 years of evolution. New Microbiol. 2014;37(3):387-391. Epub Jul 1, 2014.

[43] Pensel PE, Castro S, Allemandi D2, et al. Enhanced chemoprophylactic and clinical efficacy of albendazole formulated as solid dispersions in experimental cystic echinococcosis. Vet Parasitol. 2014;203(1-2):80-86.

[44] Alvela-Suárez L, Velasco-Tirado V, Belhassen-Garcia M, et al. Safety of the combined use of praziquantel and albendazole in the treatment of human hydatid disease. Am J Trop Med Hyg. 2014;90(5):819-22.

[45] Larrieu E, Zanini F. Critical analysis of cystic echinococcosis control programs and praziquantel use in South America, 1974-2010. Rev Panam Salud Publica. 2012;31(1): 81-87.

[46] Thompson RC. Neglected zoonotic helminths: Hymenolepis nana, Echinococcus canadensis and Ancylostoma ceylanicum. Clin Microbiol Infect. 2015:S1198-743X(15)00184-6. doi: 10.1016/j.cmi.2015.01.004. [Epub ahead of print]

[47] Zheng H, Zhang W, Zhang L, et al. The genome of the hydatid tapeworm Echinococcus granulosus. Nat Genet. 2013;45(10):1168-1175. doi: 10.1038/ng.2757.

[48] D'Alessandro A, Rausch RL, Morales GA, Collet S, Angel D. Echinococcus infections in Colombian animals. Am J Trop Med Hyg. 1981;30(6):1263-1276.

[49] ICA. Sistema de información y vigilancia epidemiológica. Sanidad Animal 2008. Situación epidemiológica en Colombia con respecto de las enfermedades. 2008. Available at: http://www.ica.gov.co/getattachment/e205da92-1991-4de4-b412-29d6dae2ae40/2008-(1).aspx.

[50] World Health Organization. Distribution of Echinococcus granulosus and cystic echinococcosis (hydatidosis), 2009. 2010. Available at: http://gamapserver.who.int/mapLibrary/Files/Maps/Global_echinococcosis_2009.png.

[51] World Health Organization Office International des Epizooties. WHO/OIE Manual on Echinococcosis in Humans and Animals: A Public Health Problem of Global Concern. 2001; Paris, France: World Organization for Animal Health.

[52] Eckert J, Deplazes P. Biological, epidemiological, and clinical aspects of echinococcosis: A zoonosis of increasing concern. Clin Microbiol Rev. 2004;17(1):107-135.

[53] Martínez S, Restrepo CS, Carrillo JA, et al. Thoracic manifestations of tropical parasitic infections: A pictorial review. Radiographics. 2005;25(1):135-155.

[54] Lichtember E. Equinococosis humana (quiste hidatídico) dos casos. Revista de la Facultad de Medicina (Bogotá). 1957; 25(3-4):119-127.

[55] D'Alessandro A, Lega J, Vera MA. Cystic calcifications of the liver in Colombia. Echinococcosis or calcified abscesses? Am J Trop Med Hyg. 1966;15(6):908-913.

[56] D'Alessandro A, Rausch RL, Morales GA, Collet S, Angel D. Echinococcus infections in Colombian animals. Am J Trop Med Hyg. 1981;30(6):1263-1276.

[57] Rausch RL, D'Alessandro A, Rausch VR. Characteristics of the larval Echinococcus vogeli Rausch and Bernstein, 1972 in the natural intermediate host, the paca, Cuniculus paca L. (Rodentia: Dasyproctidae). Am J Trop Med Hyg. 1981;30(5):1043-1052.

[58] Wells EA, D'Alessandro A, Morales GA, Angel D. Mammalian wildlife diseases as hazards to man and livestock in an area of the Llanos Orientales of Colombia. J Wildl Dis. 1981;17(1):153-162.

[59] D'Alessandro A, Rausch RL, Cuello C, Aristizabal N. Echinococcus vogeli in man, with a review of polycystic hydatid disease in Colombia and neighboring countries. Am J Trop Med Hyg. 1979;28(2):303-317.

[60] Cataño J. Cardiac echinococcosis, an unusual echocardiographic finding. Am J Trop Med Hyg. 2010;82(2):173.

[61] Gómez G, Córdoba E, Córdoba A. Quiste hidatídico hepático. Rev Colomb Gastroenterol. 2003;18:183-186.

[62] Morales GA, Guzman VH, Wells EA, Angel D. Polycystic echinococcosis in Colombia: The larval cestodes in infected rodents. J Wildl Dis. 1979;15(3):421-428.

[63] Bolívar-Mejía A, Rodríguez-Morales AJ, Paniz-Mondolfi AE, Delgado O. Cardiovascular manifestations of human toxocariasis. Arch Cardiol Mex. 2013;83(2):120-129.

[64] Hidron A, Vogenthaler N, Santos-Preciado JI, et al. Cardiac involvement with parasitic infections. Clin Microbiol Rev. 2010;23(2):324-349.

[65] Franco-Paredes C, Rouphael N, Méndez J, et al. Cardiac manifestations of parasitic infections. Part 1: Overview and immunopathogenesis. Clin Cardiol. 2007;30(4): 195-199.

[66] Franco-Paredes C, Rouphael N, Méndez J, et al. Cardiac manifestations of parasitic infections. Part 2: Parasitic myocardial disease. Clin Cardiol. 2007;30(5):218-222.

[67] Franco-Paredes C, Rouphael N, Méndez J, et al. Cardiac manifestations of parasitic infections. Part 3: Pericardial and miscellaneous cardiopulmonary manifestations. Clin Cardiol. 2007;30(6):277-280.

[68] Pastore R, Vitali LH, Macedo Vde O, Prata A. A serological survey of the infection by Echinococcus sp. in the municipality of Sena Madureira, AC. Rev Soc Bras Med Trop. 2003;36(4):473-477.

[69] Rodrigues-Silva R, Peixoto JR, de Oliveira RM, MagalhãesPinto R, Gomes DC. An autochthonous case of Echinococcus vogeli Rausch & Bernstein, 1972 polycystic echinococcosis in the state of Rondônia, Brazil. Mem Inst Oswaldo Cruz. 2002;97(1): 123-126.

[70] Thatcher VE. Neotropical echinococcosis in Columbia. Ann Trop Med Parasitol. 1972;66(1):99-105.

[71] Howells RE, Schnur LF. Hydatid cysts in spiny rats in Amazonas, Colombia. Ann Trop Med Parasitol. 1978;72(4):395-396.

[72] Bastidas A, Velásquez JC, Pérez CE. Derrame pleural eosinofílico por hidatidosis hepática: presentación de caso clínico y revisión de la literatura. Revista Med. 2008;16(1):45-55.

[73] De la Hoz F, Alvis N, Narváez J, et al. Potential epidemiological and economical impact of two rotavirus vaccines in Colombia. Vaccine. 2010;28(22):3856-3864.

[74] Mezones-Holguín E, Bolaños-Díaz R, Fiestas V, et al. Cost-effectiveness analysis of pneumococcal conjugate vaccines in preventing pneumonia in Peruvian children. J Infect Dev Ctries. 2014;8(12):1552-1562.

[75] Branci S, Ewertsen C, Thybo S, et al. Cystic echinococcosis of the liver: Experience from a Danish tertiary reference center (2002-2010). J Travel Med. 2012;19(1):28-34.

[76] Hellgren U, Botero-Kleiven S, Jansson A, Isaksson B. [Cystic echinococcosis. An imported severe parasitic disease.] Lakartidningen. 2012;109(1-2):30-33.

[77] Ito A, Budke CM. Culinary delights and travel? A review of zoonotic cestodiases and metacestodiases. Travel Med Infect Dis. 2014;12(6 Pt A):582-591.

[78] Rodriguez-Morales AJ, Schlagenhauf P. Zoonoses and travel medicine: "one world--one health". Travel Med Infect Dis. 2014;12(6 Pt A):555-556.

[79] Cascio A, Bosilkovski M, Rodriguez-Morales AJ, Pappas G. The socio-ecology of zoonotic infections. Clin Microbiol Infect. 2011;17(3):336-342.

[80] Pappas G, Cascio A, Rodriguez-Morales AJ. The immunology of zoonotic infections. Clin Dev Immunol. 2012;2012:208508.

[81] Otero-Abad B1, Torgerson PR. A systematic review of the epidemiology of echinococcosis in domestic and wild animals. PLoS Negl Trop Dis. 2013;7(6):e2249.

[82] Mayor P, Baquedano LE, Sanchez E, et al. Polycystic echinococcosis in Pacas, Amazon region, Peru. Emerg Infect Dis. 2015;21(3):456-459.

[83] Grozavu C, Ilias M, Pantile D. Multivisceral echinococcosis: Concept, diagnosis, management. Chirurgia (Bucur). 2014;109(6):758-768.

[84] Wuestenberg J, Gruener B, Oeztuerk S, et al. Diagnostics in cystic echinococcosis: Serology versus ultrasonography. Turk J Gastroenterol. 2014;25(4):398-404.

[85] Gomez I, Gavara C, López-Andújar R, et al. Review of the treatment of liver hydatid cysts. World J Gastroenterol. 2015;21(1):124-131.

4

Current Research Advance on Echinococcosis

Shukun Yang, Yumin Zhao,
Don Peter McManus and YuRong Yang

Abstract

Echinococcosis is caused by infection with larva (metacestode) of the tapeworms of the genus *Echinococcus*. Within genus *Echinococcus*, two species are known as public health concern worldwide: *Echinococcus guanulosus* causing cystic echinococcosis (CE) and *Echinococcus multilocularis* causing alveolar echinococcosis (AE). The co-evaluation due to the interaction between parasites and their hosts has been well known to be able to allow tolerating to maintain parasitism as long as possible. With many research advanced findings, scientists have been much interested in using either those molecules from parasites producing due to invading and surviving or those cytokines from hosts responding due to defenses to carry out immunotherapeutic practice that is not only against parasitic infection but also for cancer or other immunological related disorders. Taken advance of knowledge on *Echinococcus* genome research outcomes, recent attentions regarding the discoveries of targeting antiparasitic drug and/or vaccine were extensively discussed in this review.

Keywords: *Echinococcus* species, parasitism, interactions between parasites and hosts, immunotherapy agents, drug and vaccine discoveries

1. Introduction

The echinococcosis in human occurs as a result of infection by the larval stages of taeniid cestodes of the genus *Echinococcus*. Originally, four species have been recognized as the public health concern: *Echinococcus granulosus* [agent of cystic echinocococcosis (CE)], *Echinococcus multilocularis* [agent of alveolar echinococcosis (AE)], and *Echinococcus vogeli* and *Echinococcus oligarthrus* [both are the agents of polycystic echinococcosis (PE)] [1]. Recently, two new species have been identified: *Echinococcus shiquicus* [2] in small mammals from the Tibetan plateau and *Echinococcus felidis* [3] in African lions though these two new species infective to human are still unknown [4]. A couple of studies have provided augments that these diseases are an increasing public health concern and showing emerging or re-emerging diseases [4, 5].

Among recognized four public health concerned species, *E. multilocularis* and *E. granulosus* are important for human health and economic welfare [4]. The disease occurs in most areas of the world, and currently about 4 million people are infected and another 40 million people are at risk [4, 6, 7]. The economic cost of the disease is estimated to be around 3 billion USD a year. It is classified as a neglected tropical disease [4].

The knowledge on the geographical distribution of the environmental factors for the persistence of the lifecycle is scarce [8, 9]. Studies to improve the knowledge on epidemiological risk factors should be encouraged to enable risk-based sampling. *Echinococcus* notification should always be done at species level in order to discriminate between the more severe alveolar and the cystic echinococcosis [10, 11]. Updated knowledge on the *Echinococcus* parasitism was also discussed for the potential application in immunotherapeutic against parasites and other immune disorders.

2. Transmission

The life cycle of *Echinococcus* species requires a predator-prey relationship between the definitive and intermediate hosts.

E. granulosus is adapted to an environment in which livestock farming plays a central role, completing its cycle through dogs or wild carnivorous animals (as definitive host) and a variety of livestock species, mainly sheep, cattle, pigs, horses, goats, and camels as well as the several wild ungulate species serve as intermediate hosts for the different lineages of the *E. granulosus* species complex [12]. In contrast, several wild rodent species (typically rodents of the families *Arvicolidae* and *Cricetidae*) are the natural intermediate host for *E. multilocularis* [12, 13].

The intermediate hosts become infected through ingestion of eggs in contaminated food or water [12]. The host digestive enzymes dissolve the egg's shell, releasing the oncosphere, which burrows through the host's gut wall and is transported via blood or lymph to the target organ of liver for AE, but mainly liver and lungs, as well other organs for CE [14]. While the life cycle of *E. multilocularis* is completed after a fox or canine consumes a rodent infected with alveolar echincoccosis [8]. Once again adults begin to release a new gravid proglottid, which usually carries some 1500 eggs [15], to be passed to the outside environment with their feces. The adult worms are hermaphroditic. *E. granulosus* becomes prepatent in 32–80 days in the definitive hosts [16], this period varies with the species or strain. While *E. multilocularis* usually becomes prepatent in foxes or dogs in 28–35 days [17], the life cycle of *E. multiloculcaris* is predominantly sylvatic [18].

Humans can serve as an aberrant intermediate host, acquiring the infection by accidental ingestion of eggs, due to handling of infected animals or ingesting contaminated food, vegetable, and water. Except in rare cases, where infected humans are eaten by canines [19], humans are a deadend for *Echinococcus* species, which means that this kind of intermediate host does not allow transmission to the definitive host [20].

Briefly, the disease is spreading when food or water contains the eggs of the parasite, which may be eaten by intermediate animals (such as sheep for *E. granulosus* and rodents for *E. multilocularis*), or due to close contact with an infected definitive animal (carnivorous animals, e.g., dogs, foxes), while the definitive animals, to become infectious, they must eat the organs of an intermediate animal that contains the valid cysts.

3. The parasitism establishment

Generally, selective pressure between host and parasite (parasitism relationship) provides chance for coevolution [21, 22]. A constant adaptation occurs in both populations due to an accumulation of the genetic changes that results in the development of new parasitic strategies and new host defenses [21].

Parasites with complex life cycles often behave differently in their intermediate and definitive hosts [1, 23]. *Echinococcus* species presents strongly affected its intermediate hosts (moose or and small mammals, and rodents) due to high virulence but low virulence in the definitive hosts (such as wolf, fox, or dog). The strong effect makes the intermediate hosts to be more severe sick and easily be captured/hunted by the carnivorous animals [9, 18], thus, benefit parasitic life-cycle and increase transmission dynamics.

The relationship between *Echinococcus* species and their intermediate hosts leads to the necessity for the pathogen to have the virulent alleles to infect the organism and for the host to have the resistant alleles to survive parasitism. Variation in the pathogenicity of strains/species of *Echinococcus* is well known to influence the prognosis in patients with echinococcosis [23]. Increasing epidemiological evidence suggests that certain strains of *E. granulosus* (such as those adapted to horses and pigs) may not be commonly infective to humans [1], and the transmission of parasite strain differs (genetically) geographically and host-adaptively [24]. Therefore, estimates of gene flow between populations in different intermediate hosts or geographic areas can have valuable epidemiological applications [1, 11]. In the genomes of cestodes, considerable gene gain and gene loss associated with the adaptation to parasitism has been found in recent genome parasitic programs [21, 22]. Although, the different morphologies of their metacestode stages caused by *E. multilocularis* and *E. granulosus* are clinically often regarded as "distinctly different entities" [25], they are highly similar concerning gene structure and gene content [22]. Salient differences were so far only observed in the *Echinococcus*-specific apomucin gene family [21]. This is presumably associated with one of the few clear morphological differences between two species of *E. multilocularis* and *E. granulosus*, the thickness of the laminated layer, since the apomucin gene family encodes important components of this structure [26].

4. Interaction between *Echinococcal* parasites and their hosts

During echinococcosis infections (including AE and CE), the distinguishing feature of the host-parasite interaction is that chronic infection coexists with detectable humoral and cellular responses against the parasite [27]. It is well known that the *Echinococcus* species can actively interact with host's both innate and acquired immune systems to maintain their survival with successful evasion from host's immune attacks [28]. The disease spectrum is clearly dependent on the genetic background of the host, as well as on the acquired disturbances of Th1-related immunity [29], such as pregnancy [30], malnutrition [4], severe stress due to work or life [4], coinfection (e.g., HIV) [31, 32], or using immune-suppressing drugs [4, 28]; thus, this kind of circumstances can provide an opportunity to allow the pathogen invading. Human AE appears to be an example of "opportunistic infection", when you make your immunity capability weakness [28, 30]. The genetic constitution of both hosts and pathogens is involved, host genes controlling resistance or susceptibility to infection, genes of the pathogen determining characters such as virulence [23].

In order to establish a successful infection, parasite releases molecules that directly modulate the host immune responses favoring and perpetuating parasite survival in the host [33]. Recent experimental evidence suggests that parasites can not only evade immune responses actively but also exploit the hormonal microenvironment within the host to favor their establishment and growth [34]. Hormonal host parasite cross communication facilitated by the relatively close phylogenetic relationship between *E. multilocularis* and its mammalian hosts, thus appears to be important in the pathology of AE [35]. *E. multilocularis* metacestode metabolic pathway cascades can be activated by host's cell signaling [13, 36], resulting in the larvae development [37]. Conversely, the larval *Echinococcus* can also influence their host immunity response and metabolic signaling mechanisms through the secretion of various molecules [24]. Therefore, immunomodulatory activities of *Echinococcus* and pathological consequences on the host's tissues were attracted by many research concerns for decades [38].

The laminated layer could also play a role similar to that of the placenta at the materno-fetal interface [39]: ensuring parasite growth and infected tissue cell homeostasis while ensuring proper immune tolerance. Tolerance is essential to ensure growth and development of the larval stages of *Echinococcus* species in their hosts [27]. It has been recognized that a series of host-adapted species in the genus *Echinococcus* fits in nicely with observations on host range [1], life cycle, and transmission patterns in areas where echinococcosis is endemic [23]. The ability of hosts to regulate parasites through innate and adaptive immune responses is one of the most important determinants affecting levels of infection, both in the individual and the population [1]. Immunomodulation and, to some extents, immune tolerogenic role have been a great interest of researchers during echinococcosis infection both in human and in animal studies. Many reports have described the worms achieve to switch in the host's response by releasing molecules that share epitopes (and possibly functional activity) with host cytokines [40]. The high relevance for host parasite interaction mechanisms is also found that the presence of evolutionarily conserved signaling systems in *Echinococcus,* such as components of the epidermal growth factor (EGF), fibroblast growth factor (FGF), transforming growth factor ß (TGF-ß), and insulin signal transduction cascades [40, 41], though the signaling systems in animals are also known to be primarily influenced by both factors of the genetic heritage and living environments [42].

The host-derived EGF is known to induce the *Echinococcus* mitogen-activated protein kinase (MAPK) cascade, probably through direct interaction with parasite EGF-receptors [13]. Parasitic components, and not only factors from host origin, were actually acting on hepatocyte metabolic pathways. Recent report indicated that host insulin acts as a stimulant for parasite development within the host liver and that *E. multilocularis* senses the host hormone through an evolutionarily conserved insulin signaling pathway [13, 35].

Although both parasites and hosts benefit from the dynamic balance that grantees parasite-induced damage to hosts at a reasonable level and in turn [42], to some extent, provide parasites nutrients, in some cases of human echinococcosis, spontaneous healing of the disease was observed [20, 27]. Such abortive cases are characterized by calcified parasite lesions suggesting the generation of immune responses which are able to limit parasite growth in humans [27].

5. Disease in animal hosts

A carnivore animal is the definitive host—where the adult worms live in the intestines; and almost any mammal, including humans, can be the intermediate host—where the worms form cysts in various organs for CE but mainly in liver for AE.

5.1. Infection in definitive hosts (mainly implication for dogs)

It is much more difficult to tell when a dog is infected with *Echinococcus* compared to other tapeworms such as *Taenia* or *Dipylidium* [16, 17]. An adult *Echinococcus species* is tiny—only a few millimeters long. Dog infection generally does not show any signs of illness at all even though the hundreds or thousands of tapeworms live in its intestine. Despite the difficult differentiation of the eggs between *Echinococcus* and *Taenia* species under microscopy through fecal examinations [16, 17], the diagnosis of dog infection is an important and useful through dog-copro-DNA assays [16, 17, 43]. So, dog fecal examinations should be performed regularly.

5.2. Infections in intermediate animal hosts

For AE: the primary metacestodes are found in rodent's liver. The germinal membrane of *E. multilocularis* proliferates externally, rather than internally, to form a multilocular structure with many small cysts. These vesicles are usually 1–10 mm in diameter. Hundreds to thousands of protoscolices develop from the germinal membrane in some animal intermediate hosts (small mammals). These multilocular cysts have semisolid matrix and resemble malignant tumors. The center of lesion may be necrotic. The lesion can completely infiltrate an organ, and spread to other organs and tissues nearby. The cysts can also metastasize to distant sites. Although, the tumor-like cysts can kill rodents within a few weeks of infection, this parasite has recently evolved into an experimental model system by use of rodent species to study larval cestode development and associated host-parasite interaction mechanisms.

For CE: the intermediate hosts include a large number of domesticated and wild animals, particularly herbivores. The rate of development varies with the intermediate host and species of parasite, but the cysts usually grow slowly. Their diameter generally increases from less than 1 to 5 cm every year. The parasitic cyst comprises of two walls of an outer laminated membrane and an inner membrane called the germinal layer. All the brood capsules can be produced from the germinal membrane. If the cyst contains protoscolices, it will be named as fertility cyst. Some cysts are sterile, since protoscolices are not produced or killed by bacterial infection. The percentage of sterile cysts varies with the different intermediate host and its susceptibility to a particular strain/species of parasite. The cysts in livestock also seem to be asymptomatic, probably due to the relatively short lifespan of these animals. Because the cyst grows slowly and the symptoms can only appear until its size can effect on adjacent tissues and organs. Occasionally, symptoms have been reported in sheep [5]. But mostly the infected livestock shows poor growth, weakness, and lameness. Therefore, the economic loss assessment modeling due to livestock infections (mainly in sheep) has attracted some extensive attentions in endemic regions and countries worldwide.

6. Disease in humans

Epidemiological studies have demonstrated that the majority of human individuals exposed to infection with *Echinococcus* spp. eggs exhibit resistance to disease as shown by either seroconversion to parasite specific antigens or the presence of "dying out" or "aborted metacestodes" [4]. Seroconversion proving infection, but lack of any lesion indicating the failure of the parasite to establish and further develop within human tissues (mainly in liver) or resistance as shown by the presence of fully calcified lesion [44]; while the developing parasite can be partially controlled by host immunity in those susceptibility individuals where infection leads to disease, as found in the AE and CE patients who experience clinical signs and symptoms approximately 5–15 years after infection [20, 30].

If untreated or uncontrolled, the hyper proliferation of the metacestode due to an impaired immune response could be resulted by immune modulation of host immunity toward energy that can be triggered by parasite metabolites [38], and/or be resulted by additional clinical conditions, such as AIDS or any other reason to induce the immune deficiencies [20, 27, 30]. The disease often starts without symptoms, and this may last for years. The symptoms and signs can occur depend on the lesion location and size for CE. While, AE usually begins in the liver but can spread to other parts of the body.

Cystic echinococcosis (CE) can cause very severe symptoms, if the cyst bursts (e.g., from sudden trauma) or even fatal. The released protoscolices can spread the parasite to other parts of the body to form many new cysts [20].

Alveolar echinocococcis (AE) ranges in size from a sesame seed to a large melon [45]. Although, the mass lesions grow slowly, the tumor-like growth manner tends to invade neighbor organs or tissues, making treatment very difficult [30].

Fibrosis is an important component of the pathophysiology of each disease caused by *Echinococcus* species. However, this role differs markedly in CE and AE. In CE, the rapidly established periparasitic fibrosis surrounding the laminated layer contributes to the unicystic feature of the disease and to limit cyst growth [46]. In AE, the slow fibrogenesis in an extensive and partially unsuccessful periparasitic granuloma does not prevent germinal layer budding.

In the long term, it eventually leads to a dense and irreversible fibrosis, responsible for the main complications of the diseases, such as bile duct, vessel obstruction, and secondary biliary cirrhosis [47–49].

7. Human disease diagnosis

Echinococcal lesions may grow for years, depending on their location, without causing any signs of illness in people [4]. The signs of illness do occur in late stages of diseases, such as abdominal pain and jaundice due to obstruction of bile ducts (in liver), chest pain and difficulty in breathing (in lungs) [4], neurological signs, and seizures (in brain) [30]. Cysts/lesions are sometimes found occasionally when tests are performed for other reasons [4]. Generally, the clinical symptoms and image presentations, e.g., radiographs, ultrasound, CT, or MRI, need to combine the evidences from a blood test for antibodies to the parasite or biopsy for histopathological examination or PCR assay to confirm the diagnosis [4]. Screening individuals living in high-risk areas by ultrasound and serological investigation [44] can catch the infection early and can make treatment much easier and more effective [44].

Therefore, diagnosis requires a combination of tools that involve imaging, histopathology, or nucleic acid detection, and serology. The ultrasound though computer tomography (CT) or magnetic resonance imaging (MRI) may be used commonly. Serology methods for antibodies against the parasite detection can be some certain supplemental tool for imaging/clinical diagnosis. The histopathology or nucleic acid using biopsy after invading methods could provide the final confirmation [4, 20].

8. Management of echinococcosis in human

The growth of larva of *Echinococcus* spp. and the proliferation of the larva are similar to a slow-growing tumor. If the lesion occurs in liver, it can damage liver function. Sometimes, it is difficult to differentiate it from liver cancer because of invasion to biliary and vascular tissue of the liver [50]. Early diagnosis and radical surgery provide the best chance for treatment and cure. Although, treatment of AE is less effective than treatment of CE, the general approach for both types of echinococcosis treatment remains to be surgery with the purpose of complete resection of infected parts of involved organs [4]. Antiparasitic drugs cannot kill cysts if the lesions have already established. However, if untreated, patient survival time is very limited. Therefore, early detection and treatment are important ways to improve patients' survival [4, 20].

Although treatment of cystic echinococcosis by surgery to remove the hydatid cyst was always a risk that the cyst would burst during the procedure, resulting in a very severe, even fatal reaction in the patient to the spilled fluid, drug therapy alone is usually not enough to eliminate cysts, but it can help reduce lesion size and operation risks. More recently, treatment with antiparasitic drugs and drainage of the fluid from the cyst using a needle has been used to treat the disease in certain cases without surgery. Briefly, with proper care, 96–98% of CE patients survive [20].

9. *Echinococcus* species infective risk to humans

The risk of infection with *E. granulosus* or *E. multilocularis* to humans from most pets is very low, but it is higher risks for those residents living in endemic areas. Their work or recreational activities involve direct contact with contaminated water, soil, and their dogs for a long time or life time [10]. Those dogs may allow to roam, hunt, and eat raw tissues from potentially infected animals (e.g., rodents, rabbits, sheep, moose) [8].

The risks for the susceptible of infection with *Echinococcus* spp. can occur in those peoples with immune-compromised conditions (e.g., HIV/AIDS patients, transplant recipients, cancer patients) or with other complications because their immune systems cannot fight infections efficiently [20]. Mostly, ingestion of *Echinococcal* eggs occurred in early ages, if they have chance to contact with contaminated environments, but the disease may appear until they are adults [44].

10. Prevention and control program

Dogs if allowed to enter *Echinococcus*-free areas from potential endemic areas need to be treated with anthelmintic agents (e.g., Praziquantel). Routine inspection of the potential parasitic intermediate host animals before permitting for importing could also prevent the parasite into a country [15].

In endemic areas, dogs should not be allowed to eat the carcasses, particularly the viscera of potential intermediate hosts. Dogs should also be kept from hunting wild rodents and small mammals [6]. Regular examination and treatment of dogs [8] can decrease echinococcosis in domesticated livestock [14].

Prevention of *Echinococcus* species spreading is by treating dogs that may carry the disease and vaccination of sheep. Health education programs focused on echinococcosis and its agents, and improvement of the water sanitation attempt to target poor economic living condition and poor drinking water sources. Educational material should include information about proper disposal of sheep viscera in abattoirs and proximity to dogs and sources of transmission [15].

11. Parasitism perspective applications

11.1. Treatment parasitic infections

In the absence of fully effective antiparasitic chemotherapy for AE and CE, modulation of the host's immune response could be envisaged to fight against the parasite and to prevent the disease and/or its complications such as using IFN-a2a immunological treatment [28] and some parasitic antigens as potential vaccination to prevent disease occurrence such as using Em14-3-3, Em 95, EMY162, and EmTetraspanin [24]. Additionally, current picture on *Echinococcus* signaling systems will be given and the potential to exploit these pathways as targets for antiparasitic chemotherapy [51].

11.2. Using parasite productions for cancer treatment

The presence of Tn antigen in larval and adult tissues of *E. granulosus* was reported [52], this finding is interested in cancer-associated mucin-type because this parasite produced peptides can act on the nonspecific natural killer cell to express cytokines that are effective agents against tumor growth; therefore, the family of Tn antigens might be useful targets for antitumor immunotherapy [41, 53, 54]. These evidences may contribute to the design of tumor vaccines and open new horizons in the use of parasite-derived molecules that can fight against cancer [55, 56].

Cancer vaccination is an important and promising approach in cancer immunotherapy. Obstacles for clinical success may include immune tolerance to TAAs [57], the weak antigenic nature of TAAs, and active immune evasion mechanisms employed by progressing tumors [58]. Vaccination with TAAs coming from evolutionary distant organisms (such as *E. granulosus*) should be useful to override tolerance problems encountered with human TAA-based cancer therapeutic approaches [58].

11.3. Echinococcosis diagnosis

Additionally, the high level of the O-glycosylated Tn antigens generated from larvae of *E. granulosus* are found in the sera of the patients with cystic echinococcosis (CE), providing a pathway that a series of Tn antigens might be sort as a biomarker for this parasitic disease diagnosis, but the hypothesis needs more work to verify the clinical values regarding those antigens [59].

12. Conclusions

Overall, genus *Echinococcus* can be thought an example of successful adaptation to their hosts extensively. Taken advance of recent research outcomes, the parasite immunotherapy for human echinococcosis has been discussed widely by scientific literatures, but importantly, the advanced outcomes may also be interested in terms of using parasites' productions for treatment of other diseases, including cancer.

Acknowledgments

We acknowledge financial support by the National Health and Medical Research Council (NHMRC) of Australia of a NHMRC Project Grant (APP1009539). National Science Foundation of China (NSFC) of the NSFC Project Grants (30960339 and 81460311).

Author details

Shukun Yang[1], Yumin Zhao[2], Don Peter McManus[3] and YuRong Yang[4*]

*Address all correspondence to: yangyurong@hotmail.com

1 Image Diagnosis Department, The First Peoples' Hospital of Yinchuan City, Ningxia Hui Autonomous Region (NHAR), P.R. China

2 Human Pathological Department of Guiling Medical College, Guilin City, Guangxi Province, P.R. China

3 Molecular Parasitology Laboratory, QIMR Berghofer Medical Research Institute, Brisbane, Australia

4 Human Pathology & Immunology Department, Ningxia Medical University, Yinchuan City, Ningxia Hui Autonomous Region (NHAR), P.R. China

References

[1] McManus DP, Thompson RC. Molecular epidemiology of cystic echinococcosis. Parasitology. 2003;**127**(Suppl):S37-S51

[2] Xiao N, Qiu J, Nakao M, Li T, Yang W, Chen X, Schantz PM, Craig PS, Ito A. *Echinococcus shiquicus* n. sp., a taeniid cestode from Tibetan fox and plateau pika in China. International Journal for Parasitology. 2005;**35**:693-701. DOI: 10.1016/j.ijpara.2005.01.003

[3] Hüttner M, Nakao M, Wassermann T, Siefert L, Boomker JD, Dinkel A, Sako Y, Mackenstedt U, Romig T, Ito A. Genetic characterization and phylogenetic position of *Echinococcus felidis* (Cestoda: Taeniidae) from the African lion. International Journal for Parasitology. 2008;**38**:861-868. DOI: 10.1016/j.ijpara.2007.10.013

[4] McManus DP, Gray DJ, Zhang W, Yang Y. Diagnosis, treatment, and management of echinococcosis. British Medical Journal. 2012;**344**:e3866. DOI: 10.1136/bmj.e3866

[5] Carmena D, Cardona GA. Echinococcosis in wild carnivorous species: Epidemiology, genotypic diversity, and implications for veterinary public health. Veterinary Parasitology. 2014;**202**:69-94. DOI: 10.1016/j.vetpar.2014.03.009

[6] Craig PS, McManus DP, Lightowlers MW, Chabalgoity JA, Garcia HH, Gavidia CM, Gilman RH, Gonzalez AE, Lorca M, Naquira C, Nieto A, Schantz PM. Prevention and control of cystic echinococcosis. Lancet Infectious Diseases. 2007;**7**:385-394. DOI: 10.1016/S1473-3099(07)70134-2

[7] Carmena D, Sánchez-Serrano LP, Barbero-Martínez I. *Echinococcus granulosus* infection in Spain. Zoonoses and Public Health. 2008;**55**:156-165. DOI: 10.1111/j.1863-2378.2007.01100.x

[8] Craig PS, Li T, Qiu J, Zhen R, Wang Q, Giraudoux P, Ito A, Heath D, Warnock B, Schantz P, Yang W. Echinococcosis and Tibetan communities. Emerging Infectious Diseases. 2008;**14**:1674-1675. DOI: 10.3201/eid1410.071636

[9] Pleydell DR, Yang YR, Danson FM, Raoul F, Craig PS, McManus DP, Vuitton DA, Wang Q, Giraudoux P. Landscape composition and spatial prediction of alveolar echinococcosis in southern Ningxia, China. PLoS Neglected Tropical Diseases. 2008;**2**:e287. DOI: 10.1371/journal.pntd.0000287

[10] Yang YR, Craig PS, Sun T, Vuitton DA, Giraudoux P, Jones MK, Williams GM, McManus DP. Echinococcosis in Ningxia Hui Autonomous Region, northwest China. Transactions of the Royal Society of Tropical Medicine and Hygiene. 2008;**102**:319-328. DOI: 10.1016/j.trstmh.2008.01.007

[11] Yang YR, Rosenzvit MC, Zhang LH, Zhang JZ, McManus DP. Molecular study of Echinococcus in west-central China. Parasitology. 2005;**131**:547-555. DOI: 10.1017/S0031182005007973

[12] Eckert J, Deplazes P. Biological, epidemiological, and clinical aspects of echinococcosis, a zoonosis of increasing concern. Clinical Microbiology Reviews. 2004;**17**:107-135. DOI: 10.1128/CMR.17.1.107-135.2004

[13] Spiliotis M, Konrad C, Gelmedin V, Tappe D, Brückner S, Mösch HU, Brehm K. Characterisation of EmMPK1, an ERK-like MAP kinase from *Echinococcus multilocularis* which is activated in response to human epidermal growth factor. International Journal for Parasitology. 2006;**36**:1097-1112. DOI: 10.1016/j.ijpara.2006.05.008

[14] Cleary E, Barnes TS, Xu Y, Zhao H, Clements AC, Gray DJ, McManus DP, Atkinson JA, Williams GM, Yang Y. Impact of "Grain to Green" Programme on echinococcosis infection in Ningxia Hui Autonomous Region of China. Veterinary Parasitology. 2014;**205**:523-531. DOI: 10.1016/j.vetpar.2014.08.023

[15] Yang YR, McManus DP, Huang Y, Heath DD. Echinococcus granulosus infection and options for control of cystic echinococcosis in Tibetan communities of Western Sichuan Province, China. PLoS Neglected Tropical Diseases. 2009;**3**:e426. DOI: 10.1371/journal.pntd.0000426

[16] Ni XW, McManus DP, Lou ZZ, Yang JF, Yan HB, Li L, Li HM, Liu QY, Li CH, Shi WG, Fan YL, Liu X, Cai JZ, Lei MT, Fu BQ, Yang YR, Jia WZ. A comparison of loop-mediated isothermal amplification (LAMP) with other surveillance tools for *Echinococcus granulosus* diagnosis in canine definitive hosts. PloS One. 2014;**9**:e100877. DOI: 10.1371/journal.pone.0100877

[17] Ni XW, McManus DP, Yan HB, Yang JF, Lou ZZ, Li HM, Li L, Lei MT, Cai JZ, Fan YL, Li CH, Liu QY, Shi WG, Liu X, Zheng YD, Fu BQ, Yang YR, Jia WZ. Loop-mediated isothermal amplification (LAMP) assay for the identification of *Echinococcus multilocularis* infections in canine definitive hosts. Parasites & Vectors. 2014;**7**:254. DOI: 10.1186/1756-3305-7-254

[18] Yang YR, Liu TX, Bai XL, Boufana B, Craig PS, Nakao M, Ito A, Zhang JZ, Giraudoux P, McManus DP. Natural infection of the ground squirrel (*Spermophilus* spp.) with *Echinococcus granulosus* in China. PLoS Neglected Tropical Diseases. 2009;**3**:e518. DOI: 10.1371/journal.pntd.0000518

[19] Kenny JV, MacCabe RJ. Sero-epidemiology of hydatid disease in the non-intervention area of north-east Turkana. Annals of Tropical Medicine and Parasitology. 1993;**87**: 451-457

[20] Brunetti E, Kern P, Vuitton DA; Writing Panel for the WHO-IWGE. Expert consensus for the diagnosis and treatment of cystic and alveolar echinococcosis in humans. Acta Tropica. 2010;**114**:1-16. DOI: 10.1016/j.actatropica.2009.11.001

[21] Tsai IJ, Zarowiecki M, Holroyd N, Garciarrubio A, Sanchez-Flores A, Brooks KL, Tracey A, Bobes RJ, Fragoso G, Sciutto E, Aslett M, Beasley H, Bennett HM, Cai XP, Camicia F, Clark R, Cucher M, De Silva N, Day TA, Deplazes P, Estrada K, Fernández C, Holland PW, Hou JL, Hu SN, Huckvale T, Hung SS, Kamenetzky L, Keane JA, Kiss F, Koziol U, Lambert O, Liu K, Luo XN, Luo YF, Macchiaroli N, Nichol S, Paps J, Parkinson J, Pouchkina-Stantcheva N, Riddiford N, Rosenzvit M, Salinas G, Wasmuth JD, Zamanian M, Zheng YD; Taenia solium Genome Consortium, Cai JP, Soberón X, Olson PD, Laclette JP, Brehm K, Berriman M. The genomes of four tapeworm species reveal adaptations to parasitism. Nature. 2013;**496**:57-63. DOI: 10.1038/nature12031

[22] Zheng H, Zhang W, Zhang L, Zhang Z, Li J, Lu G, Zhu Y, Wang Y, Huang Y, Liu J, Kang H, Chen J, Wang L, Chen A, Yu S, Gao Z, Jin L, Gu W, Wang Z, Zhao L, Shi B, Wen H, Lin R, Jones MK, Brejova B, Vinar T, Zhao G, McManus DP, Chen Z, Zhou Y, Wang S. The genome of the hydatid tapeworm *Echinococcus granulosus*. Nature Genetics. 2013;**45**:1168-1175. DOI: 10.1038/ng.2757

[23] Thompson, RC and Lymbery AJ, Genetic variability in parasites and host-parasite interactions. Parasitology. 1996;**112**(Suppl):S7-S22

[24] Zhang S, Hüe S, Sène D, Penfornis A, Bresson-Hadni S, Kantelip B, Caillat-Zucman S, Vuitton DA. Expression of major histocompatibility complex class I chain-related molecule A, NKG2D, and transforming growth factor-beta in the liver of humans with alveolar echinococcosis: New actors in the tolerance to parasites? Journal of Infectious Diseases. 2008;**197**:1341-1349. DOI: 10.1086/586709

[25] Stojkovic, M and Junghanss T. Cystic and alveolar echinococcosis. Handbook of Clinical Neurology, 2013;**114**:327-334. DOI: 10.1016/B978-0-444-53490-3.00026-1

[26] Díaz A, Casaravilla C, Allen JE, Sim RB, Ferreira AM. Understanding the laminated layer of larval Echinococcus II: Immunology. Trends in Parasitology. 2011;**27**:264-273. DOI: 10.1016/j.pt.2011.01.008

[27] Vuitton DA, Zhang SL, Yang Y, Godot V, Beurton I, Mantion G, Bresson-Hadni S. Survival strategy of *Echinococcus multilocularis* in the human host. Parasitology International. 2006;**55**(Suppl):S51-S55. DOI: 10.1016/j.parint.2005.11.007

[28] Vuitton, DA and Gottstein B. *Echinococcus multilocularis* and its intermediate host: A model of parasite-host interplay. Journal of Biomedicine & Biotechnology. 2010;**2010**: 923193. DOI: 10.1155/2010/923193

[29] Brehm K *Echinococcus multilocularis* as an experimental model in stem cell research and molecular host-parasite interaction. Parasitology. 2010;**137**:537-555. DOI: 10.1017/S0031182009991727

[30] Yang YR, Vuitton DA, Jones MK, Craig PS, McManus DP. Brain metastasis of alveolar echinococcosis in a hyperendemic focus of *Echinococcus multilocularis* infection. Transactions of the Royal Society of Tropical Medicine and Hygiene. 2005;**99**:937-941. DOI: 10.1016/j.trstmh.2005.04.020

[31] Sailer M, Soelder B, Allerberger F, Zaknun D, Feichtinger H, Gottstein B. *Alveolar echinococcosis* of the liver in a six-year-old girl with acquired immunodeficiency syndrome. Journal of Pediatrics. 1997;**130**:320-323

[32] Ran B, Shao Y, Guo Y, Yimiti Y, Aji T, Jia J, Shayiding P, Jiang T, Cheng L, Li J, McManus DP, Zhang W, Wen H. Surgical treatment of hepatic cystic echinococcosis in patients co-infected with HIV/AIDS. Journal of Helminthology. 2016;**90**:125-128. DOI: 10.1017/S0022149X15000188

[33] Coakley G, Buck AH, Maizels RM. Host parasite communications-messages from helminths for the immune system: Parasite communication and cell-cell interactions. Molecular and Biochemical Parasitology. 2016;**208**:33-40. DOI: 10.1016/j.molbiopara.2016.06.003

[34] Escobedo G, Roberts CW, Carrero JC, Morales-Montor J. Parasite regulation by host hormones: An old mechanism of host exploitation? Trends in Parasitology. 2005;**21**:588-593. DOI: 10.1016/j.pt.2005.09.013

[35] Hemer S, Konrad C, Spiliotis M, Koziol U, Schaack D, Förster S, Gelmedin V, Stadelmann B, Dandekar T, Hemphill A, Brehm K. Host insulin stimulates *Echinococcus multilocularis* insulin signalling pathways and larval development. BMC Biology. 2014;**12**:5. DOI: 10.1186/1741-7007-12-5

[36] Gelmedin V, Caballero-Gamiz R, Brehm K. Characterization and inhibition of a p38-like mitogen-activated protein kinase (MAPK) from *Echinococcus multilocularis*: Antiparasitic activities of p38 MAPK inhibitors. Biochemical Pharmacology. 2008;**76**:1068-1081. DOI: 10.1016/j.bcp.2008.08.020

[37] Brehm K, Spiliotis M, Zavala-Góngora R, Konrad C, Frosch M. The molecular mechanisms of larval cestode development: First steps into an unknown world. Parasitology International. 2006;**55**(Suppl):S15-S21. DOI: 10.1016/j.parint.2005.11.003

[38] Wang J, Zhang C, Wei X, Blagosklonov O, Lv G, Lu X, Mantion G, Vuitton DA, Wen H, Lin R. TGF-beta and TGF-beta/Smad signaling in the interactions between *Echinococcus multilocularis* and its hosts. PloS One. 2013;**8**:e55379. DOI: 10.1371/journal.pone.0055379

[39] Szekeres-Bartho, J. Immunological relationship between the mother and the fetus. International Reviews of Immunology. 2002;**21**(6):471-495

[40] Brehm K, Spiliotis M. The influence of host hormones and cytokines on *Echinococcus multilocularis* signalling and development. Parasite. 2008;**15**:286-290. DOI: 10.1051/parasite/2008153286

[41] Koziol U and Brehm K. Recent advances in Echinococcus genomics and stem cell research. Veterinary Parasitology. 2015;**213**(3-4):92-102. DOI: 10.1016/j.vetpar.2015.07.031

[42] Wang X, Ding J, Guo X, Zheng Y. Current understandings of molecular biology of *Echinococcus multilocularis*, a pathogen for alveolar echinococcosis in humans – A narrative review article. Iranian Journal of Parasitology. 2015;**10**:329-337.

[43] Liu CN, Lou ZZ, Li L, Yan HB, Blair D, Lei MT, Cai JZ, Fan YL, Li JQ, Fu BQ, Yang YR, McManus DP, Jia WZ. Discrimination between *E. granulosus* sensu stricto, *E. multilocularis* and *E. shiquicus* using a Multiplex PCR Assay. PLoS Neglected Tropical Diseases. 2015;**9**:e0004084. DOI: 10.1371/journal.pntd.0004084

[44] Yang YR, Craig PS, Vuitton DA, Williams GM, Sun T, Liu TX, Boufana B, Giraudoux P, Teng J, Li Y, Huang L, Zhang W, Jones MK, McManus DP. Serological prevalence of echinococcosis and risk factors for infection among children in rural communities of southern Ningxia, China. Tropical Medicine & International Health. 2008;**13**:1086-1094. DOI: 10.1111/j.1365-3156.2008.02101.x

[45] Vuitton DA, Benzimidazoles for the treatment of cystic and alveolar echinococcosis: What is the consensus? Expert Review of Anti-Infective Therapy. 2009;**7**(2):145-149. DOI: 10.1586/14787210.7.2.145

[46] Godot V, Harraga S, Deschaseaux M, Bresson-Hadni S, Gottstein B, Emilie D, Vuitton DA. Increased basal production of interleukin-10 by peripheral blood mononuclear cells in human alveolar echinococcosis. European Cytokine Network. 1997;**8**:401-408

[47] Godot V, Harraga S, Beurton I, Deschaseaux M, Sarciron E, Gottstein B, Vuitton DA. Resistance/susceptibility to *Echinococcus multilocularis* infection and cytokine profile in humans. I. Comparison of patients with progressive and abortive lesions. Clinical and Experimental Immunology. 2000;**121**:484-490. DOI: 10.1046/j.1365-2249.2000.01308.x

[48] Reuter S, Buck A, Manfras B, Kratzer W, Seitz HM, Darge K, Reske SN, Kern P. Structured treatment interruption in patients with alveolar echinococcosis. Hepatology. 2004;**39**:509-517. DOI: 10.1002/hep.20078

[49] Konrad C, Kroner A, Spiliotis M, Zavala-Góngora R, Brehm K. Identification and molecular characterisation of a gene encoding a member of the insulin receptor family in *Echinococcus multilocularis*. International Journal for Parasitology. 2003;**33**:301-312

[50] Garcea G, Rajesh A, Dennison AR. Surgical management of cystic lesions in the liver. ANZ Journal of Surgery. 2013;**83**(7-8):E3-E20. DOI: 10.1111/j.1445-2197.2012.06096.x

[51] Brehm K. The role of evolutionarily conserved signalling systems in *Echinococcus multilocularis* development and host-parasite interaction. Medical Microbiology and Immunology. 2010;**199**(3):247-259. DOI: 10.1007/s00430-010-0154-1

[52] Esendagli G, Abbasoglu O. Immune system in cancer and hydatid disease: Cross-reactivity vs. immune modulation. Parasite Immunology. 2015;**37**(8):427-428.DOI: 10.1111/pim.12200

[53] Turhan N, Esendagli G, Ozkayar O, Tunali G, Sokmensuer C, Abbasoglu O. Co-existence of *Echinococcus granulosus* infection and cancer metastasis in the liver correlates with reduced Th1 immune responses. Parasite Immunology. 2015;**37**:16-22. DOI: 10.1111/pim.12152

[54] Yousofi Darani H, Yousefi M, Safari M, Jafari R. Parasites and immunotherapy: With or against? Journal of Parasitic Diseases. 2016;**40**:217-226. DOI: 10.1007/s12639-014-0533-4

[55] Gundogdu SB, Saylam B, Tez M. Cyst hydatid and cancer: The myth continues. Clinical Chemistry and Laboratory Medicine. Published in Association with the European Federation of Clinical Chemistry and Laboratory Medicine (EFLM), 2016. DOI: https://doi.org/10.1515/cclm-2016-0626.

[56] Daneshpour S, Bahadoran M, Hejazi SH, Eskandarian AA, Mahmoudzadeh M, Darani HY. Common antigens between hydatid cyst and cancers. Advanced Biomedical Research. 2016;**5**:9. DOI: 10.4103/2277-9175.175242

[57] Berriel E, Russo S, Monin L, Festari MF, Berois N, Fernández G, Freire T, Osinaga E. Antitumor activity of human hydatid cyst fluid in a murine model of colon cancer. Scientific World Journal. 2013;**2013**:230176. DOI: 10.1155/2013/230176

[58] Noya V, Bay S, Festari MF, García EP, Rodriguez E, Chiale C, Ganneau C, Baleux F, Astrada S, Bollati-Fogolín M, Osinaga E, Freire T. Mucin-like peptides from *Echinococcus granulosus* induce antitumor activity. International Journal of Oncology. 2013;**43**:775-784. DOI: 10.3892/ijo.2013.2000

[59] Alvarez Errico D, Medeiros A, Míguez M, Casaravilla C, Malgor R, Carmona C, Nieto A, Osinaga E. O-glycosylation in Echinococcus granulosus: Identification and characterization of the carcinoma-associated Tn antigen. Experimental Parasitology. 2001;**98**:100-109. DOI: 10.1006/expr.2001.4620

Section 2

Biological and Clinical Aspects

5

Echinococcosis — Rare Locations and Uncommon Clinical Manifestations

Antonio Di Cataldo[#], Giuseppe Petrillo[#], Claudia Trombatore[#], Stefano Palmucci[#], Antonella Agodi[#], Martina Barchitta, Annalisa Quattrocchi, Nunzio Crimi, Silvia Fichera, Stefano Puleo, Amy Giarrizzo, Martina Calabrini, Rosalia Latino and Rosanna Portale

Abstract

Echinococcosis is a zoonotic infection caused by tiny tapeworms of the genus Echinocococcus. Cystic Echinococcosis, also known as hydatid disease, is caused by Echinococcus granulosus and rarely by Echinococcus multilocularis.

Although the worldwide incidence and prevalence of Echinococcosis dramatically decreased in the last decades, it remains a major public health issue in several countries, where the infection is currently considered an endemic disease.

The disease is characterized by cystic lesions especially in the liver and lungs. If the parasites go beyond the lung filter, it can spread to other locations that are classified as rare, very rare, or extremely rare locations.

In these rare locations, the disease is often asymptomatic and is frequently incidentally diagnosed.

Usually, there are mechanical clinical features that will be different according to the organ where the cyst is located. Serological tests, ultrasound, and imaging radiological studies are generally used in order to make the correct diagnosis.

Keywords: Echinococcosis, surgical procedures, operative, diagnostic imaging, parasitic diseases, infection

1. Introduction

Hydatid disease is a parasitic infection that is endemic in Mediterranean countries, but it is worldwide present in consequence of the migratory phenomena. The disease is characterized by cystic lesions especially located in the liver and in the lungs. If the parasite goes beyond the pulmonary filter, it can spread to other localizations that are classified rare, very rare, or extremely rare locations [1].

2. Epidemiology of Echinococcosis

Hydatid disease is known since the ancient times and Hippocrates first described it as being located in the liver. *Echinococcosis* is a major parasitic zoonosis, of public health importance worldwide, that in humans occurs in two main forms depending on the causative species: cystic *Echinococcosis* (CE, also known as hydatidosis) and alveolar *Echinococcosis* (AE), caused by the tapeworms *Echinococcus granulosus* and *E. multilocularis,* respectively. Both diseases can cause serious morbidity and death [2, 3] if the management is not correct, and both can be regarded as emerging or re-emerging diseases [4].

CE is globally distributed, with highly endemic areas mostly found in the eastern part of the Mediterranean region, northern Africa, southern and Eastern Europe, at the southern tip of South America, in Central Asia, Siberia, and western China. AE is confined to the northern hemisphere, in particular to regions of western and northern China, the Russian Federation, most countries of continental Europe, and northern countries of North America [3]. CE occurs commonly in Bulgaria, Poland, Slovenia, and in Spain and elsewhere in Eastern and Central Europe, it is considered a serious public health problem in Turkey. AE has also emerged in Central and Eastern Europe in association with increases in fox populations. The infection has been reported in Germany, Lithuania, Slovakia, Slovenia, and Switzerland [5].

CE has a renewed importance in Europe, as reemerging cases have been documented [6]. Furthermore, CE is reported in immigrants or persons with a history of travel to endemic areas [7]. Several national surveillance systems for CE and AE exist in European countries based on voluntary data entry or on compulsory notification [8].

The recent Annual epidemiological report on food and waterborne diseases and zoonoses of the European Centre for Disease Prevention and Control (ECDC) [8] relates that in 2012 the case rate of *Echinococcosis* was 0.19 cases per 100,000 population in the European Union and European Economic Area (EEA) countries. The rate of *Echinococcosis* has been fairly stable in the last years and the number of cases reported with AE has increased, most likely reflecting the increasing spatial distribution of the parasite in animals. The highest population-based risk was noted in Bulgaria, where the notification rate in 2012 was 23 times higher than the overall EU/EEA case rate (4.37 cases per 100,000 population; 39% of the reported number of cases in Europe). No significant differences were found in *Echinococcosis* rates by gender (male-to-female ratio: 0.98:1 in 2012). The highest case rate was in males aged 65 years old and over (0.22

per 100,000) followed by females aged 65 years old and over (0.17 per 100,000). Rates were generally higher in males than in females for cases aged 25 years and older. Notably, the higher rates observed in the elderly can be explained by the extensive incubation period of several years. Furthermore, no seasonality has been observed for *Echinococcosis*, as expected for a disease with a very long incubation period. The most frequently isolated species was *E. granulosus* (81%), followed by *E. multilocularis* (18%), and by other *Echinococcus* species (1%). Over the last five years, an increasing number of cases infected with *E. multilocularis* (AE) was observed and this is an important issue since untreated disease is often fatal. Notably, as highlighted by the ECDC [8], most European surveillance systems capture only a proportion of the cases occurring in their countries and some cases of disease remain undiagnosed or are diagnosed but not reported to public health authorities. Furthermore, the direct comparison of *Echinococcosis* rates between countries should be undertaken with caution. In fact, in most cases, differences in case rates reflect not only differences in the occurrence of the disease, but also in systematic differences in health and surveillance systems [8].

Mandatory notification of CE to the Italian Ministry of Health has been discontinued since 1991 (D. Min. San. 15.12.1991), and thus, the data on CE occurrence have only produced by the regional cases summaries. Therefore, information on CE distribution in Italy is still incomplete and insufficient and no data has been submitted for the European surveillance. However, an Italian Registry of CE was established by the Istituto Superiore della Sanità (http://www.iss.it/riec/). In Italy, the prevalence of the CE is high on the islands and medium in the central and southern regions of Italy [9–10] where farming and raising sheep are frequent activities, confirming that the disease is often an occupational one, and farming and raising sheep seem to be risk factors [11–12]. Data from the Italia registry reports that up to 75% of sheep and goats can be infected and up to 14 cases per 100,000 inhabitants (1,400 cases/year estimated) (http://www.iss.it/riec/).

As suggested, compulsory notification of *Echinococcosis* and harmonization of the data entry system are essential instruments for the surveillance of human diseases in order to make both clinical and epidemiological data accessible to clinicians, epidemiologists, and policymakers [12]. In fact, surveillance data are useful to assist policymakers and health leaders in making evidence-based decisions to plan and improve programs, services, and interventions for preventing, managing, and treating these diseases [8].

In 2013, the EchinoWorld website (www.echinoworld.org), sponsored by the International Association of Hydatidology, was developed. It provides a feasible and effective platform for professionals and scholars around world in the field of hydatid disease, with the aim to help prevention, diagnosis, and treatment especially in endemic countries and globally.

CE can be prevented by periodic deworming of dogs; improved hygiene in the slaughtering of livestock, including proper destruction of infected offal; and public education campaigns. Vaccination of livestock offers encouraging prospects for prevention and control. The World Health Organization reports that a program combining vaccination of lambs, deworming of dogs, and culling of older sheep could lead to the elimination of human cystic *Echinococcosis* in less than 10 years [3]. Because of the unique sylvatic nature of AE, it is one of the few helminth infections in Europe that is not linked to poverty and inadequate sanitation [1–5]. Prevention and control of AE is particularly complex as the cycle involves wild animal species as both definitive and intermediate hosts. Regular deworming of domestic carnivores that have access to wild rodents should help to reduce the risk of infection to humans. However, sustainability and cost–benefit effectiveness of such campaigns are controversial [3].

3. Unusual locations of echinococcosis

About 90% of the hydatid cysts occur in the liver (65%–75%) and lungs (15%–20%), organs that can be affected simultaneously in about 5%–13% of the cases. If the cyst goes beyond the hepatic and pulmonary filters, it can spread to other organs. A possible dissemination through lymphatic channels could explain the presence of the cysts in uncommon sites [13].

The diameter of the parasite is about 25 microns–35 microns, and it can pass through the hepatic sinusoids (10 microns–100 microns), depending on the biophysical and structural features of the parasite, which has ameboid movements and different dimensions in the different stages of its biological cycle. It is as an emulsoid that adapts itself to the different diameters of the anatomic structures. Other factors such as pH, surface tension, and the presence of the colloids are also involved in explaining the passage of the parasite through the hepatic sinusoids. However, it is also possible that the parasite reaches the peripheral locations by passing the hepatic sinusoids through the presence of arteriovenous anastomoses or through anastomoses between the portal and hepatic veins. Furthermore, we should believe that the parasite is able to bypass the pulmonary capillary vessels in a similar way, otherwise, the incidence of the parasite in the lungs should be higher than in the liver [14].

In 1964, Grassi classified the peripheral locations of the hydatid disease into three groups:

a. rare locations: spleen, kidney, bone, muscle;

b. very rare locations: diaphragm, pancreas, thyroid, brain, salivary glands, subcutaneous tissue;

c. extremely rare locations: thymus, lymphatic nodes, adrenal gland, hypophysis, tonsils [1].

The percentage of site involvement varies and the exact incidence in unusual locations is about 8%–10%, but it is difficult to ascertain, as they are only reported as case reports [4].

Previous data reported that incidence of CE involving the spleen, kidney, peritoneal cavity, skin, and muscles was about 2-3% each and incidence of the heart, brain, vertebral column, ovaries, pancreas, gall bladder, thyroid gland, bones, and breast involvement was about 1% or less, each [15]. Figure 1 summarizes updated data on frequencies of unusual locations of CE as reported in different scientific articles.

A recent meta-analysis conducted in Iran where *Echinococcosis* is endemic, focused on the unusual locations (i.e., other than the liver and lung) diagnosed in the last 20 years (1990–2011). About 463 cases of the hydatid cyst located in different parts of the body, excluding the liver and lung, have been published from Iran. The most common locations were

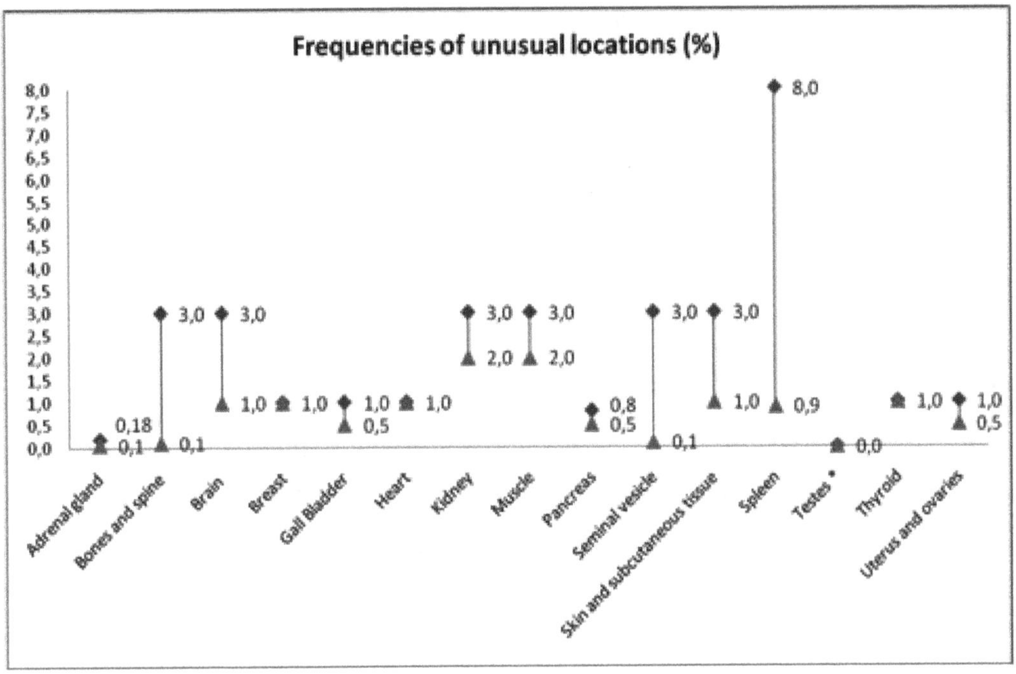

* Only five case reports of testicular location

(Adrenal gland: Akcay et al., 2004 [42]; Bones and spine: Drimousis et al., 2006 [43]; Brain: Greenberg SM, 2001 [44]; Altas et al., 2010 [45]; Breast: McManus et al., 2003 [15]; Gall Bladder: Raza et al., 2003 [46]; Mushtaque et al., 2011 [47]; Heart: McManus et al., 2003 [15]; Kidney: Gogus et al., 2003 [48]; Muscle: Verasaci et al., 2005 [49]; Arora et al., 2011 [50]; Pancreas: Palaivelu C, 2007 [51]; Moosavi et al., 2007 [52]; Seminal vesicle: Vasileios et al., 2002 [53]; Safioleas et al., 2006 [54]; Skin and subcutaneous tissue: Zulfikaroglu et al., 2005 [55]; Dirican et al., 2008 [56]; Spleen: Polat et al., 2003 [57]; Testes: Tlili et al., 2014 [58]. Thyroid: McManus et al., 2003 [15]; Uterus and ovaries: Arora et al., 2005 [59]; Palaivelu C, 2007 [59])

Figure 1. Frequencies of unusual locations of cystic *Echinococcosis* as reported in different scientific articles.

the central nervous system (brain, spinal cord, and orbit), musculoskeletal system, heart, and kidney, whereas some less common locations were the spleen, pancreas, appendix, thyroid, salivary gland, adrenal gland, breast, ovary, retroperitoneum, and mediastinum [16].

With the advent of modern DNA-based methods, the genetic variability of *E. granulosus* was confirmed and a number of genotypes were recognized (named G1–G10). *E. granulosus* comprises several intraspecific variants or strains that have substantial variation at the genetic level. By contrast, there seems to be very limited genetic variation within *E. multilocularis* [17]. A recent study has reported results of analyses conducted on agents responsible for causing 10 cases of cerebral hydatid disease. Strain differentiation was possible for eight cases and all were found to be of the G6 genotype, suggesting that this genotype may have a propensity for infecting the brain [18]. Further genetic investigations in unusual localizations are recommended to evaluate a possible cluster of genotypes and or subtypes by different location in order to support differential diagnosis of *Echinococcosis* for any cystic mass found in patients, especially from endemic areas [4].

4. Diagnostic serological tests

Immunodiagnosis is an important tool for diagnosis of hydatid infection. The increase in serum IgE is characteristic for helminthic disease and is stimulated by the synthesis of IL-4 from Th2 lymphocites [19]. Different serological tests were developed and applied. Usually, they detect anti-Echinococcus IgG, but there are also methods for examination of IgE in serum such as RAST (RIA), ELISA, and Western blot. The sensitivity of the ImmunoCAP system, in some studies, is significantly lower than the sensitivity of both the ELISA and Western blot. In contrast, the ImmunoCAP system demonstrated increased specificity and decreased cross-reactivity compared with the ELISA. Western blot remains the principle method for the detection of CE because of its significantly higher sensitivity. The lower sensitivity of the ImmunoCAP system for detecting anti-Echinococcus IgE compared with the tests for specific IgG can be explained by the stronger IgG response in CE. Comparison of anti-Echinococcus IgE in hepatic and pulmonary CE showed significant differences in the immune response that were not only qualitative (more often positive in hepatic CE) but also quantitative (lower antibody levels in pulmonary CE). While there was a detectable difference in anti-Echinococcus IgG by ELISA and Western blot, the discrepancy was not significant. In rare locations of the disease, that are often peripheric locations, serological tests have shown a lower sensitivity. In conclusion, detection of anti-Echinococcus IgE could be applied as an additional confirmatory method when false-positive results are suspected from other immunological tests [20].

5. Imaging features

Radiological signs of *Echinococcosis* are usually non-specific, and the serologic tests are necessary to confirm the diagnosis [21]. The liver (75%) and lungs (15%) are the most commonly involved organs, but the disease can be seen anywhere in the body (10%) [21–22]. Most typical imaging findings of the hydatid disease are cystic lesions in the affected organs; namely, imaging features vary according to the stage of cyst development [23]. In the early stage, the cysts usually show as a simple cyst, with a homogeneous fluid content with both CT attenuation values and MRI signal similar than water. Cystic content is generally hypointense on T1-weighted images, and homogeneously hyperintense on T2-weighted sequences. Then, imaging appearance may be slightly different due to the presence of intracystic debris, hydatid sand, and inflammatory cells. During the natural evolution of the hydatid cyst, a ring-like calcification of the cystic wall can be seen and this sign is more common in the liver, spleen, and kidney. However, calcification of the pericyst does not necessarily indicate death of parasite. It is, instead, highly likely when the cyst is completely calcified [24]. The endocyst may detach partially or completely from the pericyst causing "floating membranes" inside the cavity, a finding that is highly specific for hydatid disease. When there are daughter cysts inside the hydatid cyst, it appears multi-vesicular with a "honeycomb pattern" [22] (Figure 2); daughter vesicles are located peripherally and they usually contain fluid with a lower attenuation than that of the fluid in the mother cyst [24].

In addition to the liver and lungs, echinoccosis could be also found in different other organs; in these cases, the diagnosis could be difficult, and differential diagnosis is generally required.

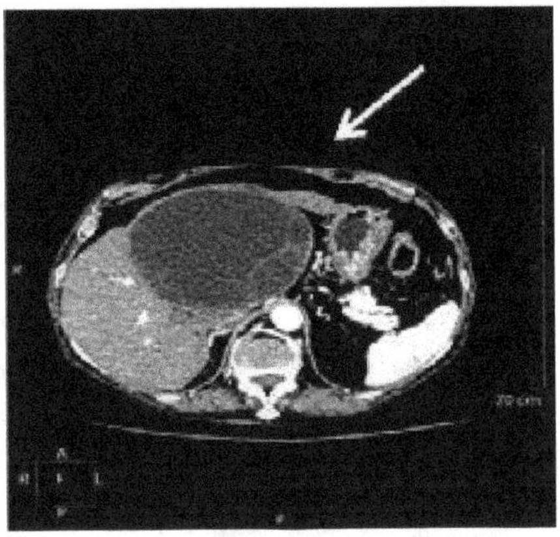

Figure 2. Typical hydatid cyst of the liver, with some peripheral daughter cysts (arrow).

Uncommon locations are briefly discussed, emphasizing imaging features.

Spleen is the most common affected organ after the liver and lungs and its involvement ranges from 0.9% to 8%. Primary splenic hydatidos is rare (less than 2%) [22].

Splenic cysts are commonly solitary and often develop secondary to systemic dissemination or intraperitoneal spread from ruptured liver hydatid cysts. Differential diagnosis includes epidermoid cyst, pseudocyts, abscess, or hematoma; also cystic neoplasms should be differentiated from hydatid splenic disease [21].

Pancreas is involved very rarely (0.25% of the cases). Patients could aspecific symptoms as abdominal discomfort, nausea, and vomiting. In a case report described by Szanto et al., an hydatic pancreatic cyst was found on the tail of the pancreas, causing portal hypertension and splenic veins congestion [25]. In cases of pancreatic locations, lesions show typical imaging findings: cystic appearance, sometimes with wall calcifications and daughter cysts. Clear fluid content is generally represented hypodense on CT images. Additionally, signs of vascular compression could be detected on CT and MR imaging. Differential diagnosis from other pancreatic cystic lesions (pseudocyst, serous cystadenoma, and mucinous cystic neoplasm) may be difficult; it is based on the presence of a more thickened and laminated cystic wall, often with thin calcifications.

Kidney is a rare location of Echinoccosis. Symptoms are often nonspecific and, when the cysts are intact and the antigenic stimulation is too low, imaging is crucial for a correct diagnosis [26]. Renal cysts are usually unilateral and located in the cortex of the upper or lower pole; they appear unilocular or multilocular if there are daughter cysts inside the parental cyst. Three types of cysts have been described by Ishimitsu [27]:

- type 1: unilocular cysts (initial stage of parasite development)

- type 2: multiple daughter cysts within the mother cyst (intermediate stage of parasitic development)
- type 3: completely calcified cysts (death of the parasite)

In type 1 and type 2 cysts, the cyst wall may be thick or calcified (Figure 3), and both the wall and the internal septa may show enhancement after e.v. administration of the contrast agent. In up to 18% of cases, the cyst may rupture into the collecting system and at imaging several round filling defects may be seen due to the migration of daughter cysts within calices and renal pelvis [24]. Differential diagnosis of renal hydatidosis includes simple or infected renal cyst, abscess, and cystic or necrotic neoplasms [22].

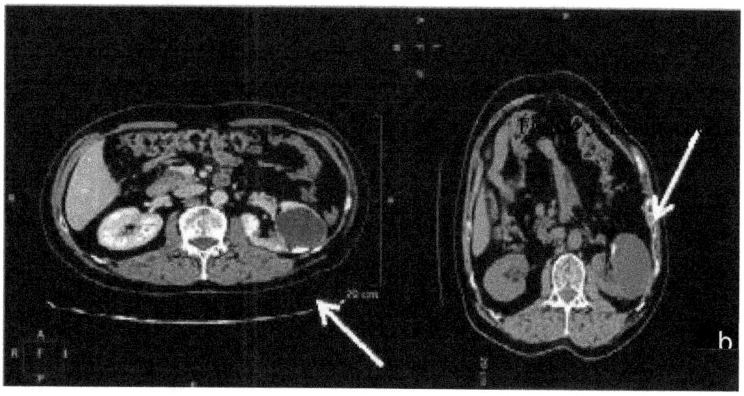

Figure 3. Unilocular hydatid cyst of the left kidney with internal calcifications that move (arrows) changing patient's decubit: supine (a) and on the right flank (b).

Hydatid cysts of the *adrenal gland* are very rare, with an incidence at autopsy of 0.06%–0.18%. They are usually secondary to a systemic *Echinococcosis* beyond the hepatic and the pulmonary filters.

Organs of female genital tract are rarely involved; first articles have been reported more than 50 years ago. It is generally associated to the developing of other parasitic cysts in the pelvis after the rupture of a primary lesion located in an abdominal organ (Figure 4). Ovaries are more affected than the uterus; differential diagnosis includes all the other ovarian cystic lesions.

Involvement of the *peritoneum* represents about the 13% of all abdominal hydatidosis [22]. Primary peritoneal disease is extremely rare. Peritoneal cysts generally develop as a consequence of seeding from either spontaneous rupture or prior surgery of hepatic, splenic, or mesenteric cysts [28]. Peritoneal cysts may be multiple and located anywhere in the peritoneal cavity [24]; they can enlarge and cause abdominal distension or obstruction [21]. Isolated retroperitoneal hydatid cysts of *retroperitoneum* are rare; they usually are secondary to the involvement of the liver [22]. The invasion of the *abdominal wall* by liver hydatid cysts has already been reported in literature. A cyst usually passes through a small orifice and develops within the abdominal wall, keeping communication with its hepatic component and showing a typical "hourglass" configuration.

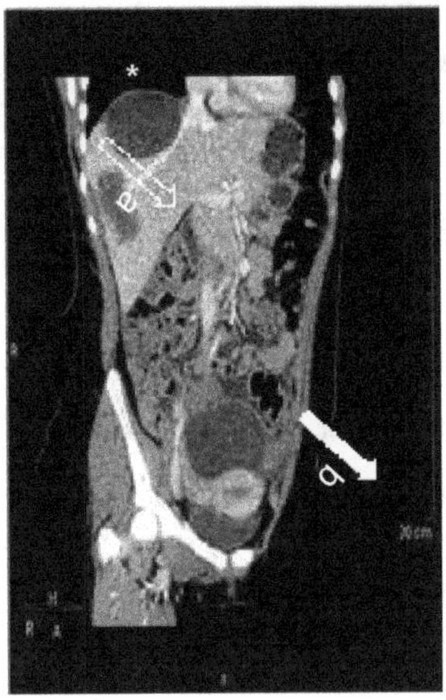

Figure 4. Pelvic hydatid cyst above the uterus (arrow), formed after the rupture of a liver cyst (open arrow). Asterisk shows another cyst at the hepatic dome.

Primary *soft-tissue* involvement is extremely rare and represents 0.5%–4.7% of patients. Clinical manifestation often consists of a palpable mass. Imaging findings are nonspecific and may include unilocular or multilocular cysts and complex solid lesions if some inflammatory changes overlap.

Diaphragmatic localization has an incidence of 1% and is often associated with liver disease. It is believed that the lack of peritoneum in the bare area of the liver is usually the weak point, which favors the transdiaphragmatic migration of a liver hydatid cyst. Diaphragma may appear thickened and lobulated with unilocular or multilocular cysts. When the chest is reached, possible complications may be represented by a rupture into the pleural cavity, seeding in the pulmonary parenchyma and chronic bronchial fistula.

6. Clinical presentation

The unusual anatomic locations may cause difficulties in making the differential diagnosis, as *E. granulosus* is usually not suspected in some locations of the body [29]; signs and symptoms may be easily confused with those of other illnesses [30]. In these peripheral locations the clinical picture is extremely variable and depends upon the involved organs. Mechanical symptoms on adjacent structures are often present, in other cases complications arise, due to secondary infection or rupture with unforeseeable anaphylactic reactions [3].

It is not easy, neither simple, to describe the clinical manifestations of a hydatid cyst located in a peripheric organ, very often each case presents different clinical features, as it appears from our series. In the rare localizations the hydatid disease in the beginning is almost always asymptomatic, due to the slow growth of the cyst, and frequently is incidentally diagnosed. While the clinical signs of the hepatic cysts depend on its size and location inside the liver, when it is located in the peripheric organs, after an initial period during which the cyst is asymptomatic, clinical signs appear only when the diameter of the cyst increases and determines "mechanical" clinical features, which will be different according to the organ where the cyst is located. Splenic hydatid disease is mainly produced by systemic dissemination or intraperitoneal spread from a ruptured liver cyst [24].

The clinical manifestations include abdominal pain, enlarged spleen, and fever [21]. In renal hydatid disease, patients may be asymptomatic or refer non-specific clinical manifestation (flank mass, renal colic, persistent fever, hematuria, dysuria, pyuria, or hypertension) [21].

In *Echinococcosis* of the adrenal gland, when symptoms are present, they are related to local visceral compression. In the patient present in our personal series, abdominal pain and dispeptic symptoms were present [14].

6.1. Personal series

In the Department of General Surgery of the University of Catania, Italy, from 1974 to 2014, 434 patients underwent surgical treatment for hydatid disease: in 319 cases (73.50%) the cyst was located in the liver, while in 79 cases (18.20%) it was located in the lungs. The remaining 36 patients (8.29%) presented a rare localization of the disease: in 3 patients (0.69%) the cyst was in the mediastinum, in 3 patients (0.69%) in the diaphragm, in one case (0.23%) in the dorsal muscle, and in 1 case (0.23%) in the subcutaneous tissue of the right lumbar region. In 28 cases (6.45%) the rare localization of the hydatid cyst was in the abdominal cavity: 11 cysts (2.53%) were in the peritoneal serosa, 9 (2.07%) in the spleen, 6 (1.38%) in the kidney, 1 (0.23%) in the adrenal gland, and 1 (0.23%) in the retroperitoneal region.

In the patients in whom the cyst was located in the peritoneal serosa, pain was present in 6 cases, a palpable mass in 4 cases, while in the other cases the cyst was incidentally diagnosed in an asymptomatic phase. Nine patients had a splenic localization and in 3 of them a hepatic cyst was also present. In 4 patients, a palpable mass in the left hypochondrium was present, 3 patients complained of a painful clinical picture, while 2 patients were asymptomatic. The patient with a cyst in the retroperitoneal space complained of a continuous pain in the right gluteal region with diffusion to the iliac bone and the omolateral thigh. A palpable mass was present in the mesogastrium. The patient with an adrenal cyst had perceived abdominal pain and dyspeptic symptoms with nausea [14]. The patient with the localization in the dorsal muscle was a woman who had noticed a mass in the lower lateral part of the axilla, which had increased until it reached a diameter of 12 cm.

6.2. Atypical manifestations

Absolutely unexplainable was the growth pattern of the cyst located in the subcutaneous tissue of the lumbar region in a 77-year-old woman that we observed in 2007. The diameter of the mass was about 8 cm, and clinical examination revealed that the mass had a smooth surface with distinct margins (Figure 5a). Absolutely unusual, the report of CT that displayed the atypical behaviour of the cyst that seemed to originate from the liver through a little peduncle and then went into the muscle layer and reached the subcutaneous tissue of the lumbar region (Figure 5b) [31]. These data were confirmed at surgery but a clear explanation of this atypical case has not been obtained. If a hydatid cyst develops into the liver, usually it grows inside the liver and outside it towards the peritoneal cavity, it can reach a great dimension but does not go over the abdominal wall muscles as an infiltrating tumor. A similar growth pattern may occur in cysts located in the liver cupola when, in consequence of an inflammatory process, go into the diaphragm and open to the bronchial tubes. However, in our case, infective processes were not present and so this case remains unexplainable.

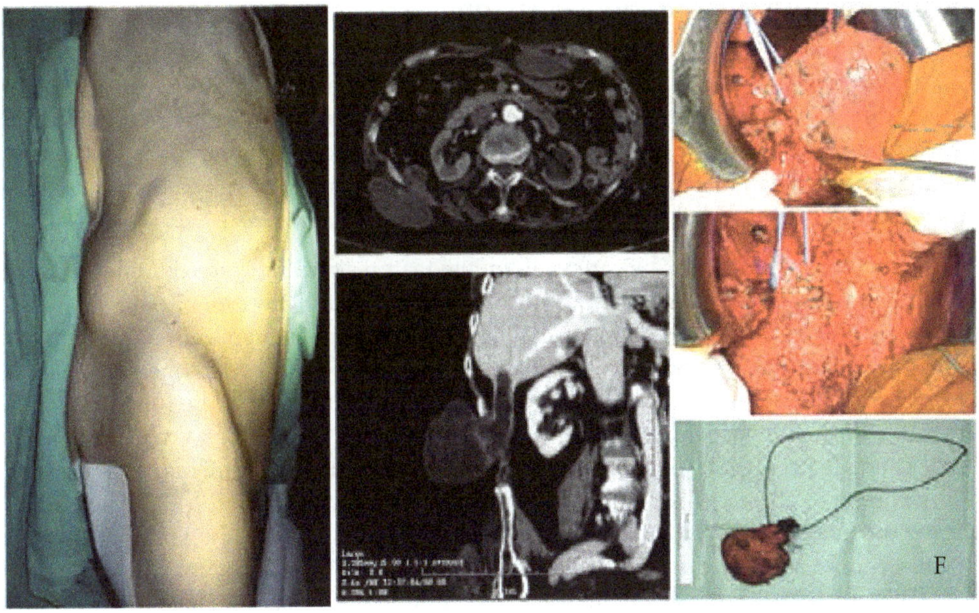

Figure 5. Clinical (a), radiological (b) and surgical (c) appearance of a rare hydatid cyst of the subcutaneous tissue of the lumbar region, correlated to the liver through a little peduncle [31].

6.3. Diagnostic evaluation and surgical treatment

In our experience, immunological tests have been very useful when the hydatid cyst was located in the liver, but have not showed the same diagnostic profit in patients affected by rare locations of the disease. In these cases, globally considered, echinotest has been positive in about one third of the cases. Diagnostic tools that have been essential to obtain the diagnosis were ultrasound and CT. The surgical treatment of the hydatid cysts peripherically located is not standardized, usually they are cases sporadically reported and the same great experience gained in the surgical treatment of the hepatic cysts is lacking. In hepatic cysts, a considerable reduction of the conservative surgical approaches has been reported and nowadays an increase in radical surgery is the preferred treatment.

In peripheric locations, the radical surgical removal without spreading the disease due to spillage of cystic fluid has been the treatment of choice, and this method has been applied to the cysts located in the peritoneum. In the splenic localization, splenectomy has always been performed and the patients underwent the standardized protocols to avoid the consequences of the overwhelming postsplenectomy infection [32]. In the renal localizations it has been possible to avoid nephrectomy and realize a partial pericystectomy and no recurrences have been observed. The cyst located in the adrenal gland was treated by surrenectomy and the cysts located in the dorsal muscle and in the subcutaneous tissue of the lumbar region (Figure 5c) were easily removed.

7. Echinococcosis and allergy — Anaphylaxis

Echinococcus granulosus and *E. multilocularis* are involved in parasitic disease in humans: cystic *Echinococcosis* (CE) ("hydatid diseas") and alveolar *Echinococcosis* (AE), respectively. Both diseases and parasites have tight links with allergy because of the immunological characteristics that contribute to maintaining the larva in its human host, as well as their potential in inducing clinical anaphylactic reactions in some patients [19].

Allergic reactions and anaphylaxis are well-known features of CE. Elevated total IgE, as well as occurrence of specific IgE against Echinococcus antigens in the serum of patients with CE are also key biological features of the disease [33–34]. IgE-dependent immune reactions were long neglected in AE; obviously, anaphylactic reactions are far less frequent than in CE. However, specific IgE antibodies against *E. Multilocularis* antigens may be found in patients with AE [19]. Anaphylactic reactions have been reported in cystic *Echinococcosis* for several decades and are usually observed in case of overt or unapparent rupture of the parasitic cyst [19]. A variety of allergic symptoms has been described in patients with CE. They include urticaria that may be only mild or present as chronic and apparently "idiopathic" urticaria, or as giant urticaria associated with systemic signs and symptoms. Respiratory symptoms may also be observed; asthma may be the first manifestation of hepatic hydatidosis and acute bronchospasm may occur when the cyst is manipulated at surgery. Anaphylactic shock is the most impressive and severe clinical presentation of IgE-dependent allergic reactions in CE. It may occur spontaneously and precede any other symptoms. Recurrent life-threatening anaphylactic shocks, with or without laryngospasm, may be due to small, incomplete rupture of the cyst [35–36]. Overt rupture of the cyst, however, is a much more frequent cause of anaphylaxis; it may be observed after trauma, even trivial, such as that derived from a sport (football) accident. Sometimes, however, intraperitoneal perforation of a hepatic hydatid cyst can happen without anaphylactic reaction, confirming the inaccurate knowledge of the mechanisms that control the allergic phenomena produced by the parasite [37]. The most usual circumstance is surgery, however, even in the immediate postoperative period, or laparoscopy. As for other etiologies of anaphylactic shock, tryptase measurement is of help for diagnosis [19]. In AE, the low rate of anaphylactic symptoms could be related to a more "masked" form of Echinococcus antigens in patients with AE than in those with CE: the extremely fibrotic lesions of AE cannot rupture, and the echinococcal fluid may never be in contact with mast cell-bound IgE [38].

8. Medical treatment

In patients treated for liver and/or lung hydatid cysts, the possibility of secondary *Echinococcosis* can be minimized by concurrent treatment with benzimidazoles [39].

Mebendazole (MBZ) and albendazole (ABZ) are the benzimidazole (BMZ) agents used for the treatment of hepatic CE. They interfere with the absorption of glucose through the wall of the parasite, causing glycogen depletion, and degenerative changes in echinococcal mitochondria and endoplasmic reticulum. BMZ may be favorably used alone for the treatment of small (<5 cm) CE liver cysts or for inoperable patients; BMZ is also usually associated with PAIR or surgery to prevent secondary CE. BMZ is not indicated for the treatment of inactive or calcified asymptomatic cysts, unless they are complicated lesions. Both ABZ and MBZ are effective, but ABZ is considered the drug of choice. The usual dose of orally administered ABZ is 10–15 mg/kg/day in two divided doses; if using MBZ, the daily dose is 40–50 mg/kg in three divided doses. Treatment with BMZ should be administered continuously for 3–6 month. Praziquantel has been used (40 mg/kg once a week) with ABZ for combined treatment of CE; this therapeutic association seems to be more effective than ABZ alone [40–41]. Usual adverse effects include nausea, hepatotoxicity, neutropenia, and occasionally alopecia [39]. In patients treated for rare peripheric locations, in our opinion, treatment with BMZ should be especially recommended. In these patients, hepatic and pulmonary filters have been bypassed, so the disease should be considered systemic and chemotherapy should be promising in preventing further recurrences.

9. Conclusions

Although the incidence of *Echinococcosis* has dramatically reduced in recent decades, many cases can still be found in daily medical practice. The surgeon must keep in mind that this parasitosis can occur even in uncommon locations and therefore it should be regarded as a potentially systemic disease. In these cases the diagnosis is challenging and can be achieved only through a complete interdisciplinary evaluation of clinical, laboratory, and radiological data.

Acknowledgements

Part of the text of paragraph 6.2. "Atypical manifestations" and Figure 5 are used with kind permission of the publisher for World Journal of Gastroent erology. The Authors wish to thank Bench srl for the technical support. Main Authors (Antonio Di Cataldo, Giuseppe Petrillo, Claudia Trombatore, Stefano Palmucci, Antonella Agodi) did study conception, acquisition and interpretation of data, wrote the manuscript and performed the final critical revision. Other Authors cooperated in the writing the manuscript, according to their competence and specific knowledge.

Author details

Antonio Di Cataldo[1 * #], Giuseppe Petrillo[2 #], Claudia Trombatore[2 #], Stefano Palmucci[2 #], Antonella Agodi[1 #], Martina Barchitta[1], Annalisa Quattrocchi[1], Nunzio Crimi[3], Silvia Fichera[3], Stefano Puleo[1], Amy Giarrizzo[1], Martina Calabrini[1], Rosalia Latino[1] and Rosanna Portale[1]

*Address all correspondence to: dicataldoa@tiscali.it

1 Department of Medical and Surgical Sciences, Advanced Technologies GF Ingrassia, University of Catania, Italy

2 Radiodiagnostic and Radiotherapy Unit, University Hospital Policlinico-Vittorio Emanuele, Catania, Italy

3 Department of Respiratory Diseases and Allergology, University of Catania, Italy

#Principal authors

References

[1] Grassi G: Contributo allo studio di alcune localizzazioni rare delle cisti d'echinococco. Gazz San 9: 428-433, 1965.

[2] Craig PS, McManus DP, Lightowlers MW: Prevention and control of cystic echinococcosis. Lancet Infectious Diseases 7: 385–394, 2007.

[3] Sachar S, Goyal S, Sangwan S: Uncommon locations and presentations of hydatid cyst.Ann Med Health Sci Res 204:447-522014.

[4] World Health Organization. About echinococcosis. Available online at: http://www.who.int/echinococcosis/about_disease/en/.

[5] Hotez PJ, Gurwith M: Europe's neglected infections of poverty. Int J Infectious Diseases 15: e611–e619, 2011.

[6] Rojo-Vazquez FA, Pardo-Lledias J, Francos-Von Hunefeld M: Cystic echinococcosis in Spain: Current situation and relevance for other endemic areas in Europe, PLoS Neglected Tropical Diseases 5: article e893, 2011.

[7] Polat P, Kantarci M, Alper F: Hydatid Disease from Head to Toe. Radiographics 23: 475-494, 2003.

[8] European Centre for Disease Prevention and Control. Annual epidemiological report 2014—food and waterborne diseases and zoonoses. Stockholm: ECDC; 2014.

[9] Garippa G: Updates on Cystic Echinococcosis (CE) in Italy. Parassitologia 48: 57–59, 2006.

[10] Garippa G, Manfredi MT: Cystic Echinococcosis in Europe and in Italy. Veterinary Research Communications 33: supplement S35–S39, 2009.

[11] Moro P, Schantz PM: Echinococcosis: A review. Int J Infectious Diseases13: 125–133, 2009.

[12] Petrone L, Cuzzi G, Colace L: Cystic Echinococcosis in a Single Tertiary Care Center in Rome, Italy. BioMed Res Int, Article ID 978146, 2013.

[13] Wani RA, Wani I, Malik AA, Parray FQ, Wani AA, Dar AM: Hydatid disease at unusual sites. IJCR 3:1–6, 2012.

[14] Di Cataldo A, Trombatore G, Greco R, Lanteri R, Li Destri G, Licata A: Hydatid disease in a very unusual location: The adrenal gland. A case report. Chir. Ital. 55: 275–278, 2003.

[15] McManus DP, Zhang W, Li J, Bartley PB: Echinococcosis. Lancet 362:1295-304, 2003

[16] Geramizadeh B: Unusual locations of the hydatid cyst: A review from Iran. Iran J Med Sci. 38:2–14, 2013.

[17] Alvarez Rojas CA, Romig T, Lightowlers MW: Echinococcus granulosus sensu lato genotypes infecting humans—Review of current knowledge. Int J Parasitol. 44:9–18, 2014.

[18] Sadjjadi SM, Mikaeili F, Karamian M, Maraghi S, Sadjjadi FS, Shariat Torbaghan S, Kia EB: Evidence that the Echinococcus granulosus G6 genotype has an affinity for the brain in humans. Int. J. Parasitol. 43: 875–877, 2013.

[19] Vuitton A: Echinococcosis and allergy. Clin Rev Allergy Immunol 26: 93–104, 2004.

[20] Marinova I, Nikolov G, Michova A, Kurdova R, Petrunov B: Quantitative assessment of serum-specific IgE in the diagnosis of human cystic echinococcosis. Parasite Immunol. Jul; 33(7): 371–6, 2011.

[21] Gossios KJ, Kontoyiannis DS, Dascalogiannaki M, Gourtsoyiannis NC: Uncommon locations of hydatid disease: CTappearances. Eur Radiol 7: 1303–1308, 1997.

[22] Ilica A, Kocaoglu M, Zeybek N, Guven S, Adaletli I, Basgul A, Coban H, Bilici A, Bukte Y: Extrahepatic abdominal hydatid disease caused by echinococcus granulosus: Imaging findings. AJR 189:337–343, 2007.

[23] Ortega CD, Ogawa NY, Rocha MS, Blasbalg R, Motoyama Caiado AH, Warmbrand G, Cerri GG. Helminthic diseases in the abdomen: An epidemiologic and radiologic overview. RadioGraphics 30:253–267, 2010.

[24] Pedrosa I, Saíz A, Arrazola J, Ferreirós J, Pedrosa CS: Hydatid disease: Radiologic and pathologic features and complications. RadioGraphics 20: 795–817, 2000.

[25] Szanto P, Goian I, Al Hajjar N, Badea R, Seicean A, Manciula D, Serban A: Hydatic cyst of the pancreas causing portal hypertension. Maedica (Buchar). 5(2): 139–41, 2010.

[26] Volders WK, Gelin G, Stessens RC: Hydatid cyst of the kidney: Radiologic-pathologic correlation. RadioGraphics 21: S255–S260, 2001.

[27] Ishimitsu DN, Saouaf R, Kallman C, Balzer BL: Best cases from the AFIP: Renal hydatid disease. RadioGraphics 30: 334–337, 2010.

[28] Pickhardt PJ, Bhalla S: Unusual non-neoplastic peritoneal and subperitoneal conditions: CT findings. RadioGraphics 25: 719–730, 2005.

[29] Yuksel M, Demirpolat G, Sever A, Bakaris S, Bulbuloglu E, Elmas N: Hydatid disease involving some rare locations in the body: A pictorial essay. Korean J Radiol 8: 531–540, 2007.

[30] Yildirim M, Erkan N, Vardar E: Hydatid cyst with unusual localizations: Diagnostic and treatment dilemmas for surgeons. Ann Trop Med Parasitol 100: 137–142, 2006.

[31] Di Cataldo A, Latino R, Cocuzza A, Li Destri G: Unexplainable development of a hydatid cyst. World J Gastroenterol 15: 3309–3311, 2009.

[32] Di Cataldo A, Puleo S, Li Destri G, Racalbuto A, Trombatore G, Latteri F, Rodolico G: Splenic trauma and overwhelming post-splenectomy infection. Br J Surg 74: 343–345, 1987.

[33] Guisantes JA, Vincente-Garcia F, Abril JM, Eraso E, Martinez J: Total and specific IgE levels in human hydatid disease determined by enzyme immunoassay: Serological follow-up after surgery. J Investig Allergol Clin Immunol 4: 301–304, 1994.

[34] Riganò R, Ioppolo S, Ortona E, Margutti P, Profumo E, Ali MD, Di Vico B, Teggi A, Siracusano A: Long-term serological evaluation of patients with cystic echinococcosis treated with benzimidazole carbamates. Clin Exp Immunol 129: 485–492, 2002.

[35] Boyano T, Moldenhauer F, Mira J, Joral A, Saiz F: Systemic anaphylaxis due to hepatic hydatid disease. J Investig Allergol Clin Immunol 4: 158–159, 1994.

[36] Saenz de San Pedro B, Cazaña JL, Cobo J, Serrano CL, Quiralte J, Contreras J, Martinez F: Anaphylactic shock by rupture of hydatid hepatic cyst. Follow-up by specific IgE serum antibodies. Allergy 47: 568–570, 1992.

[37] Di Cataldo A, Lanteri R, Caniglia S, Santangelo M, Occhipinti R, Li Destri G: A rare complication of the hepatic hydatid cyst: Intraperitoneal perforation without anaphylaxis. Int Surg 90: 42–44, 2005.

[38] Vuitton DA, Bresson-Hadni S, Lenys D, Flausse F, Liance M, Wattre P, Miguet JP, Capron A: IgE-dependent humoral immune response in Echinococcus multilocularis infection: circulating and basophil-bound specific IgE against Echinococcus antigens in patients with alveolar echinococcosis. Clin Exp Immunol 71: 247–252, 1988.

[39] Nunnari G, Pinzone MR, Gruttadauria S, Celesia BM, Madeddu G, Malaguarnera G, Pavone P, Cappellani A, Cacopardo B: Hepatic echinococcosis: Clinical and therapeutic aspects. World J Gastroenterol 18: 1448–1458, 2012.

[40] Kumar A, Lal BK, Chattopadhyay TK: Hydatid disease of the liver non-surgical options. J Assoc Physicians India 41: 437–443, 1993.

[41] Vutova K, Mechkov G, Vachkov P, Petkov R, Georgiev P, Handjiev S, Ivanov A, Todorov T: Effects of mebendazole on human cystic echinococcosis: The role of dosage and treatment duration. Ann Trop Med Parasitol 93: 357–365, 1999.

[42] Akcay MN, Akcay G, Balik AA, Boyuk A: Hydatid cysts of the adrenal gland: Review of nine patients. World J Surg 28: 97–99, 2004.

[43] Drimousis PG, Stamou KM, Koutras A, Tsekouras DK, Zografos G: Unusual site of recurrent musculoskeletal hydatid cyst: Case report and brief review of the literature. World J Gastroenterol 12: 5577–5578, 2006.

[44] Greenberg SM: Handbook of Neurosurgery. 1st ed. New York: Thieme Medical Publisher 2001. p. 238-239.

[45] Altas M, Aras M, Serarslan Y, Davran R, Evirgen O, Yilmaz N: A medically treated multiple cerebral hydatid cyst disease. J Neurosurg Sci 54: 79–82, 2010.

[46] Raza MH, Harris SH, Khan R: Hydatid cyst of gall bladder. Indian J Gastroenterol 22: 67–68, 2003.

[47] Mushtaque M, Malik AA, Malik RA: Hydatid cyst of the gall bladder: A rare location. East J Med 16: 83–86, 2011.

[48] Gogus C, Safak M, Baltaci S, Turkolmez K: Isolated renal hydatidosis: Experience with 20 cases. J Urol 169: 186–189, 2003.

[49] Verasaci A, Scuderi G, Rosato A: Rare localizations of echinococcosis; personal experience. ANZ J Surg 75: 986–991, 2005.

[50] Arora M, Gupta CR, Jindal S, Kapoor N: An unusual case of hydatid cyst of broad ligament. J Indian Acad Clin Med 6: 86–87, 2005.

[51] Palaivelu C: Laparoscopic management of hydatid cysts of liver. Art of Laparoscopic surgery. Textbook and Atlas. Dehli Jaypee Publishers; 2007. p. 757–783.

[52] Moosavi SR, Kermany HK: Epigastric mass due to a hydatid cyst of the pancreas. A case report and review of the literature. JOP 8: 232–234, 2007.

[53] Vasileios R, Athanasios P, Stavros T: Echinococcal cyst of the seminal vesicles: A case report and literature review. Int Urol Nephrol 34: 527–530, 2002.

[54] Safioleas M, Nikiteas N, Stamatakos M: Echinococcal cyst of the subcutaneous tissue: A rare case report. Parasitol Int 57: 236–238, 2008.

[55] Zulfikaroglu B, Koc M, Ozalp N, Ozmen MM: A rare primary location of echinococcal disease: Report of a case. Ups J Med Sci 110:167–171, 2005.

[56] Dirican A, Unal B, Kayaalp C, Kirimlioglu V: Subcutaneous hydatid cysts occurring in the palm and the thigh: Two case reports. J Med Case Rep 2: 273, 2008.

[57] Polat P, Kantarci M, Alper F, Suma S, Koruyucu MB, Okur A: Hydatid disease from head to toe. Radiographics 23: 475–494, 2003.

[58] Tlili G, Bouassida K, Slama A, Tlili T, Ziadi S, Taher MA: Hydatid cyst of the scrotum miming a testicular tumor. J Case Reports 4: 151–154, 2014.

[59] Arora V, Nijjar IS, Gill KS, Singh G: Case report: Primary hydatid cyst of muscle—A rare site. Indian J Radiol Imaging 16: 239–241, 2006.

6

Brain Hydatid Cyst

Said Hilmani

Abstract

Brain echinococcosis is the most common brain parasitic infection in the world. It happens in a very rare location, representing 1% to 2% all cases with hydatid disease. It is more common by approximately 50–70% in pediatric population and young adultswith a male predominance. The definite hosts of echinococcus are various carnivores; man is an accidental host. The growth of hydatid cysts is usually slow and asymptomatic, and clinical manifestations are caused by compression of the involved organ. CT provides definitive results of diagnosis. It shows hydatid cyst as a spherical, well defined, thin walled, homogeneous and non-enhancing cystic lesion without peripheral oedema. Dowling technic is the most commonly done procedure designed to give birth to the intact cyst by irrigating saline between cyst wall-brain interfaces. Medical treatment can be indicated in multiple locations and in cases with peroperative rupture. Prognosis is often good, but same complications can occur after surgery and depend on the location, the size, the number of cysts and the technique used.

Keywords: Brain hydatid cyst, Echinococcosis, CT, Dowling technic

1. Introduction

Echinococcosis, also referred to as hydatid disease, is a general term used to define zoonosis caused by Echinococcus tapeworms, or cestodes. There are four types of Echinococci, the most common seen worldwide is Echinococcus granulosis whose adult form parasite the dog's small intestine and the larval form that develops in humans, and alveolar echinococcosis, caused by *Echinococcus multilocularis* and restricted to the northern hemisphere (12). Echinococcosis of the central nervous system is the most common brain parasitic infection in the world. It is a cosmopolitan anthropozoonosis and represents a significant public health problem. Humans are the accidental intermediate host in the life cycle of this genus. Intracranial pressure, seizure and focal deficit are common signs. CT scan and MRI are the choice exams. Surgery is the radical treatment.

2. Epidemiology

Hydatid disease is endemic in Mediterranean countries, Middle East, South America, North Africa and Australia (14). The achievement pulmonary pleura is the second frequency (15–40%) after the liver and associated to brain localization in 30% (7). Intracranial hydatid disease is rare, with reported incidence of 1–2% of all cases with hydatid disease (1,5). There are less than 5 cases per year in our practice (15). Cerebral hydatid disease is more common in pediatric population and young adults approximately 50–70%, with a male predominance. Sixty percent of our patients were males (9,15). Patients with cerebral hydatid cysts may have hydatid cysts in other organs in 10% to 28% of the cases, especially hepatic, pulmonary abut other organs. In general abdominal ultrasound and chest X-ray are sufficient to determine those locations.

3. Pathophysiology

Hydatid disease is due to the larval form of Taenia dog. The definite hosts of echinococcus are various carnivores, the common being the dog, which develop the adult worm in the gut following ingestion of the larvae that are present in the tissues of the intermediate host (typically sheep and goats and occasionally, humans) and then go on to develop in the visceral tissue, particularly in the liver and lungs. Man is an accidental host. He gets infected through the faeco-oral route by ingestion of food contaminated by dog faeces containing ova of the parasite or by direct contact with dogs. The embryos pass through the wall of the gut into the portal system and are carried to the liver where most larvae get entrapped and encysted. Some may reach the lungs and occasionally, some may pass through the capillary filter of the liver and lungs and get entry into the systemic circulation, to the brain or bone (6). The cerebral hydatid cysts are slow growing and present late when they increase in size and become large. There is no consensus on the growth rate of the hydatid cysts of the brain and has been variably reported between 1.5 and 10 cm/year (5). Intracranial hydatid cyst may also be classified as primary or secondary. The primary cysts are formed as a result of direct infestation of the larvae in the brain without demonstrable involvement of other organs. In the human host, a hydatid cyst can lead to life-threatening complications, such as cyst rupture, with the spread of new cysts, and bacterial infection.

There are some risk factors. Rural origin of adult patients was reported in over 70% of cases (1). Exposure may be the result of contact with dogs from breeders, farmers, butchers, veterinarians, or during recreational activities (hunting). Comorbidity is observed in some adults patients such as hypertension, diabetes, chronic lung disease or hepatitis.

4. Pathology

Hydatid cyst is formed by two membranes. First is an outer circular membrane made of concentric layers acidophilic, soft and acellular, milky characteristic appearance. And another is an internal germinal membrane, thin, grainy and nucleate. The cyst contains a liquid compound NaCl, carbohydrate, protein and lipid. This liquid has a spring water appearance if the cyst is healthy, opalescent or purulent if infected. Daughter vesicles fertile cyst containing 10 to 100 scolex, born of the germinal membrane and bathed in liquid hydatid. This explains the interest to evacuate the block cyst to avoid dissemination. Between brain tissue and cyst volume increase, forms a third membrane or adventitious, easy peel and helps to better remove the cyst fluid (3).

5. Clinical presentation

The growth of hydatid cysts is usually slow and asymptomatic, and clinical manifestations are caused by compression of the involved organ. The average time before diagnosis is 7 months (15 days to 3 years). The patients with intracranial hydatid cysts usually present with features of raised intracranial pressure may be complicated by blindness or loss consciousness; focal neurological deficit and seizure. Papilloedema is usually present in patients with intracranial hydatid cysts at the time of diagnosis.

6. Diagnosis

6.1. Imagery

CT provides definitive results of diagnosis. The exact location, size and number of hydatid cysts in the brain can be determined with a CT scan. However, MR is becoming more and more widely used as a diagnostic tool as it can show details that cannot be seen on CT (18). CT scan and MRI characteristically show hydatid cyst as a spherical, well defined, thin walled, homogeneous and non-enhancing cystic lesion without peripheral oedema. The fluid density is generally equal to that of CSF. The cyst wall usually show a rim of low signal intensity on both T1- and T2-weighted images (Figures 1 and 2). The presence of daughter cysts is considered pathognomonic but has been rarely reported (18). Compression of the midline structures and ventricles are seen in most of the cases, however surrounding oedema is usually absent in uncomplicated cases.

Intracranial hydatid can occur anywhere within the brain, but are more frequently located in the supratentorial compartment, especially in the middle cerebral artery territory. The parietal lobe is the most common site with 69% (11). Cerebellar location (Figure 3) is rare and serious with the risk of cerebral herniation and very rarely in the ventricles (18).

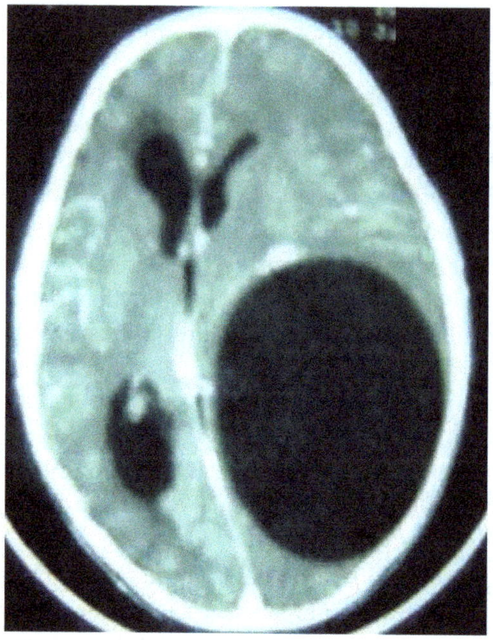

Figure 1. CT scan of solitary cerebral hydatid cyst.

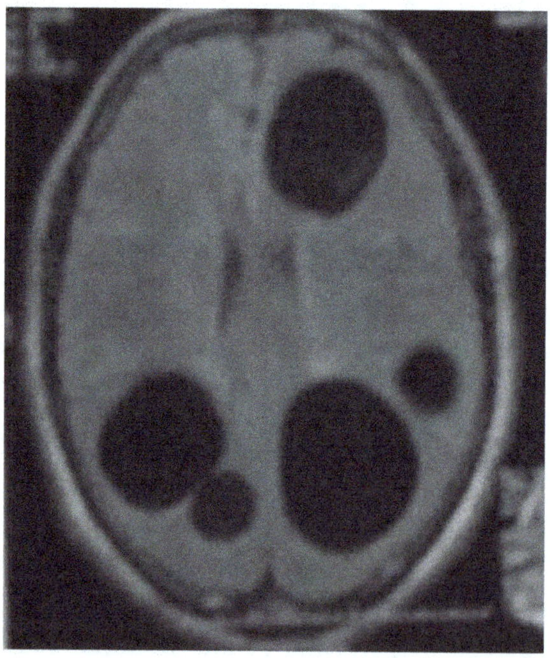

Figure 2. MRI T1 weighted image of multiple cerebral hydatid cyst.

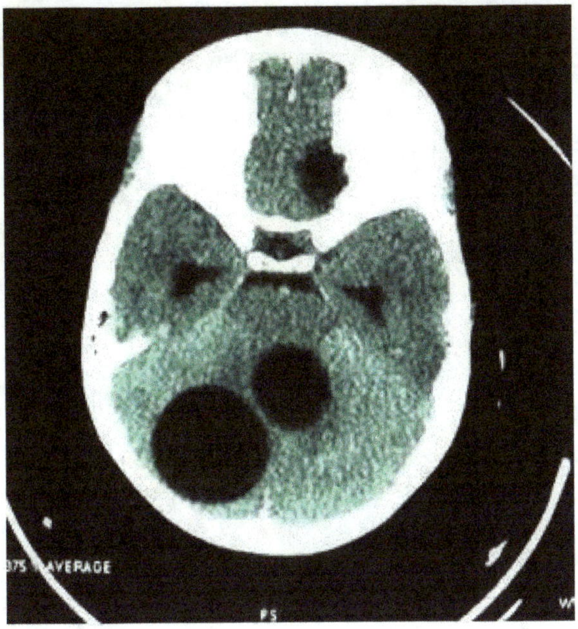

Figure 3. CT scan of double cerebellar hydatid cyst.

Exceptionally the skull can be reached after meningeal invasion (10). Cysts may be single or multiple (Figure 4), uni-or multiloculated. Intracranial hydatid cysts are commonly solitary in 93% (11). Multiple intracranial cysts are rare (18). We have reported 3.4% of each multiple and multiloculated hydatid cysts (15). They result from spontaneous, traumatic or surgical rupture of a solitary primary cyst or as a consequence of a cyst rupture elsewhere and embolization of hydatids to the brain. In those cases it necessary to search a cardiac location (2). A few cases of calcified or infected cyst were reported in the literature as in our series (10,11). The differential diagnosis of intracerebral hydatid cysts includes cystic lesions such as arachnoid cyst, cystic tumor of the brain and pyogenic abscess. In contrast to hydatid cysts, arachnoid cysts are not spherical in shape and not surrounded entirely by brain substance. Arachnoid cysts are extra-axial masses that may deform adjacent brain. Cystic tumors of the brain could be differentiated by the enhancement of the mural nodule. When a pyogenic abscess shows a cyst-like central necrotic area, peripheral oedema is almost always present and the rim enhances intensely following contrast administration (18). Proton MR spectroscopy and diffusion-weighted MR imaging have been used to distinguish between cerebral abscess and cystic or necrotic brain tumor. Shukla-Dave et al. (16) reported three cases of hydatid cysts demonstrated an increase in lactate, acetate and succinate.

6.2. Biology

The definitive diagnosis is by physical imaging methods – CT and MRI. Immunodiagnosis can also play an important complementary role. It is useful not only for primary diagnosis but also for follow-up of patients after surgical or pharmacological treatment. The enzyme-linked

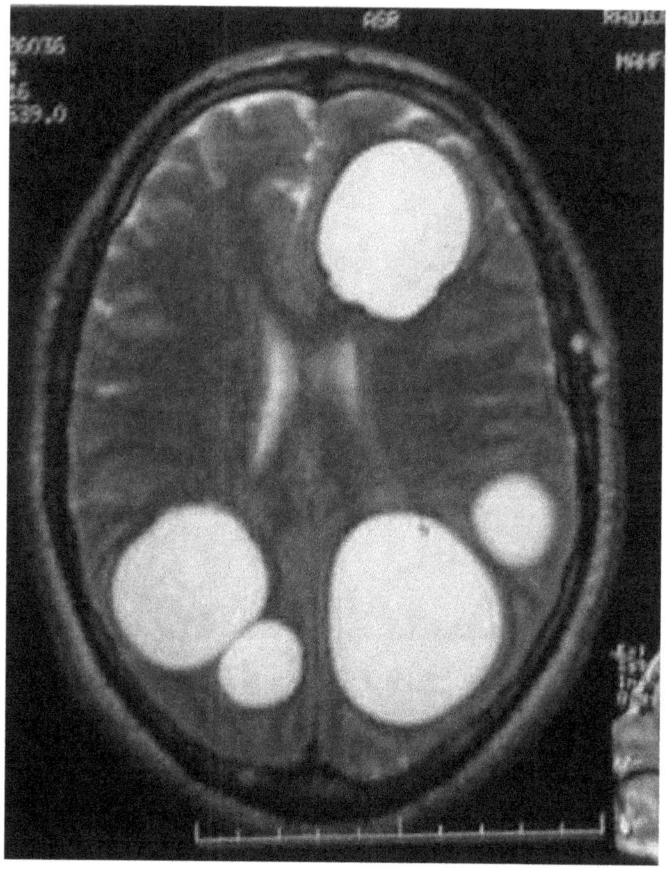

Figure 4. MRI T2 weighted image of multiple cerebral hydatid cyst.

immunosorbent assay (ELISA), the indirect immunofluorescence antibody test, immunoelectrophoresis, and immunoblotting are the hydatid serological testing in laboratory application (12,17). ELISA for specific anti-echinococcus IgG and IgE titer detection is frequently used in cystic echinococcosis serological diagnosis and screening, as it requires a short preparation time, and shows a sensitivity and specificity of 95%. (11). But in primary brain location, it is rarely positive. It was positive in less than 4% in our series. Hyper-eosinophilia can be observed in cases with other visceral location bone. In the literature, cystic echinococcosis diagnosis and follow-up eosinophil cell counts have usually been considered of limited value because it is significantly high in no more than half of CE affected patients (6). Sedimentation rate is normal in healthy cyst, and can be accelerated if infected.

7. Treatment

The treatment of hydatid cyst is surgical and the aim of surgery is to excise the cyst in toto without rupture to prevent recurrence and anaphylactic reaction.

7.1. Surgery

The most commonly done procedure designed to give birth to the intact cyst by irrigating saline between cyst wall-brain interfaces (Figure 5). This technique, reported by Dowling and improved by Arana-Iniguez, is possible because of minimal adhesions around the cyst wall (4). Aspiration of the cystic contents through puncturing during the surgery for deep-seated cyst or cysts which located in critical areas is an alternative method, especially as multiple hydatid cysts resulting from the rupture of a primary cyst are infertile and have no broad capsule witch permits the use of Dowling technique. Scolicide product use, as hypertonique saline serum, is essential to protect the brain parenchyma and the risk of dessiminisation in cases of intraoperative ruptured. For multiple and bilateral hydatid cysts the surgery must be done in several times.

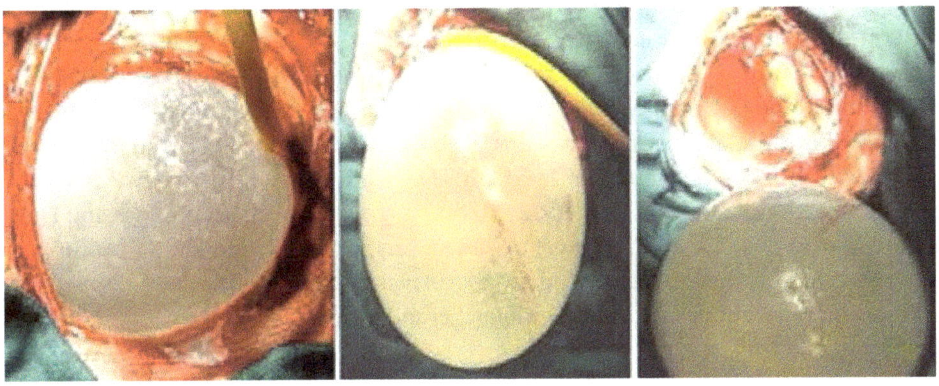

Figure 5. Dowling technique of solitary cerebral hydatid cyst.

7.2. Medical treatment

Only a few reports are available mentioning the efficacy of drug therapy. Albendazole therapy in a daily dose of 10 mg/kg, taken for four months, is a broad spectrum oral antihelminthic drug, which act by blocking glucose uptake of the larvae and the adult worm. The glycogen storage is depleted and thereby decreasing the ATP formation resulting in the death of the parasite (8). We think that medical treatment can be indicated in multiple locations and in cases with peroperative rupture.

8. Post-operative complications

Same complications can occur after surgery and depend on the location, the size, the number of cysts and the technique used. Hyperthermia within non meningitis or superinfection of the residual cavity, can be related to the translational phenomenon of brainstem during the evacuation of the cyst. It can be avoided by keeping the head turned to the opposite side of the lesion.

9. Evolution

Total recovery of the neurological deficit occurs in the majority of cases "90% in our practice". The risk of recurrence is about 19% and is correlated with the rate of intraoperative rupture of the cyst (6). The mortality is about 9% and is not negligible. Morbidity associated to hydatid cyst boils down a focal deficit or seizure (13).

10. Conclusion

Cerebral hydatid cyst is a rare disease that occurs in children with a history of contact with dogs. The definite hosts of echinococcus are various carnivores – man is an accidental host. It is most often manifested by intracranial hypertension, seizures and focal neurological deficit. The diagnosis is strongly suspected to brain CT scan. It show hydatid cyst as a spherical, well defined, thin walled, homogeneous and non-enhancing cystic lesion without peripheral oedema. MRI is especially useful in cases of hydatid cyst revamped to make the differential diagnosis with other cystic intracranial process. The positive hydatid serology is only suggestive. The treatment of choice is surgery with total removal without rupture, using Dowling technic, except in deep location. Medical treatment can be indicated in multiple locations and in cases with peroperative rupture. The prognosis is usually good if early diagnosis and out of multiple brain locations that pose a serious therapeutic problem.

Author details

Said Hilmani*

Address all correspondence to: hilmani.said@yahoo.fr

Neurosurgical Department, Hassan II University, Casablanca, Morocco

References

[1] Abbassioun K, Amirjamshidi A. Diagnosis and management of hydatid cyst of the central nervous system: Part 2 : hydatid cysts of the skull, orbit and spine. Neurosurgery, Vol. 11, March 2001: 10–16.

[2] Ait Ben Ali S, Hilmani S, Choukri M, Sami A, El Azhari A, Achouri M, Ouboukhlik A, El Kamar A, Boucetta M. Multiple cerebral hydatid cysts of cardiac origin. Neurochirurgie. 1999 Dec;45(5):426–429.

[3] Alzain TJ, Alwitry SH, Khalili HM. Multiple intracranial hydatidosis. Acta Neurochirurgica. 2002, 144, 1179–1185.

[4] Arana Iniquez R. Echinococcus. Infection of the Nervous System. Hand Book of Clinical Neurology, Part III, Eds. Vinken PJ, Bruyn GW, Elsevier/North Holland Biomedical Press, Amsterdam 1978; 175–208.

[5] Bouaziz M. Calcified cerebral hydatid cyst: a case report. Sante. 2005 Apr–Jun; 15.

[6] Cappello E, World J. Gastroenterol. 2013 December 28; 19(48): 9351–9358

[7] Ciurea AV, Vasilescu G, Nuteanu L, Carp N. Cerebral hydatid cyst in children. Experience of 27 cases. Childs Nerv Syst. 1995 Dec; 11(12): 679–685.

[8] Golematis B, Lakiotis G, Pepsidou GP et al. Albendazole in the conservative treatment of multiple hydatid disease. Sinai J Med. 1989; 56: 53–55.

[9] Haliloglu M, Saatci I, Akhan O, Ozmen MN, Besim A. Spectrum of imaging findings in pediatric hydatid disease. AJR Am J Roentgenol. 1997;169:1627–1631.

[10] Hilmani S, Bertal A, Lakhdar A, Ouboukhlik A, Elkamar A, Elazhari A. Craniocerebral hydatid cyst. J Neurosurg. 2006 Jul;105(1 Suppl):77.

[11] Iacona A, Pini C, Vicari G. Enzyme-linked immunosorbent assay (ELISA) in the serodiagnosis of hydatid disease. *Am J Trop Med Hyg.* 1980; 29: 95-102.

[12] McManus D. P, W. Zhang, J. Li, and P. B. Bartley. Echinococcosis. *The Lancet.* 2003, 362, 9392, 1295–1304.

[13] Nur A, Murad B, Hakan H, Bülent E. Central nervous system hydatidosis in Turkey: a cooperative study and literature analysis of 458 cases. J. Neurosurgery. 2000, July, Vol.93: 1-8.

[14] Onal C, Orhan B, Metis O et al. Three unusual cases of intracranial hydatid cysts in paediatric age group. Pediatr Neurosurg. 1997; 26 : 208-213.

[15] Salaou O, Ibahioin Kh, Chellaoui A, Hilmani S, LAakhdar A, Ouboukhlik A, EL kamar A, EL Azhari. AIntracerebral hydatid cyst: 104 cases. AJNS. 2007 Vol. 26, No 1.

[16] Shukla-Dave A, Gupta RK, Roy R, Husain N, Paul L, Venkatesh SK, Rashid MR, et al. Prospective evaluation of in vivo proton MR spectroscopy in differentiation of similar appearing intracranial cystic lesions. Magn Reson Imaging. 2001; 19:103–10.

[17] Wenbao Zhang, Jun Li, and Donald P. McManus. Concepts in immunology and diagnosis of hydatid disease. Clinical Microbiology Reviews. Jan. 2003, 18–36.

[18] Yas, A, Serdar K, Hasan N, Umit O, Adnan C, Masum S. Cerebral hydatid disease: CT and MR imaging findings. Swiss Med Wkly. 2004; 134: 459–467.

7

Radiological Characteristics of Pulmonary Hydatid Cysts

Dilek Emlik, Kemal Ödev, Necdet Poyraz and
Hasan Emin Kaya

Abstract

Hydatid disease is a parasitic infection caused by *Echinococcus granulosus* (EG), characterized by cystic lesions in the liver, lungs, and rarely in other parts of the body. Lungs and liver are the most frequent sites involved. Simultaneous lung and liver cysts are observed in less than 10% of the cases. Hydatid cysts are found more frequently in the lungs of children and adolescents than in their liver, while most cysts in adults are hepatic and relatively few are in the lungs. The hydatid serology results are often negative in patients with isolated pulmonary hydatidosis, and hence may not be helpful in problematic cases. Radiologic approach to the intact, complicated, or ruptured pulmonary hydatid cysts includes a CT scan following the chest radiograph. Thoracic CT may be supplemented with magnetic resonance (MR) imaging and occasionally with ultrasound (US) in clarifying a pleural-based hydatid cyst as extrapleural, pleural, or parenchymal.

Keywords: Thoracic hydatid disease, radiography, CT, MRI

1. Introduction

Echinococcus granulosus is a tapeworm of dogs and other carnivores. Eggs are passed in the feces of the dog and ingested by an intermediate host, commonly sheep or cattle, where they develop and grow into cystic structures [1]. After ingesting the cysts by carnivorous dogs, the life cycle is completed and numerous tapeworms develop in the intestine of the definitive host. Humans act as accidental intermediate hosts and harbor cysts that are most commonly found in the liver and lung but echinococcal cysts may develop in almost any part of the body except hair, teeth, and fingernails [2]. The liver is the most common site of infection followed by the lung in 15%-25% of the cases, and other sites (spleen, kidney, brain, bone) in about 10% of the cases [3-5].

Hydatid disease, caused by EG, is endemic in some countries, particularly those where sheep and cattle are raised, such as Australia, New Zealand, the Mediterranean countries, the Middle East, and South America [5-7]. Hydatid disease affects not only those living in endemic regions but also those in regions with a high rate of immigration from endemic areas [8].

The purpose of this chapter is to show the spectrum of the pathogenesis, clinical manifestations and imaging findings of pulmonary hydatid cysts in adults and children based on our experience.

2. Pathogenesis and pathology

Hydatid cyst may develop in almost any part of the body except hair, teeth, and fingernails [2]. Liver is the most frequently involved organ (60%-70%) [2, 5]. Thoracic involvement may occur via a transdiaphragmatic route (0.6%-16% of cases of hepatic disease) or by means of hematogenous spread. The former results from the migration of the parasite from the liver to the pleural cavity. Pulmonary parenchymal involvement and chronic bronchial fistula can also be found. The lung is the second most common site of involvement in adults (10%-30% of cases) and the most frequent site of involvement in children and young adults [9-11]. Compressible organs, such as the lung or brain, facilitate the growth of the cyst and this has been proposed as a reason for the high prevalence of the disease in children [12, 13].

Echinococcal cysts have three layers composed of both host and parasite tissue. A non-ruptured hydatid cyst is surrounded by the pericyst, a layer derived from compressed host tissue and chronic inflammatory cells. The true cyst wall is derived from the parasite and is arranged in two layers. The acellular outer laminated ectocyst is 1 mm-2 mm thick and is lined by a one-cell-thick germinal membrane, the endocyst [12].

3. Clinical findings

Adult patients with pulmonary hydatid cyst (PHC) present with nonspecific symptoms including cough, dyspnea, hemoptysis, pleurisy, and a bulge on the thoracic wall. The majority of the intact pulmonary cysts are known to produce no symptoms or are occasionally responsible for a non-productive cough or minimal hemoptysis. Pulmonary hydatid cyst usually remains asymptomatic until the time of rupture, and the clinic presentation in these patients is directly related to whether the cyst is intact or ruptured. The cyst may rupture spontaneously or due to antihelmintic treatment, percutaneous aspiration, or coughing and can lead to severe complications, such as massive hemoptysis and tension pneumothorax. Moreover, an acute hypersensitivity reaction or severe and life threatening problems can be encountered [14-17].

Compared with adults, PHCs in children frequently remain asymptomatic and cysts are often found by chance during physical examination or by imaging studies for other reasons. Moreover, pediatric patients may have symptoms such as chest pain, fever, purulent sputum, cough, and hemoptysis in the early period of the disease caused by compression of the surrounding tissue or perforation of the cyst [16].

4. Laboratory tests

Although the diagnosis of PHCs relies heavily on radiographic appearance and epidemiologic setting, serologic tests [e.g., immunoelectrophoresis (IEP) or electrosyneresis, indirect immunofluorescence (IIF), enzyme-linked immunosorbent assay (ELISA) or hemagglutination] can provide indirect evidence of echinococcosis. They are all sensitive methods but are compromised by nonspecific cross reactivity with other helmints [51]. The hydatid serology results are often negative in patients with isolated pulmonary hydatidosis and hence may not be helpful in problematic cases [15, 18]. Serologic tests have false-positive or false-negative rates of 15%-20% and positive tests may not revert to normal until several years after cyst removal [4].

5. Imaging findings

A brief description of the morphological characterization of PHCs is essential for the understanding of various conventional chest radiographic and CT appearances that will be discussed. In adults, the typical hydatid cyst of the lungs, when discovered by chest radiography, usually presents as a large well-demarcated, spherical, homogeneous single mass (Figure 1a, 1b), multiple nodules (Figure 2a, 2b) or masses [5, 14]. The cysts may range between 1 cm and 20 cm in diameter. Large cysts can shift the mediastinum, and peripheral cysts can produce a pleural reaction, or cause atelectasis of adjacent parenchyma [5, 14, 19]. Radiographically, the closed or simple cyst (intact cyst) may simulate carcinoma of the lung, primary sarcoma of the lung, solitary metastasis, hematoma, arteriovenous aneurysm, granuloma of different etiology, benign tumors, inflammatory masses, solid or fluid-filled cysts (e.g., bronchogenic cyst, bronchiectatic cyst, dermoid cyst), and mesothelioma [5, 19]. When the cystic opacity is localized in the juxtamediastinal area, it may look like an aneurysm of the aorta, a tumor in the mediastinum or a huge left auricula. A cyst attached to the thoracic wall may resemble a tumor, a cold abscess or loculated pleural effusion. In fact, sharply circumscribed homogeneous opacity in the lung is of great value in a country with endemic hydatid disease. Multiple cysts can be confused with pulmonary metastases. The imaging studies comprise only some of the diagnostic resources that must be used [15]. Calcifications of cysts in the liver and abdomen, and even in the rest of the body, are not uncommon but in the lung parenchyma they are extremely rare [4, 5]. However, on occasion they are found in the mediastinum including heart [5].

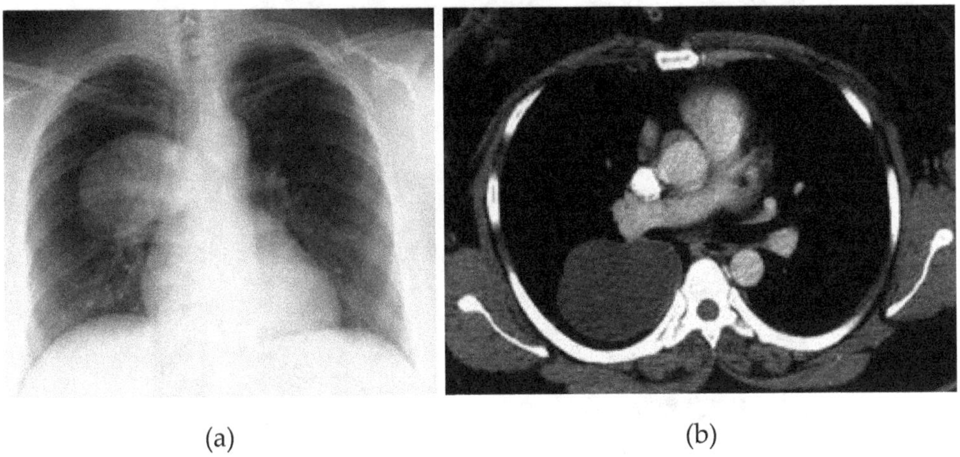

Figure 1. Intact simple cyst: (a) Chest radiograph shows a well-defined opacity located in the upper and middle zone of the right lung. (b) CT image shows that the mass has water attenuation.

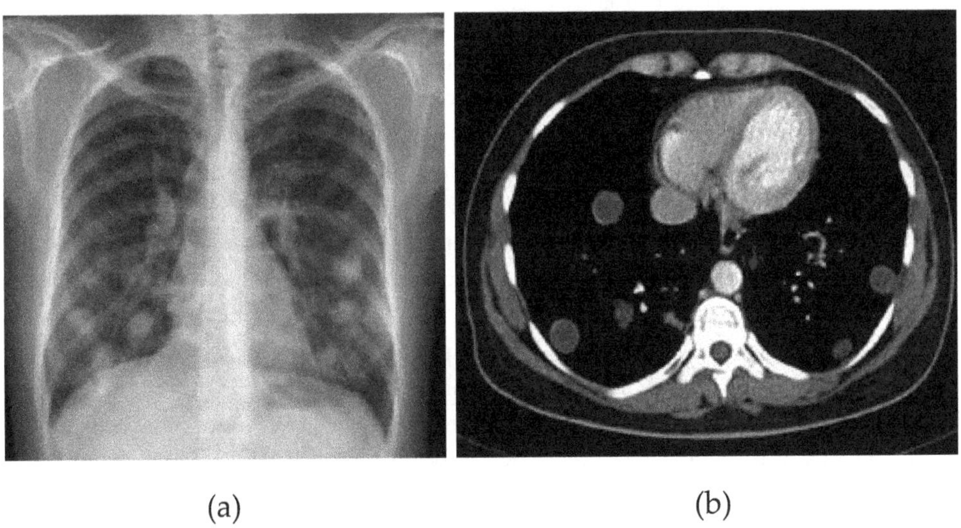

Figure 2. (a) Chest radiograph shows multiple hydatid cysts located in both lungs as well-defined lesions. (b) CT scan shows multiple hydatid cysts in both lungs as well-demarcated cystic masses.

Unlike adults, in children the rate of growth of the cyst in the lung is progressive and more constant than in the liver due to elastic capability and low resistance of the lungs. This may explain the high incidence of pulmonary disease in children [21-23]. In the literature, it has been reported that giant PHCs (greater than 15 cm) were prevalent in children (Figure 3) [22].

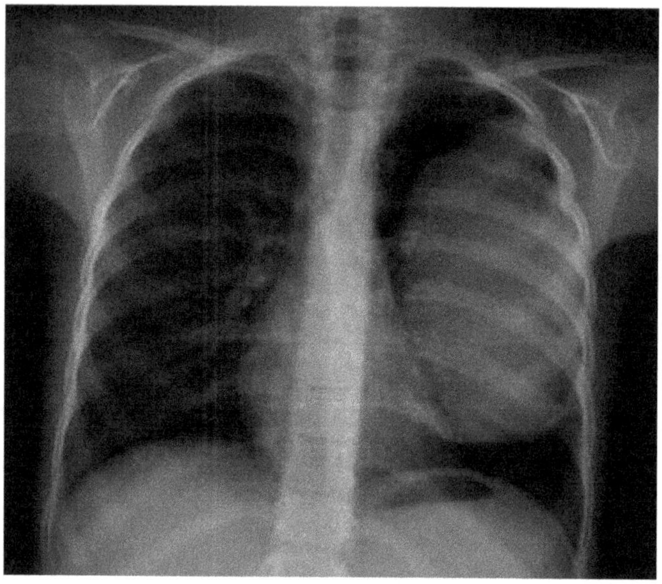

Figure 3. A 15-year-old boy. Chest radiograph shows a huge hydatid cyst located in the upper and mid-zone of the left lung causes displacement of the mediastinum to the right.

Computed tomography (CT) shows simple cysts to have smooth walls of variable thickness and homogenous internal contents of water or near-water density. The adventitious (pericyst), laminated, and germinal layers in an intact cyst are averaged together and seen as a single wall. On contrast enhanced CT, enhancement of the vascularized pericyst may not be a significant feature in intact cystic masses. However, in those cases exhibiting obvious enhancement, this finding has little or no diagnostic value [15, 18]. Chest CT can be of value in determining the presence of cysts in areas difficult to visualize with chest radiography, especially in the posterior and anterior costophrenic angles, as has been illustrated (Figure 4a, 4b) [18]. Also CT is superior to chest radiography in the cystic characterization of the parenchymal abnormality. Furthermore, determination of wall thickness is more accurate with CT, as compared with chest radiography. Multiple PHCs cause a diagnostic problem since they should be differentiated from metastatic disease, Wegener granulomatosis, and other granulomas [24]. Moreover, simple hydatid cyst cannot be differentiated from water-density lung cysts of different etiology in the basis of CT appearance alone. However, in endemic regions the CT demonstration of the cystic nature of a lung mass provides collaborative evidence in clinically suspected cases [18].

A patient with intact PHC is usually asymptomatic until the time of rupture and clinical presentation in these patients is directly related to whether the cyst is intact or ruptured. The cyst may rupture spontaneously due to trauma, degeneration by aging, or toxins. Moreover, infections, chemotherapy, or lack of nutrients may lead to the damage of the

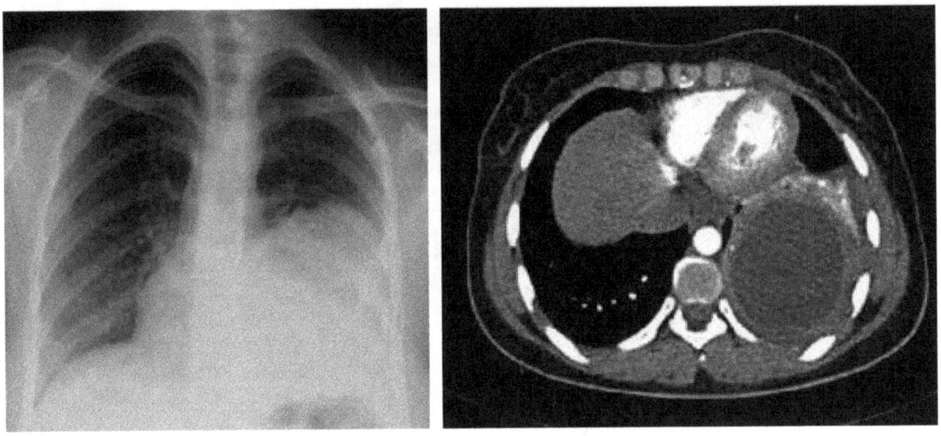

(a) (b)

Figure 4. (a) Chest radiograph shows well-defined mass in the lower zone of the left lung obscuring the left ventricular margin and costophrenic sinus. (b) Axial CT obtained through the postero-basal segment of the left lung shows a high-density cystic lesion and also parenchymal consolidation adjacent to the HC.

cystic wall with an increased risk of rupture. As a consequence, the fragile parasite membranes may split and pressure necrosis may result in a communication with a bronchiole allowing air to dissect into the cyst wall. If air enters into the potential space between the pericyst and ectocyst (laminated membrane of the parasite), the local detachment of parasitic membranes from the pericyst is called 'the sign of detachment'. This segmental peripheral radiolucency is called 'the crescent' or the 'meniscus sign' (Figure 5). Some authors have stated that when the air enters the potential space between the pericyst and endocyst and separates the parasitic membranes, air meniscus or the crescent sign is formed [4, 14, 15]. This sign is highly reliable for hydatid disease but not pathognomonic [11, 20]. In non-endemic areas, cavities with fungus balls (mycetoma) are the most common cause of the meniscus sign, but blood clots, carcinoma, pulmonary gangrene, tuberculosis, sarcoma, and aircap within a tumor may also present with pulmonary meniscus sign [20, 25].

Expanding cysts sooner or later reach a bronchiolus and after erosion of the bronchiolus, a communication between the pericyst and bronchial tree is established. This condition causes a variety of more or less characteristic radiographic signs of ruptured PHCs, which may raise suspicion about the presence of hydatid cyst(s) or even allow a specific diagnosis of the disease. In the literature, radiologic signs related to ruptured HC have been well-described [5, 14, 20, 26, 27]. Some of these signs are double-arch or cumbo sign (Figure 6a, 6b), iceberg sign, sign of the rising sun, serpent sign, and whirl sign (Figure 7). If more air is introduced to the parasitic membranes, the endocyst collapses and an air-fluid level is seen. If the parasitic membranes are floating on the fluid surface, this produces the 'water lily sign' or 'Camelot sign' resembling leaves of a water lily (Figure 8a, 8b). If all the parasitic

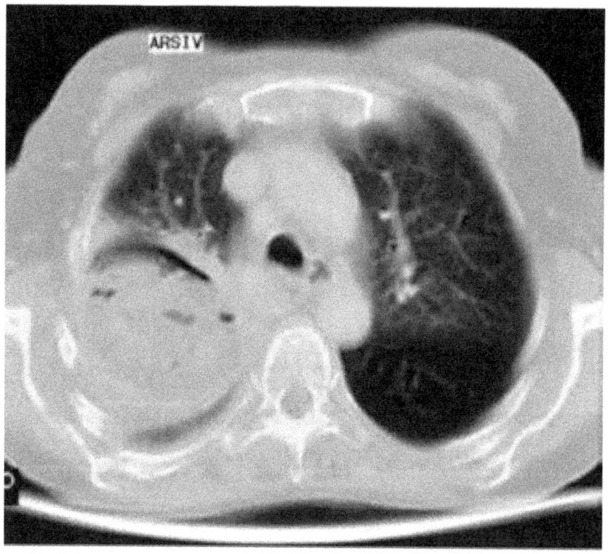

Figure 5. CT appearance of meniscus sign: A crescent shaped air is seen in the potential space between the pericyst and ectocyst of the cystic lesion.

contents are evacuated and only the pericyst produced by the host remains, it may even be filled with air. This condition is called the 'empty cyst sign' (Figure 9) [4, 14].

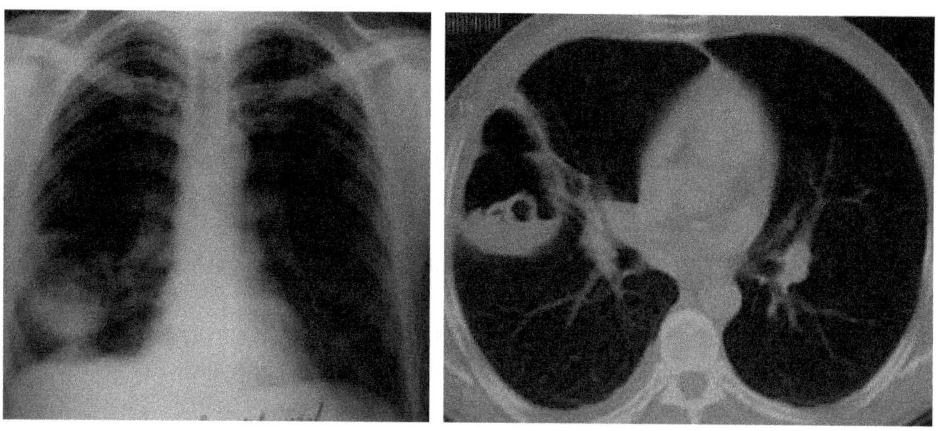

(a) (b)

Figure 6. Cumbo sign: Double air arc is seen in (a) chest radiography and (b) CT scan.

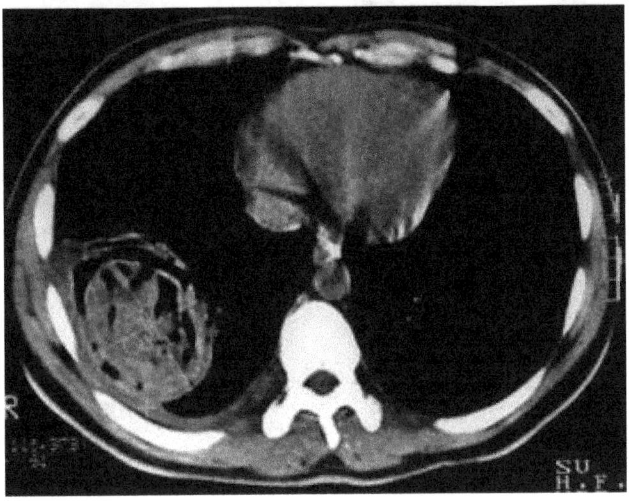

Figure 7. Whirl sign: CT scan (mediastinal window) shows floating detached membranes in the cystic cavity with minimal pleural effusion.

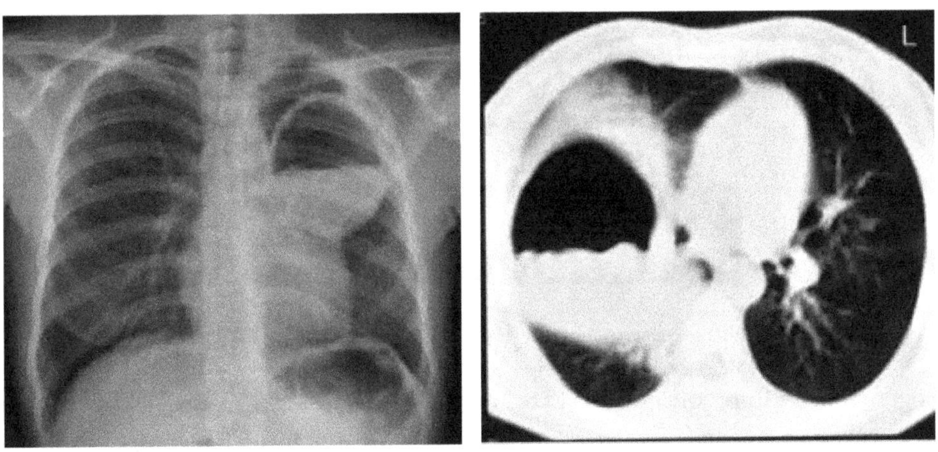

(a) (b)

Figure 8. Water lily or Camelot sign: (a) chest radiography shows a cavitary lesion with a germinative layer in the left lung. (b) On CT scan (mediastinal window), a cystic cavitary lesion with dependent wavy contour created by floated parasitic membranes is seen.

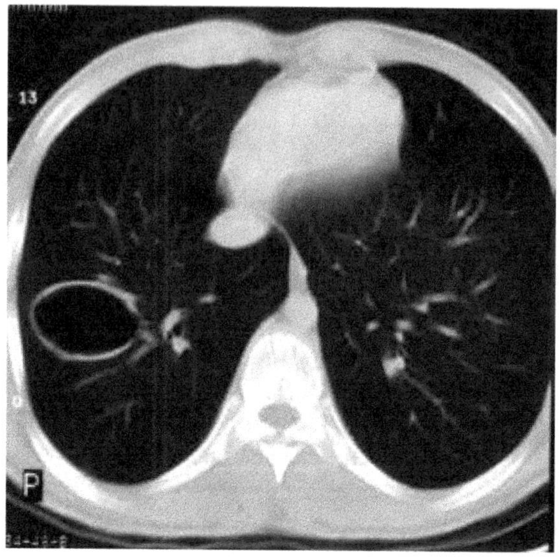

Figure 9. Empty cyst sign: CT scan of the chest shows an empty cavity with thin walls after complete evacuation of the hydatid membrane.

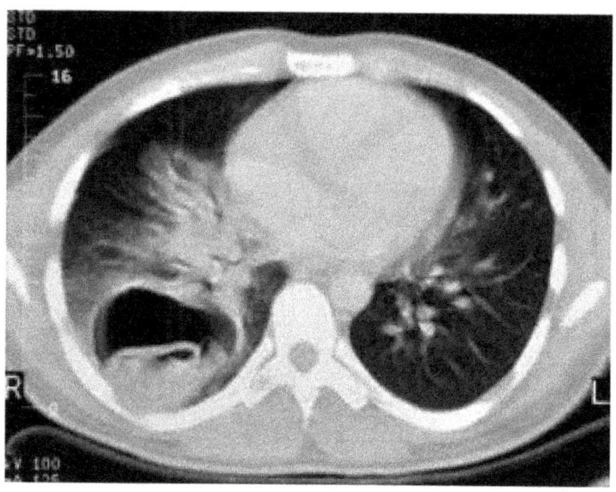

Figure 10. CT scan (mediastinal window) of the chest shows a collapsed cystic lesion.

Pathognomonic features of ruptured PHCs on CT are detached or collapsed endocyst membranes, collapsed daughter cyst membranes (Figure 10), and intact daughter cysts [18]. The most frequent complication of ruptured PHC is bacterial infection. Purulent sputum and fever are strong indicators of pneumonia or infected cyst. The presence of air pockets or air bubbles within the cyst and ring enhancement of the pericyst on contrast enhanced CT indicate either infection or communication with the bronchial tree (Figure 11a, 11b) [5, 27]. Because of the high density of infected hydatid cyst, the differentiation from a solid or fluid-filled cyts, abscess, or neoplasm is usually impossible [20, 28, 29].

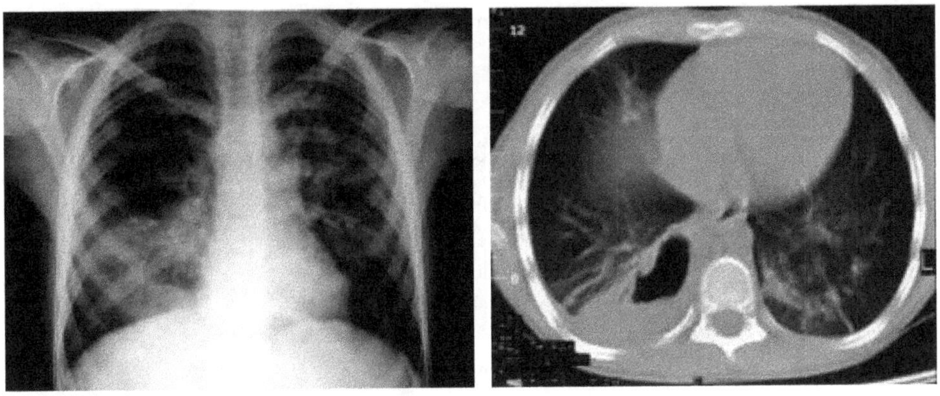

(a) (b)

Figure 11. Infected HC: (a) Chest radiograph and (b) enhanced CT scan show an infected cavitary lesion with adjacent parenchymal consolidation in the right lung.

Infected hydatid cyst may cause uncontrolled bacterial infection and hydatid lung abscess. Further disintegration of membranes and the purulent cystic content may produce an air-fluid level with no demonstrable floating membranes [14]. A hydatid cyst with such an appearance cannot be differentiated from ordinary pyogenic abscess by CT even in endemic regions and false-positive diagnosis is inevitable. Complicated PHCs, either ruptured or infected, may have higher CT attenuation numbers than that of water due to mucus, hemorrhagic content or infection (Figure 12a, 12b). These lesions are also difficult to differentiate from other cavitary lesions, such as infarctions, hemorrhage, carcinoma, benign tumors, inflammatory masses, fluid-filled cystic lesions, and active cavitary tuberculosis [24, 26, 28-31]. Thus, transthoracic aspiration or bronchoscopic biopsy can be attempted in PHCs with atypical or complicated radiologic appearances, if there is radiologic evidence of a coexisting mass [24, 30-32].

Pulmonary arteries are exceptional localizations for hydatid cysts [33]. Most frequent cause is embolism from primary cardiac locations [34, 35]. Another possibility is that the embryos of EG pass through the liver, into the inferior vena cava, and from there via the right cardiac chambers to the pulmonary arteries [33, 36]. On contrast enhanced CT, the cystic lesions within the pulmonary arteries show the typical hypodense appearance, quite similar to other cysts in the lung. These findings should be differentiated from other intraluminal filling defects such as pulmonary embolism and pulmonary artery tumors [33, 34, 37]. On MR imaging intra-arterial cyst is typical with low signal intensity on T1 weighted images and high signal intensity on T2 weighted images (Figure 13a, 13b).

Cardiac involvement of hydatid disease is very rare. It is known that cardiac involvement is approximately 0.02%-2% of all cases of human hydatidosis (Figure 14a, 14b) [11, 33, 34]. Rupture into the heart chambers may result in embolisation of hydatid tissue in the pulmonary arteries or organs of the major circulation (secondary metastatic hydatidosis) [15, 34, 38]. Infrequently, as a result of the rupture of the right ventricle and right atrium cysts into the pulmonary arteries, acute, subacute, or chronic recurrent embolization of hydatid cysts may be seen [34].

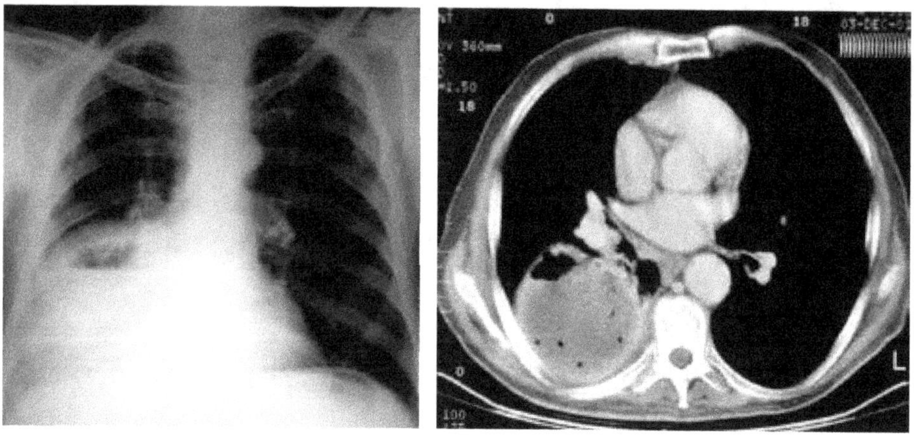

(a) (b)

Figure 12. Abscesses: (a) Chest radiograph and (b) CT image show a thick-walled cystic lesion with air-fluid level located at the right paracardiac region with surrounding consolidation.

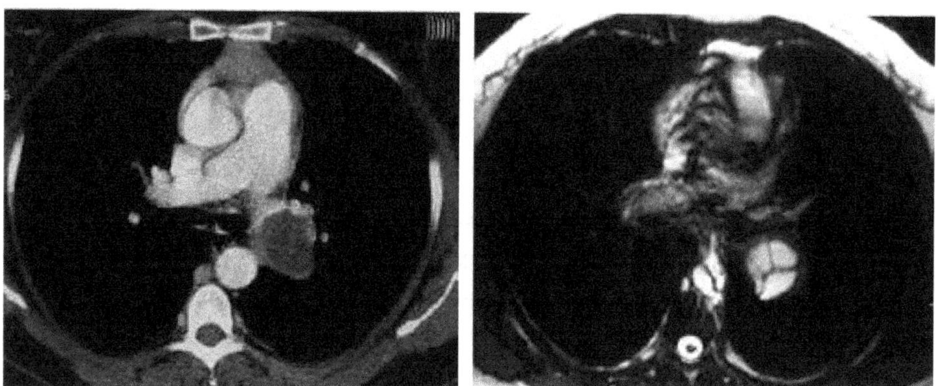

(a) (b)

Figure 13. (a) CT scan and (b) MRI of the chest show hydatid cyst with daughter cysts inside the left pulmonary artery.

Cysts that are localized in the chest wall, mediastinum, pericard, myocard, fissure, and pleura have been reported in the literature as intrathoracic extrapulmonary cysts [39, 40]. Intrathoracic extrapulmonary hydatid cysts have been reported in 7.4% of patients [39]. Primary pleural echinococcosis, including pleural fissure (Figure 15a, 15b, 15c) is relatively uncommon even in pastoral or domestic echinococcosis [41]. Rarely infection follows the primary hematogenous dissemination of larvae to the pleural tissues.

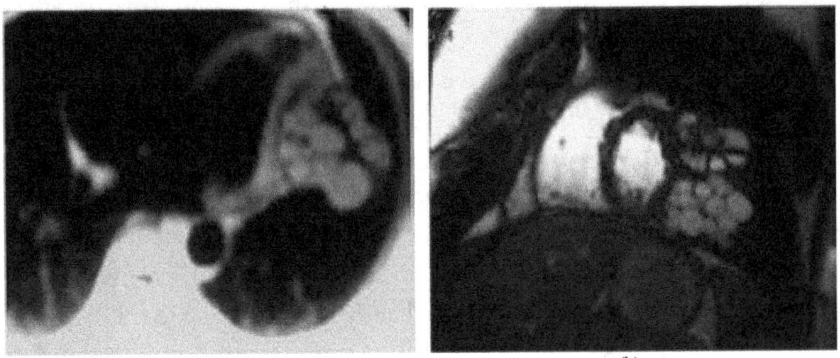

(a) (b)

Figure 14. Primary pericardial multilocular HC. (a) Proton density weighted axial MR image shows high signal intensity of the multilocular pericardial cysts with a low signal intensity capsule in the pericardium. (b) The pericardial daughter cysts are best demonstrated with T2-weighted MR image.

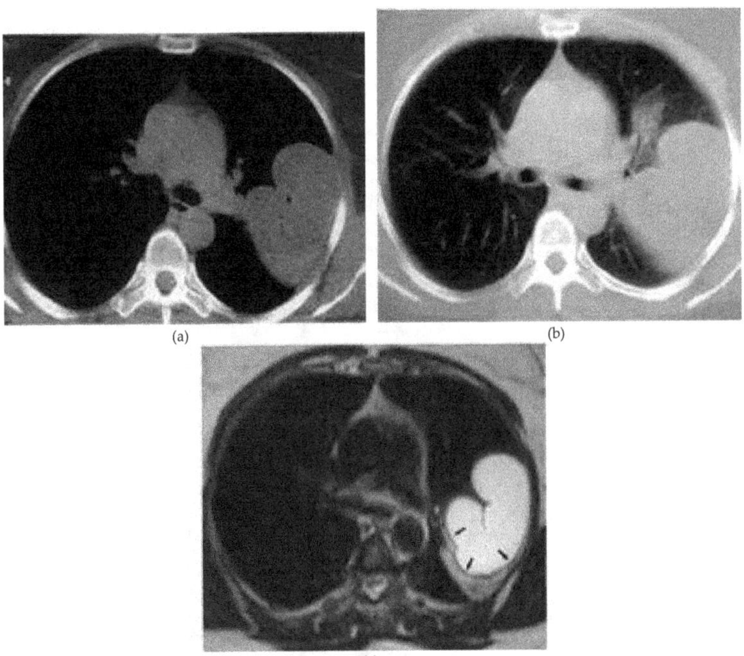

(a) (b) (c)

Figure 15. Primary hydatid cyst in the pleural fissure (a, b) Enhanced CT images show a hypodense lobulated mass in the left upper lung parenchyma on the mediastinal and lung window settings. (c) Axial T2-weighted MR image showing a high signal intensity cyst with a low signal intensity capsule in the left major fissure (arrows).

Pleural hydatid cyst is rare and usually caused by the rupture of a pulmonary or hepatic cyst into the pleural space, but on rare occasions it may be primary (Figure 16) [11]. Hydatid cyst that perforates into the pleural cavity (secondary pleural hydatidosis or SPH) can cause pneumothorax, tension pneumothorax, hydropneumothorax, pleural effusions, or empyema [15, 16, 56]. The documented rate of simple pneumothorax in patients with PHC ranges from 2.4% to 6.2% [15, 42]. Secondary pleural hydatidosis may also occur after percutaneous transthoracic needle puncture performed for diagnostic purposes. Secondary pleural hydatidosis may be due to hematogenous dissemination of the larvae of EG or by the rupture of neighboring hydatid cysts (multiple daughter cysts and scolices) along the pleura [41, 43]. This is a rare condition occurring in less than 10% of such cases. Although not frequent, involvement of the diaphragm (Figure 17) [44, 58], thoracic cavity or pleural space occurs in 0.6%-16% of cases of hepatic hydatid disease [13]. Transdiaphragmatic migration of hydatid disease from the posterior segment of the right hepatic lobe has been reported to be a common complication. This condition varies from simple adherence to the diaphragm to rupture into the pleural cavity [13, 45, 46]. Although ultrasound of the thorax and abdomen is useful for diagnosis of pulmonary hydatidosis [46], MR imaging is more useful in evaluation of cases with synchronous pulmonary and liver involvement and in depicting its close connection with thoracic lesions (Figure 18a, 18b, 18c) [47].

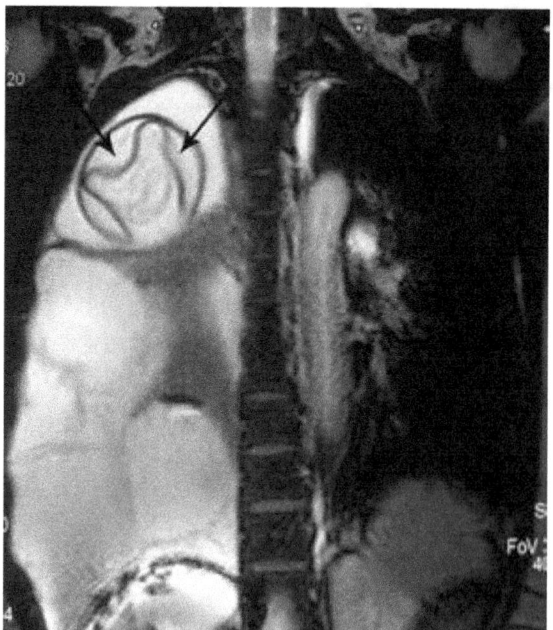

Figure 16. Ruptured primary pleural HC with diffuse pleural effusion. Coronal MRI shows a pleural HC after rupture. Detached germinal membranes are clearly seen as hypointense structures.

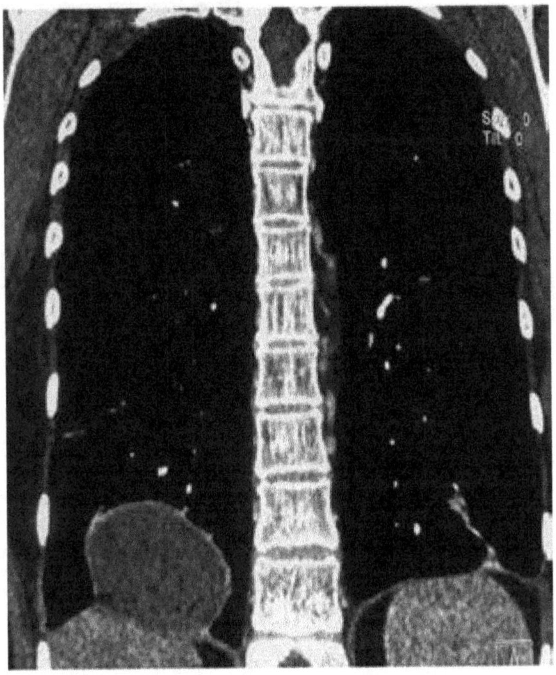

Figure 17. Primary diaphragmatic HC. Coronal and reformatted CT scans show a hydatid cyst in the right diaphragm.

Mediastinal hydatid cysts (MHCs) are very rare and are seen with an incidence ranging from 0% to 6% [11]. Several patterns of MHCs including, unilocular cyst or type 1, cyst with daughter cysts (multivesicular) or type 2 (Figure 19a, 19b), calcified cyst or type 3, and complicated cyst or type 4, have been described by using imaging techniques [47]. Characteristic finding of echinococcal cysts (e.g., floating membranes, daughter cysts, and vesicles) can usually help in establishing the diagnosis of MHCs [11, 47]. CT best demonstrates cyst wall calcification. MR imaging has the capacity of providing more information about anatomical location of MHCs. Type 2 and type 3 MHCs in the anterior mediastinum should be differentiated from cystic teratoma, thymoma, and necrotic neoplasms [11, 48].

Primary chest wall hydatid cyst is an exceptional entity. Chest wall disease presents with involvement of the anterior or lateral thoracic wall soft tissues. On contrast enhanced CT or MR imaging, the appearance of chest wall echinococcal cysts is characteristic as in other organ involvements. On contrast enhanced CT, chest wall involvement may occur as a multiloculated mass with daughter cysts in the chest wall. Multiloculated osteolytic lesion in the rib due to hydatid cyst may present as an extrapleural soft tissue mass and cause cortical expansion or destruction of the rib. This primary rib lesion slowly grows and may involve the adjacent structures such as vertebra, pleura, or subcutaneous soft tissues. The radiologic differential diagnosis includes round cell tumors, plasmacytoma, osteolytic metastases, neurofibromas, and other similar conditions that are associated with extrapleural soft tissue masses (Figure 20a, 20b) [49, 50].

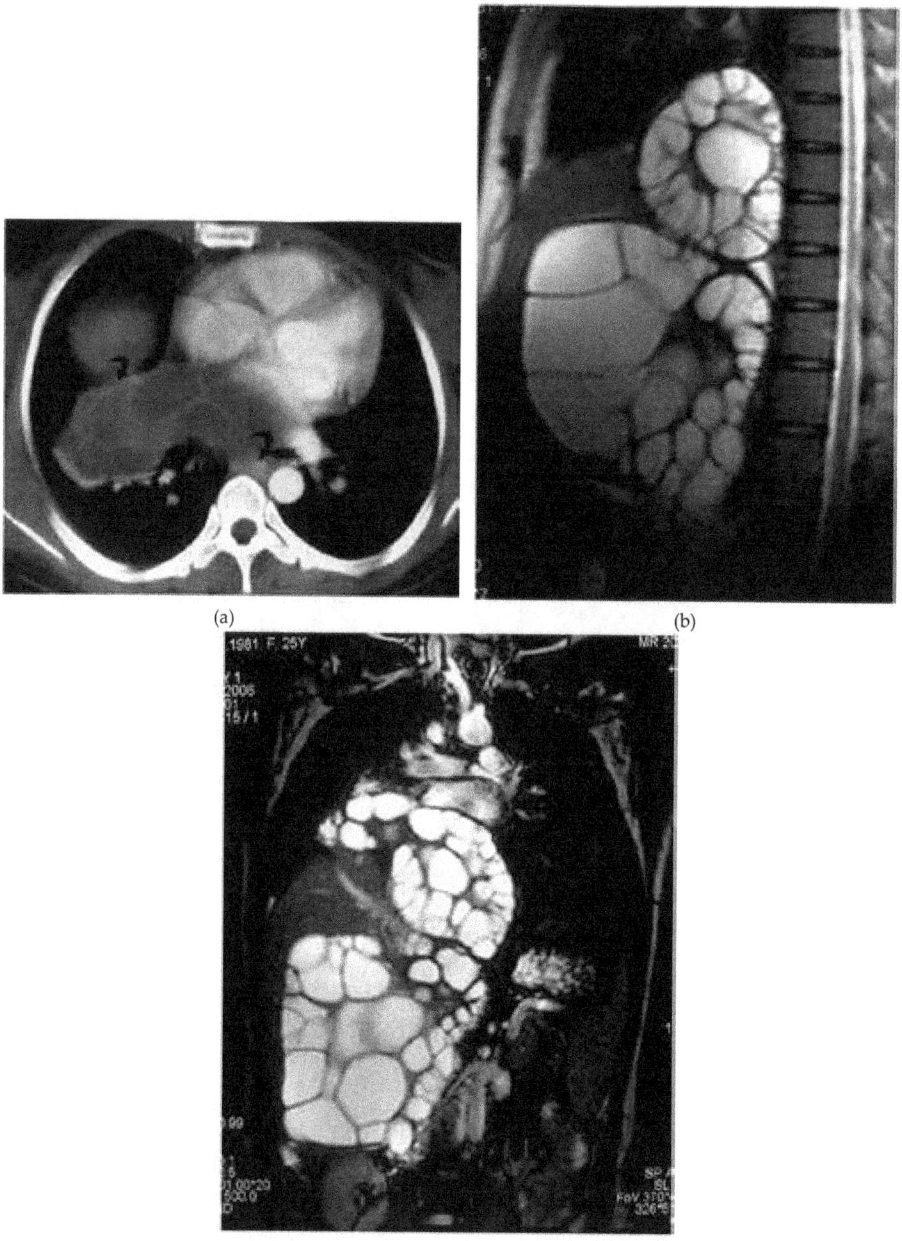

Figure 18. Posterior mediastinal HC with transdiaphragmatic extension from the abdomen. (a) Enhanced CT scan shows a large cystic mass containing multiple daughter cysts in the posterior mediastinum. (b) Sagittal and (c) coronal T2-weighted MR images show a huge cystic mass extending through the diaphragm to the posterior mediastinum from abdomen.

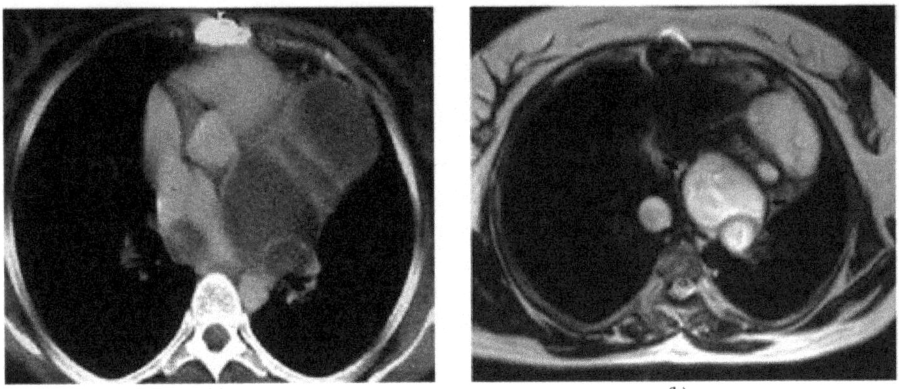

(a) (b)

Figure 19. Mediastinal multilocular HC. (a) Enhanced CT scan shows a multilocular HC with mediastinal involvement. (b) T2-weighted MRI shows multiple high signal intensity daughter cysts with a low signal intensity capsule (arrows) in the mediastinum.

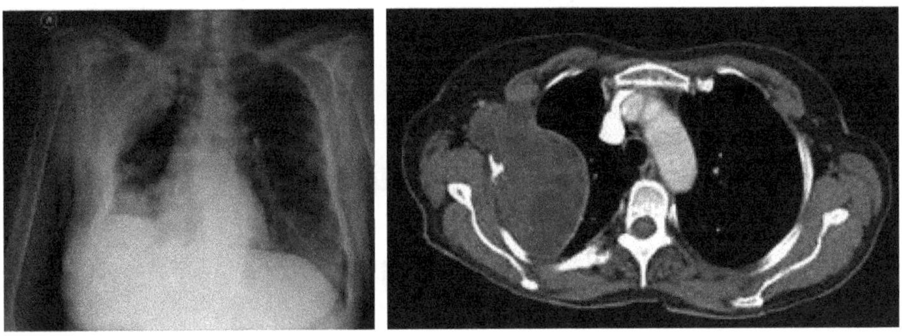

(a) (b)

Figure 20. Chest wall HC. (a) Chest radiograph shows a bulging soft tissue mass extending to the thoracic cavity. (b) CT shows multivesicular cystic lesion involving right chest wall and adjacent ribs.

6. Conclusion

Primary diagnostic method in pulmonary hydatid disease is the plain radiograph. This method is helpful for the diagnosis of intact cysts, but it may be inadequate for the assessment of complicated cyst morphology. Computed tomography depicts certain details of the lesions and can detect others that are not visible by chest radiograph. CT examination can elucidate the cystic nature of the pulmonary lesion and provide accurate localization for planning of surgical treatment of complicated cysts. Multiplanar and multiparameter imaging features of MRI facilitate comprehensive evaluation of intrathoracic but extrapulmonary hydatid cysts (e.g., chest wall, mediastinal, pericardial, fissural, and pleural localization).

Author details

Dilek Emlik*, Kemal Ödev, Necdet Poyraz and Hasan Emin Kaya

*Address all correspondence to: drdemlik@hotmail.com

Necmettin Erbakan University, Meram Medicine School, Department of Radiology, Meram, Konya, Turkey

References

[1] Neva FA, Brown HW. Intestinal helmints. In: Basic clinical parasitology. Norwalk, Conn.: Appleton & Lange. 1994;128-133.

[2] Ismail MA, Al-Dabagh MA, Al-Janabi TA, et al. The use of computerised axial tomography (CAT) in the diagnosis of hydatid cysts. Clin Radiol. 1980;31(3):287-90.

[3] Kiresi DA, Karabacakoglu A, Odev K, et al. Uncommon locations of hydatid cysts. Acta Radiol. 2003;44(6):622-36.

[4] Beggs, I. The radiology of hydatid disease. American Journal of Roentgenology. 1985; 145(3):639-648.

[5] Von Sinner W. Radiographic, CT and MRI spectrum of hydatid disease of the chest: A pictorial essay. European Radiology. 1993;3(1):62-70.

[6] Sarsam A. Surgery of pulmonary hydatid cysts. Review of 155 cases. J Thorac Cardiovasc Surg. 1971;62(4):663-8.

[7] Aytaç A, Yurdakul Y, Ikizler C, et al. Pulmonary hydatid disease: Report of 100 patients. The Annals of Thoracic Surgery. 1977;23(2):145-51.

[8] Martínez S, Restrepo CS, Carrillo JA, et al. Thoracic manifestations of tropical parasitic infections: A pictorial review 1. Radiographics. 2005;25(1):135-55.

[9] Doğan R, Yüksel M, Cetin G, et al. Surgical treatment of hydatid cysts of the lung: Report on 1055 patients. Thorax. 1989;44(3):192-9.

[10] Gottstein B, Reichen J. Hydatid lung disease (echinococcosis/hydatidosis). Clinics in Chest Medicine. 2002;23(2):397-408.

[11] Polat P, Kantarci M, Alper F, et al. Hydatid disease from head to toe 1. Radiographics. 2003;23(2):475-94.

[12] Lewall DB, McCorkell SJ. Rupture of echinococcal cysts: diagnosis, classification, and clinical implications. American Journal of Roentgenology. 1986;146(2):391-394.

[13] Pedrosa I, Saiz A, Arrazola J, et al. Hydatid disease: radiologic and pathologic features and complications 1: (CME Available in print version and on RSNA Link). Radiographics. 2000;20(3):795-817.

[14] Balikian JP, Mudarris FF. Hydatid disease of the lungs: a roentgenologic study of 50 cases. American Journal of Roentgenology. 1974;122(4):692-707.

[15] Ramos G, Orduña A, García-Yuste M. Hydatid cyst of the lung: Diagnosis and treatment. World Journal of Surgery. 2001;25(1):46-57.

[16] Kuzucu A, Soysal Ö, Özgel M, et al. Complicated hydatid cysts of the lung: Clinical and therapeutic issues. The Annals of Thoracic Surgery. 2004;77(4):1200-4.

[17] Balci AE, Eren N, Ülkü R. Ruptured hydatid cysts of the lung in children: Clinical review and results of surgery. The Annals of Thoracic Surgery. 2002.;74(3):889-892.

[18] Saksouk FA, Fahl MH, Rizk GK. Computed tomography of pulmonary hydatid disease. Journal of Computer Assisted Tomography. 1986;10(2):226-232.

[19] Morar R, Feldman C. Pulmonary echinococcosis. European Respiratory Journal. 2003; 21(6):1069-1077.

[20] von Sinner WN. New diagnostic signs in hydatid disease: Radiography, ultrasound, CT and MRI correlated to pathology. European Journal of Radiology. 1991;12(2): 150-159.

[21] Karaoglanoglu N, Kurkcuoglu IC, Gorguner M, et al. Giant hydatid lung cysts. European Journal of Cardio-thoracic Surgery. 2001;19(6):914-7.

[22] Montazeri V, Sokouti M, Rashidi H. Comparison of pulmonary hydatid disease between children and adult. Tanaffos. 2007;6(1):13-8.

[23] Tantawy IM. Hydatid cysts in children. Annals of Pediatric Surgery. 2010;6(2): 98-104.

[24] Gouliamos A, Kalovidouris A, Papailiou J, et al. CT appearance of pulmonary hydatid disease. CHEST Journal. 1991;100(6):1578-81.

[25] Reeder MM. RPC 1 of the month from the AFIP 2. Radiology. 1970;95(2): 429-437.

[26] Ramos L, Hernández-Mora M, Illanas M, et al. Radiological characteristics of perforated pulmonary hydatid cysts 1. Radiology. 1975;116(3):539-42.

[27] Odev K, Guler İ, Altinok T, et al. Cystic and cavitary lung lesions in children: Radiologic Findings with pathologic correlation. Journal of Clinical Imaging Science. 2013;3.

[28] Köktürk O, Öztürk C, Diren B, et al. "Air bubble": A new diagnostic CT sign of perforated pulmonary hydatid cyst. European Radiology. 1999;9(7):1321-3.

[29] Koul PA, Koul AN, Wahid A, et al. CT in pulmonary hydatid disease: Unusual appearances. CHEST Journal. 2000;118(6):1645-7.

[30] Köksal D, Altinok T, Kocaman Y, et al. Bronchoscopic diagnosis of ruptured pulmonary hydatid cyst presenting as nonresolving pneumonia: Report of two patients. Lung. 2004;182(6):363-8.

[31] Tor M, Özvaran K, Ersoy Y, et al. Pitfalls in the diagnosis of complicated pulmonary hydatid disease. Respiratory Medicine. 2001;95(3):237-9.

[32] Saygi A, Oztek I, Guder M, et al. Value of fibreoptic bronchoscopy in the diagnosis of complicated pulmonary unilocular cystic hydatidosis. European Respiratory Journal. 1997;10(4):811-4.

[33] Yagüe D, Lozano M, Lample C, et al. Bilateral hydatid cyst of pulmonary arteries: MR and CT findings. European radiology. 1998;8(7):1170-2.

[34] Odev K, Acikgözoglu S, Gormüs N, et al. Pulmonary embolism due to cardiac hydatid disease: imaging findings of unusual complication of hydatid cyst. European Radiology. 2002;12(3):627-33.

[35] Alper H, Yünten N, ScSener R. Intramural hydatid cysts of pulmonary arteries: CT and MR findings. European Radiology. 1995;5(6): 666-668.

[36] Oztürk C, Ağildere A, Cila A, et al. Pulmonary arterial embolism secondary to hydatid cyst of the liver. Canadian Association of Radiologists journal (Journal l'Association Canadienne des Radiologistes). 1992;43(5):374-6.

[37] Bressler EL, Nelson JM. Primary pulmonary artery sarcoma: Diagnosis with CT, MR imaging, and transthoracic needle biopsy. AJR. American Journal of Roentgenology. 1992;159(4):702-704.

[38] von Sinner W. CT and MRI findings of cardiac echinococcosis. European Radiology. 1995;5(1): 66-73.

[39] Oğuzkaya F, Akçali Y, Kahraman C, et al. Unusually located hydatid cysts: intrathoracic but extrapulmonary. The Annals of Thoracic Surgery. 1997;64(2):334-7.

[40] Burgos L, Baquerizo A, Munoz W, et al. Experience in the surgical treatment of 331 patients with pulmonary hydatidosis. The Journal of Thoracic and Cardiovascular Surgery. 1991;102(3):427-30.

[41] Xanthakis D, Efthimiadis M, Papadakis G, et al. Hydatid disease of the chest report of 91 patients surgically treated. Thorax. 1972;27(5):517-28.

[42] Aguilar X, Fernandez-Muixi J, Magarolas R, et al. An unusual presentation of secondary pleural hydatidosis. European Respiratory Journal. 1998;11(1):243-5.

[43] Skerrett SJ, Plorde JJ. Parasitic infections of the pleural space. Semin Respir Med. 1982;13:242-258

[44] Cattelani L, D'Ippolito R, Facciolongo N, et al. [Localization of hydatid cysts in the left hemidiaphragm. Description of a case]. Acta bio-medica de L'Ateneo parmense: organo della Societa di medicina e scienze naturali di Parma. 1987;59(1-2):41-7.

[45] Gómez R, Moreno E, Loinaz C, et al. Diaphragmatic or transdiaphragmatic thoracic involvement in hepatic hydatid disease: surgical trends and classification. World Journal of Surgery. 1995;19(5):714-9.

[46] Kilani T, El Hammami S, Horchani H, et al. Hydatid disease of the liver with thoracic involvement. World Journal of Surgery. 2001;25(1):40-5.

[47] Emlik D, Kiresi D, Sunam GS, et al. Intrathoracic extrapulmonary hydatid disease: Radiologic Manifestations. Canadian Association of Radiologists Journal. 2010;61(3): 170-6.

[48] Ödev K, Arıbaş BK, Nayman A, et al. Imaging of cystic and cyst-like lesions of the mediastinum with pathologic correlation. Journal of Clinical Imaging Science. 2012;2.

[49] Bonakdarpour A, Zadeh YFA, Maghssoudi H, et al. Costal echinococcosis: Report of six cases and review of the literature. American Journal of Roentgenology. 1973;118(2):371-7.

[50] Ozdemir N, Akal M, Kutlay H, et al. Chest wall echinococcosis. Chest. 1994;105(4): 1277-9.

[51] Force L, Torres JM, Carrillo A, Buscá J. Evaluation of eight serological tests in the diagnosis of human echinococcosis and follow-up. Clin Infect Dis. 1992;15:473-480.

8

Echinococcus shiquicus and *Echinococcus felidis*

Adel Spotin

Abstract

Currently, ten genotypes (G1-G10) of *Echinococcus* Sensu Lato have been explicitly identified on the basis of taxonomic criteria. These include morphometric keys, host specificity, geographical distribution, phylogenetic analysis and genome mapping. However, a few emergent species of genus *Echinococcus* have been indigenously confirmed in some autonomous regions of Tibet plateau and Africa where there is little known about their biological aspects and potential pathogenicity in intermediate and definitive hosts. This chapter is focused on the parasite history, life cycle, phenotypic aspects, epidemiology, zoonotic potential and phylogeny relationship of two enigmatic parasites namely: *Echinococcus shiquicus* and *Echinococcus felidis*. This aims to provide a better understanding of their taxonomic status, public health problems and biological features in the mentioned regions.

Keywords: *Echinococcus shiquicus*, *Echinococcus felidis*, Biological Aspects, Phylogenetic traits

1. Introduction

Currently, ten genotypes (G1-G10) of *Echinococcus* Sensu Lato have been explicitly identified on the basis of taxonomic criteria. These include morphometric keys, host specificity, geographical distribution, phylogenetic analysis and genome mapping. However, a few emergent species of genus *Echinococcus* have been indigenously confirmed in some autonomous regions of Tibet plateau and Africa where there is little known about their biological aspects and potential pathogenicity in intermediate and definitive hosts. This chapter is focused on the parasite history, life cycle, phenotypic aspects, epidemiology, zoonotic potential and phylogeny relationship of two enigmatic parasites namely: *Echinococcus shiquicus* and *Echinococcus felidis*. This aims to provide a better understanding of their taxonomic status, public health problems and biological features in the mentioned regions.

2. *Echinococcus shiquicus*

2.1. History, morphology and biology

In ~2005, *Echinococcus shiquicus* was first described by Xiao, from the Tibetan fox in Shiqu county of the Qinghai–Tibet plateau, China called the "Roof of the World" [1]. Earlier than molecular analysis, the *E. shiquicus* isolated from Tibetan fox; *Vulpes ferrilata* was considered as a morphological strain of *E. multilocularis*, whilst it is metacestode from the plateau pika; *Ochotona curzoniae*, was then recognized as *E. granulosus* because of its unilocular cystic characteristics [2].

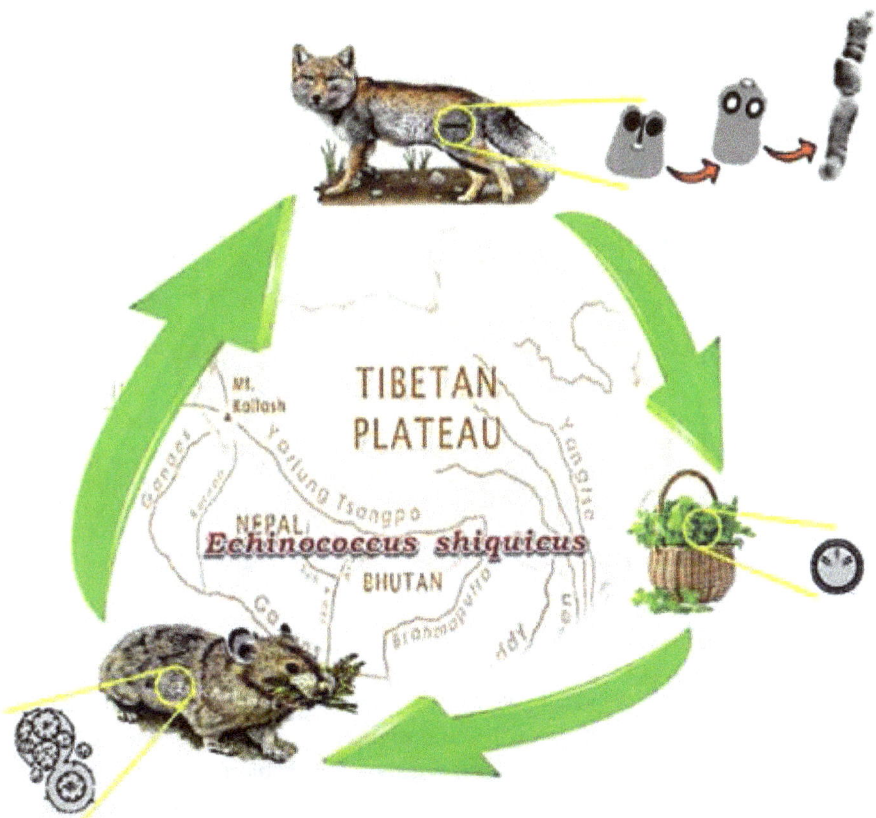

Figure 1. The life cycle of *Echinococcus shiquicus*. Credit: Image courtesy of Seyyed Ali Shariatzadeh.

Afterward, based on taxonomic criteria including morphology, host specificity, molecular characters and geographical distribution was considered as a new species of *Echinococcus* [1].

The sylvatic cycle of *E. shiquicus* is supported by the Tibetan fox and the plateau pika as the definitive and intermediate hosts, respectively, which are indigenous to the highlands of Tibet (Figure 1) [1]. However, *E. shiquicus* using copro-PCR and sequencing strategies has been naturally reported in dogs from eastern Qinghai–Tibet plateau region, China [3].

The adult worms of *E. shiquicus* are observed into two types. The majority of the samples included pre-mature and gravid proglottid which testes and ovary are placed in the pre-mature segment while the genital pore is closed (Figure 2A) [1]. The second type consisted of immature, mature and gravid proglottid (Figure 2B). The number of segments in an adult worm is limited to three. *E. shiquicus* is readily discriminated from *E. granulosus* by its shorter length, length of hooks on the rostellum, branchless gravid uterus and anterior position of genital pore in the gravid proglottid. Also, the upper position of genital pore in the mature segment, smaller rostellar hooks and the fewer eggs in gravid segment of *E. shiquicus* (less than 100) are useful for differentiation of *E. shiquicus* in compared to *E. multilocularis*.

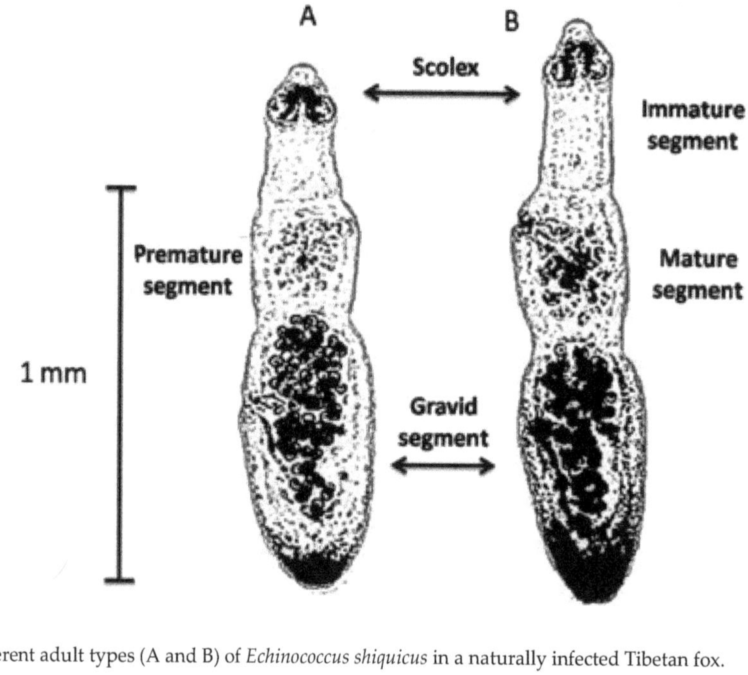

Figure 2. Different adult types (A and B) of *Echinococcus shiquicus* in a naturally infected Tibetan fox.

The metacestode stage of *E. shiquicus* is characterized by presence of unilocular minicyst containing developed brood capsules with no daughter cysts. The morphometric aspects of *E. shiquicus*, *E. multilocularis* and *E. granulosus* are shown in Table 1.

The concomitant (dual) infections of *E. shiquicus* with *E. multilocularis* have been recently identified in *O. curzoniae* and Tibetan foxes [4]. The zoonotic potential of *E. shiquicus* is still

Features	*E. shiquicus*	*E. granulosus*	*E. multilocularis*
Body Length (mm)	1.3 -1.7	2.0–11.0	1.2– 4.5
Number of segments	2–3	2– 7	2–6
Length of large hook on the rostellum (microns)	20.0– 23.0	25.0– 49.0	24.9– 34.0
Length of small hook on the rostellum (microns)	16.0–17.0	17.0– 31.0	20.4– 31.0
Number of testicles	12–20	25– 80	16– 35

Table 1. Comparison of the morphological aspects of *Echinococcus* spp.

unknown; although recently, some cases with unilocular and alveolar echinococcosis inclusive atypical ultrasound images have been characterized in Tibetans [5].

Although, no human infection of *E. shiquicus* has been reported yet, nevertheless the public health problems of *E. shiquicus* should not be neglected in control programs such as follow-up, monitoring and surveillance in an at risk population.

Therefore, additional studies are required to survey the possibility of human infections which can be employed in animal's models by serial passages using diagnostic antigens. The biological aspects of *E. shiquicus* including definitive host, intermediate hosts, genetic similarity and *etc*. are shown in Table 2.

Hydatid characters	Infectivity to humans	Genetic similarity	Distribution	Intermediate host	Definitive host	Species
Unilocular	Uncertain	*Echinococcus multilocularis*	Tibetan plateau	Pika	Tibetan fox	***Echinococcus shiquicus***
Unknown	Uncertain	*Echinococcus granulosus*	Africa	Warthog (possibly zebra, wildebeest, bush pig, buffalo, various antelope, giraffe, hippopotamus)	Lion	***Echinococcus felidis***

Table 2. A list of *Echinococcus felidis* and *Echinococcus shiquicus* features.

2.2. The evolutionary markers and molecular approaches in identifying *Echinococcus* spp.

The evolution in *Echinococcus* spp. can be considered as a combination of three major mechanisms that separately affect the composition of the genome of each species: mutation, selection and genetic drift [6].

Mutations occurred in the non-synonymous sites (called replacement sites because mutations at these sites lead to a change in the protein sequence) and the synonymous sites (called silent sites because mutations there do not lead to a change in the protein sequence) [6, 7].

It is worth noting that the nucleotide substitutions (Transition/Tranversion models) and/or indels (insertion or deletion) in the first and second positions of codons usually lead to create a new species/strain, which directly affect the frame shift of amino acids in case of any amino acid shifting or changing protein functionality while, changing in third position of codons (wobble site) is frequently leaded to creating novel haplotypes [8–11].

To date, the status of *Echinococcus* spp. is identified evidently by sequencing of nuclear DNA [12] and mitochondrial genome (mitogenome) accompanied by employing phylogenetic analysis on the basis of cladistics methods (Maximum Likelihood and Maximum Parsimony or Bayesian statistics and uses allele frequencies to study the nature and extent of genetic variation within and between populations) [13]. Although recently, a diagnostic pattern has been reported based on RFLP technique in differentiation of *Echinococcus* spp. using non-coding conserved gene [14].

It is important that the employing extra nuclear (mitochondrial) markers with low copy numbers and high variation characteristics are able to identify the unknown species/strains even haplotypes in exceptional regions where several intermediate hosts are circulating unequivocally [15].

2.3. Phylogenetic findings

Sequencing, phylogenetic and bioinformatics' analyses of mtDNA [16] and nuclear DNA [12] revealed that *E. shiquicus* and *E. multilocularis* are sister species with identical branch lengths in a specific clade and bootstrapping value of 99%.

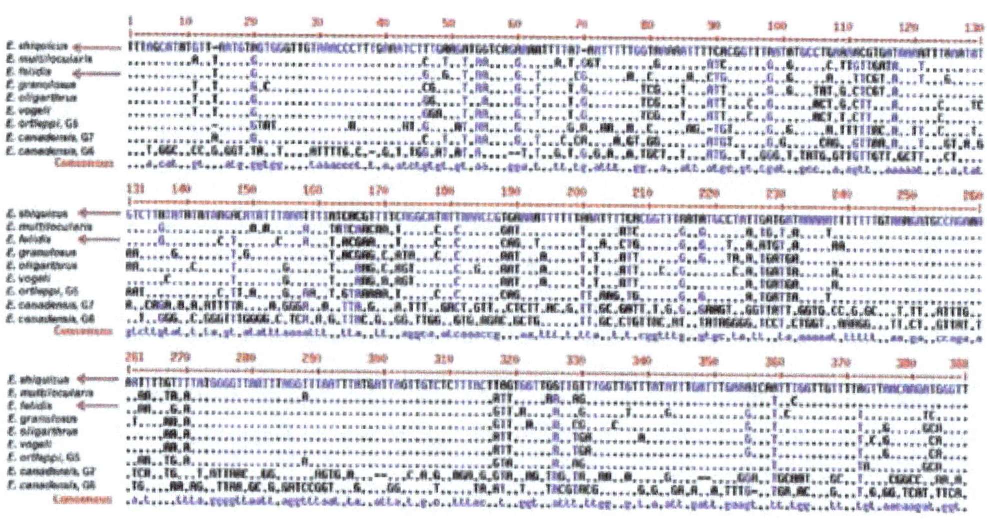

Figure 3. Nucleotide sequence alignments of Cox1 gene in *Echinococcus* spp.

The molecular characterization of *Echinococcus* spp. in the Tibetan plateau has demonstrated that the richness of genetic diversity indices of *E. shiquicus* is higher than those of *E. granulosus* s.s and *E. multilocularis* (Figure 3).

E. shiquicus, however, is placed with *E. multilocularis* in a common clade of ancestor with bootstrap value >70% (Figures 4 and 5).

This heterogeneity can be elucidated by description of three assumptions. First: presence of two turnover mechanisms, namely; unequal crossing over/transposition and slippage in the sequence length of parasite [17]. Second: lack of any bottleneck effects after its ancestor had been isolated on the Tibetan Plateau by colonizing alpine mammals (genetic drift or founder effect) [18]. And third: the long term geographic segregation into the plateau.

In a study, three polymerase chain reaction (PCR) assays based on the amplification of a fragment within the NADH dehydrogenase subunit 1 (ND1) mitochondrial gene have been optimized for the detection of *E. shiquicus*, *E. granulosus* and *E. multilocularis* in co-endemic regions of Qinghai-Tibet plateau, China [19].

3. *Echinococcus felidis*

3.1. Introduction

In *Echinococcus* species position, *E. granulosus* Sensu Lato has been categorized into *E. granulosus* Sensu Stricto (G1–G3), *E. equinus* (horse strain; genotype G4), *E. ortleppi* (cattle strain; genotype G5) and *E. canadensis* (genotypes G6–G10).

However, the taxonomic position, human infection, intermediate hosts and DNA profile of enigmatic 'lion strain' from Africa [20] has been unknown due to unavailability of suitable isolates.

3.2. History and biology

In 1937, *Echinococcus felidis* (Cestoda: Taeniidae) was first described by Ortlepp, from the lion *Panthera leo*, in South Africa [21]. Then, Rausch and Nelson (1963) declared that the taxonomic status of *E. felidis* remained to be uncertain from other *Echinococcus* spp. owing to existence of the host specificity and its rostellar hooks [22]. Verster (1965) re-checked the morphological features of *E. felidis* proglottids and proposed as a sub-specific rank of *E. granulosus felidis* [23]. Afterward, Rausch (1967) invalidated the sub-specific/strain status regarding *E. felidis* as an *E. granulosus* synonym because of lack of a valid evidence for it being a geographically isolated sylvatic cycle [24].

Many records of this parasite remained unidentified from a large variety of African mammals, due to the lack of diagnostic criteria, mainly genetic characterization and the misdiagnosis with the sympatric *Echinococcus* spp. [25] (Figure 6).

Echinococcosis is a high public health priority in the endemic areas of the world especially Africa, where more than one species of intermediate host is present and there is the possibility of interaction between cycles of transmission. Therefore the concomitant infections of *E. felidis* with other *Echinococcus* spp. may be sympatrically overlapped in under studied regions where it can be neglected.

The explicit status of *E. felidis* had not been determined until recent times. Huttner et al. (2008) presented its validity based on genetic classification and phylogenetic position [20].

The felids act as definitive hosts for enigmatic 'lion strain' however, It is still unclear which of the sympatric wild ungulates serve as intermediate hosts in life cycle of *E. felidis*. The different features of *E. felidis* are shown in Table 2. Like *E. shiquicus*, there is not enough data about human infection, hydatid feature and intermediate hosts. Therefore the zoonotic potential and public health concern among circulating isolates particularly those concomitant infections should be noticed absolutely.

3.3. Phylogenetic findings in *E. felidis*

Based on sequences of mitochondrial genes for cytochrome c oxidase subunit 1 (cox1), NADH dehydrogenase subunit 1 (nad1), cytochrome b (cob), rRNA (rrn), and nuclear genes for elongation factor 1 alpha (ef1a), ezrin-radixin-moesin (ERM)-like protein (elp) and

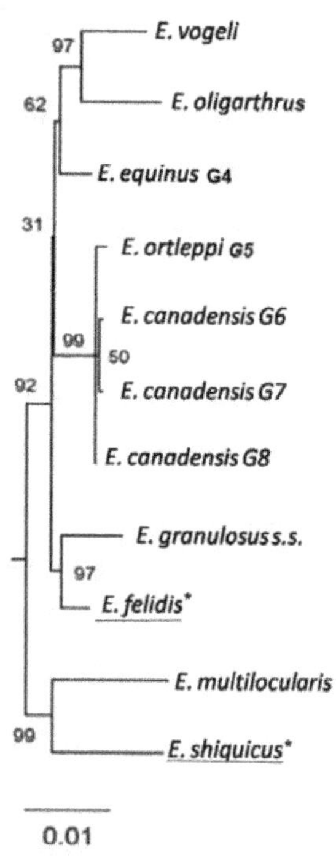

Figure 4. Phylogenetic tree of *Echinococcus* spp. inferred from nuclear protein-coding genes.

Internal transcribed spacer (ITS), *E. felidis* and *E. granulosus* Sensu Stricto are presumed to have a common ancestor from Asian Felidae [20, 26].

Considering the assumption, ancestral lineage of *Panthera leo* in Asia is refereed to late Pliocene [10], which had been invaded to Africa in the early Pleistocene [27]. Phylogenetic trees of *Echinococcus* spp. inferred from mitogenome and nuclear protein-coding genes shown that both *E. felidis* and *E. granulosus* have placed in *E. granulosus* Sensu Stricto complex (genotypes G1, G2 and G3; Figures 4 and 5). In Figure 4 the *E. felidis* and *E. granulosus* are characterized with different branch lengths in a common clade and bootstrapping value of 97%.

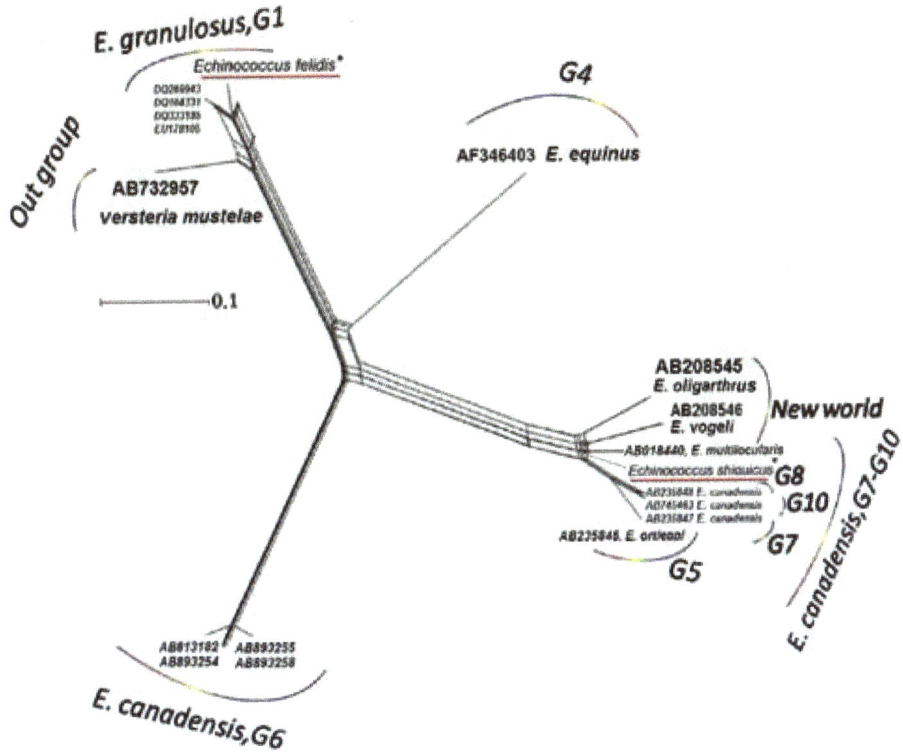

Figure 5. NeighborNet graph according to the Kimura-2 parameter model and concatenated sequences of *Cox1* gene (mitogenome) of *Echinococcus* spp. *Echinococcus felidis* and *Echinococcus shiquicus* have characterized by asterisk (*) and red underline in *E. granulosus* and *E. canadensis* complexes respectively

The tree was reconstructed by the maximum likelihood method and Kimura-2 parameter model. *Echinococcus felidis* and *Echinococcus shiquicus* have characterized by asterisk (*) and red underline.

At this time, there are no valid data on the pathogenicity of *E. felidis* to humans and livestock although its close relationship with *E. granulosus* s.s proposed a zoonotic potential [28].

On the other hand, information about intermediate hosts of this parasite is still unknown, even though a hydatid cyst was identified as *E. felidis* from warthog in Queen Elizabeth National Park, Uganda [29].

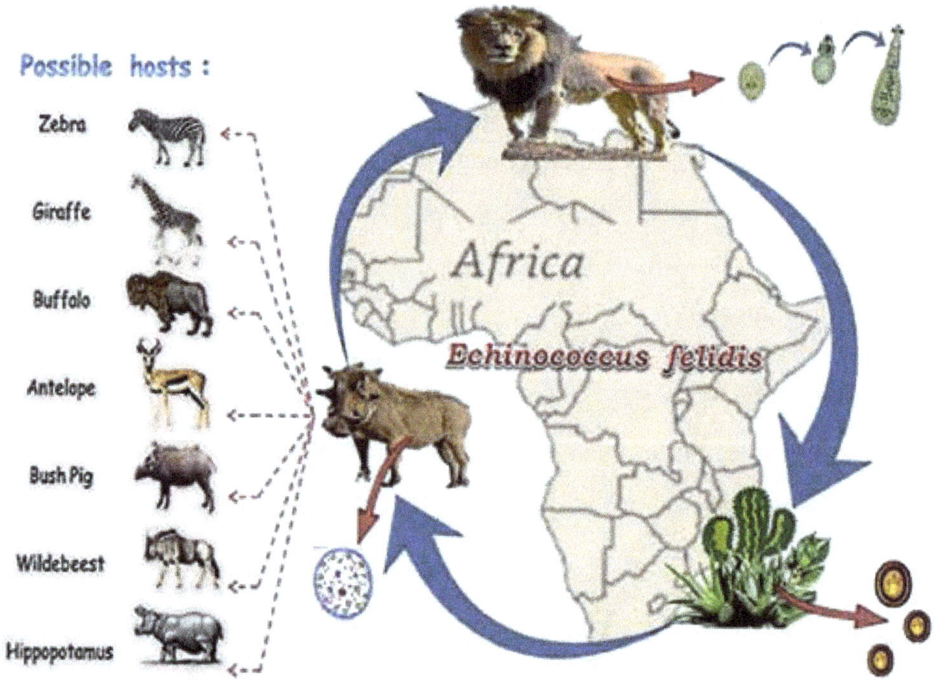

Figure 6. The life cycle of *Echinococcus felidis*. Credit: Image courtesy of Seyyed Ali Shariatzadeh.

4. Conclusion

In the past decade, *E. shiquicus* and *E. felidis* have been indigenously confirmed in some sympatric regions of Tibet plateau and Africa, however, there is no more known about their zoonotic potential, human infection and public health problems. The contents of this chapter can be useful in the parasite history, biology, morphometric aspects, epidemiology, zoonotic potential and phylogeny relationship of mentioned *Echinococcus* which is provided a better understanding of their taxonomic position, public health priority and biological aspects in the regions.

Author details

Adel Spotin

Address all correspondence to: Espotina@tbzmed.ac.ir ; Adelespotin@gmail.com

Department of Parasitology and Mycology, Tabriz University of Medical Sciences, Tabriz, Iran

References

[1] Xiao, N., Qiu, J., Nakao, M., Li, T., Yang, W., Chen, X., Schantz, P.M., Craig, P.S., Ito, A., 2005. *Echinococcus shiquicus* n. sp., a taeniid cestode from Tibetan fox and plateau pika in China. *Int. J. Parasitol.* 35, 693–701.

[2] Xiao, N., Qiu, J., Nakao, M., Li, T., Yang, W., Chen, X., Schantz, P.M., Craig, P.S., Ito, A., 2006. *Echinococcus shiquicus,* a new species from the Qinghai-Tibet plateau region of China: discovery and epidemiological implications. *Parasitol. Int.* 55 (Suppl.), S233–S236.

[3] Boufana, B., Qiu, J., Chen, X., Budke, C. M., Campos-Ponce, M., Craig, P. S., 2013. First report of *Echinococcus shiquicus* in dogs from eastern Qinghai–Tibet plateau region, China. *Acta Trop.* 127(1), 21–24.

[4] Jiang, W., Liu, N., Zhang, G., Renqing, P., Xie, F., Li, T., Wang, Z., Wang, X., 2012. Specific detection of *Echinococcus* spp. from the Tibetan fox (*Vulpes ferrilata*) and the red fox (V. vulpes) using copro-DNA PCR analysis. *Parasitol. Res.* 111, 1531–1539.

[5] Craig, P.S., Li, T., Qiu, J., Zhen, R., Wang, Q., Giraudoux, P., Ito, A., Heath, D., Warnock, B., Schantz, P., Yang, W., 2008. Echinococcosis and Tibetan communities. *Emerg. Infect. Dis.* 14, 1674–1675.

[6] Wright, S., 1951. The genetic structure of populations. *Ann Eugen.*15, 323–354.

[7] Yang, Z., Bielawski, J.P., 2000. Statistical methods for detecting molecular adaptation. *Trends Ecol Evolut.* 15, 496–503.

[8] Strachan, T., 1999. Instability of the human genome: mutation and DNA repair.Human Molecular Genetics. 2nd edition. Chapter 9.

[9] Najafzadeh, N., Sedaghat, M. M., Sultan, S. S., Spotin, A., Zamani, A., Taslimian, R.,. Parvizi, P., 2014. The existence of only one haplotype of *Leishmania major* in the main and potential reservoir hosts of zoonotic cutaneous leishmaniasis using different molecular markers in a focal area in Iran. *Rev Soc Bras Med Trop.* 47(5), 599–606.

[10] Sharbatkhori, M., Spotin, A., Taherkhani, H., Roshanghalb, M., Parvizi, P., 2013. Molecular variation in *Leishmania* parasites from sandflies species of a zoonotic cutaneous leishmaniasis in northeast of Iran. *J Vector Borne Dis.* 51, 16–21.

[11] Rouhani, S., Mirzaei, A., Spotin, A., Parvizi, P., 2014. Novel identification of Leishmania major in Hemiechinus auritus and molecular detection of this parasite in Meriones libycus from an important foci of zoonotic cutaneous leishmaniasis in Iran. *J Infect Public Health.* 7(3), 210–217.

[12] Knapp, J., Bart, J.M., Glowatzki, M.L., Ito, A., Gerard, S., Maillard, S., Piarroux, R., Gottstein, B., 2007. Assessment of use of microsatellite polymorphism analysis for

improving spatial distribution tracking of *Echinococcus multilocularis*. *J. Clin. Microbiol.* 45, 2943–2950.

[13] Bowles, J., Blair, D., McManus, D.P., 1992. Genetic variants within the genus *Echinococcus* identified by mitochondrial DNA sequencing. *Mol. Biochem. Parasitol.* 54, 165–173.

[14] Spotin, A., Gholami, S., Nasab, A.N., Fallah, E., Oskouei, M.M., Semnani, V., Shariatzadeh, S.A., Shahbazi, A., 2015. Designing and conducting in silico analysis for identifying of *Echinococcus* spp. with discrimination of novel haplotypes: an approach to better understanding of parasite taxonomic. *Parasitol. Res.* 1–7 [Epub ahead of print].

[15] Spotin, A, Rouhani, S., Parvizi, P., 2014. The associations of *Leishmania major* and *Leishmania tropica* aspects by focusing their morphological and molecular features on clinical appearances in Khuzestan province, Iran. *Biomed. Res. Int.* 2014: 1–13.

[16] Nakao, M., McManus, D.P., Schantz, P.M., Craig, P.S., Ito, A., 2007. A molecular phylogeny of the genus *Echinococcus* inferred from complete mitochondrial genomes. *Parasitology.* 134, 713–722.

[17] Van Herwerden, L., Gasser, R. B., Blair, D., 2000. ITS-1 ribosomal DNA sequence variants are maintained in different species and strains of *Echinococcus. Int. J. Parasitol.* 30, 157–169.

[18] Nakao, M., Li, T., Han, X., Ma, X., Xiao, N., Qiu, J., Wang, H., Yanagida, T., Mamuti, W., Wen, H., Moro, P.L., Giraudoux, P., Craig, P.S., Ito, A., 2010. Genetic polymorphisms of *Echinococcus* tapeworms in China as determined by mitochondrial and nuclear DNA sequences. *Int. J. Parasitol.* 40, 379–385.

[19] Boufana, B., Umhang, G., Qiu, J., Chen, X., Lahmar, S., Boué, F., Craig, P. 2013. Development of Three PCR Assays for the Differentiation between *Echinococcus shiquicus, E. granulosus* (G1 genotype), and E. multilocularis DNA in the Co-Endemic Region of Qinghai-Tibet plateau, China. *Am. J. Trop. Med. Hyg.*, 88(4), 795–802.

[20] Huttner, M., Nakao, M., Wassermann, T., Siefert, L., Boomker, J.D., Dinkel, A., Sako, Y., Mackenstedt, U., Romig, T., Ito, A., 2008. Genetic characterization and phylogenetic position of *Echinococcus felidis* (Cestoda: Taeniidae) from the African lion. *Int. J. Parasitol.* 38, 861–868.

[21] Ortlepp, R.J., 1937. South African Helminths, Part I. *Onderstepoort J. Vet. Sci. Anim. Ind.* 9, 311–336.

[22] Rausch, R.L., Nelson, G.S., 1963. A review of the genus *Echinococcus* Rudolphi, 1801. *Ann. Trop. Med. Parasitol.* 57, 127–135.

[23] Verster, A., 1965. Review of *Echinococcus* species in South Africa. Onderstepoort *J. Vet. Res.* 32, 7–118.

[24] Rausch, R.L., 1967. A consideration of intraspecific categories in the genus *Echinococcus* Rudolphi, 1801 (Cestoda: Taeniidae). *J. Parasitol.* 53, 484–491.

[25] Macpherson, C.N.L., Wachira, T.W.M., 1997. Cystic echinococcosis in Africa south of the Sahara. In: Andersen, F.L., Ouhelli, H., Kachani, M. (Eds.), Compendium of Cystic Echinococcosis in Africa and in Middle Eastern Countries with special Reference to Morocco. Brigham Young University, Provo, pp. 245–277.

[26] Johnson, W.E., Eizirik, E., Pecon-Slattery, J., Murphy, W.J., Antunes, A., Teeling, E.,O Brien, S.J., 2006. The late Miocene radiation of modern Felidae: a genetic assessment. *Science.* 311, 73–77.

[27] Werdelin, L., Lewis, M.E., 2005. Plio-Pleistocene Carnivora of eastern Africa: species Richness and turnover patterns. *Zool. J. Linn. Soc.* 144, 121–144.

[28] Jenkins, E.J., Peregrine, A.S., Hill, J.E., Somers, C., Gesy, K., Barnes, B., Gottstein, B., Polley, L., 2012. Detection of European strain of *Echinococcus multilocularis* in North America. *Emerg. Infect. Dis.* 18, 1010–1012.

[29] Huttner, M., Siefert, L., Mackenstedt, U., Romig, T., 2009. A survey of *Echinococcus* Species in wild carnivores and livestock in East Africa. Int. J. Parasitol. 39, 1269–1276.

9

Genitourinary Hydatid Disease

Santosh Kumar and Shivanshu Singh

Abstract

Genitourinary echinococcosis is an uncommon cyclo-zoonotic disease. It is caused by Echinococcus species. Kidneys are the common target organs in the genitourinary tract. Clinical presentation is usually non-specific. Pre-operative diagnosis requires a high index of suspicion. It should be considered in differential diagnosis of cystic mass of genitourinary tract, especially in endemic regions. Computed tomography, ultrasonography, and antibody testing aid in diagnosing and classifying the stage of the cyst. Although a number of operative techniques have been described, complete removal of germinal layer with daughter cysts without spillage of viable cyst contents with perioperative medical therapy provides an optimum chance of cure with minimal morbidity. Considering the benign nature of the disease, organ preservation is feasible in majority of the cases. The conventional open surgical treatment has evolved into minimally invasive laparoscopic, endoscopic, and even robotic techniques with concomitant improvement in postoperative and cosmetic outcome. Given the rarity of the disease, no randomized control trial comparing the treatment modalities for genitourinary hydatid exists. Moreover, long-term follow up in many cases is unavailable. Overall, the incidence of local and systemic recurrence is low.

Keywords: Genitourinary hydatid, echinococcosis, laparoscopic management

1. Introduction

Echinococcosis or hydatid disease in humans is caused by larval forms of cestode *Echinococcus granulosus* and rarely by *E. multilocularis* [1]. It's a cyclozoonotic parasitic infection with the liver (45%–75%) and the lung (10%–50%) being the most commonly involved organs [2]. The disease is endemic in Middle East Asia, South America, Australia, New Zealand, and Alaska where sheep and cattle rearing are common [3]. Genitourinary tract infestation is rare, with kidneys being the most common target. Renal involvement accounts for 1%–5% of all cases [4]. Cases of adrenal, prostatic, vesicle, retro-vesicle, and even testicular hydatid cyst have been reported in the literature. Imaging plays a key role in the diagnosis and staging of hydatid disease [5, 6]. Definitive therapeutic options include surgical excision or cyst aspiration with instillation of scolicidal agents. Laparoscopy and image guided percutaneous techniques have decreased the morbidity associated with open surgical excision. Medical therapy is commonly used as an adjunct in the perioperative period and as a primary modality in disseminated disease or in patients with poor surgical risk [7].

2. Etiopathogenesis and clinical presentation

Echinococcosis is a zoonotic disease. Definitive hosts are carnivores such as dogs, wolves, and foxes [8]. The adult worms mature in the small intestine of definitive hosts and shed proglottids in their feces. Upon ingestion of these eggs by intermediate hosts (herbivores such as sheep, horses, cattle, pigs, goats, camel, and humans), the oncosphere larva is released in the small intestine and penetrates the mucosa to enter the lamina propria. From there, passive transport occurs to target organs by hematogenous or lymphaticroute, disseminating primarily to the liver, secondarily to the lung, and finally to other organs where it forms the hydatid cyst. The triple layered cyst consists of an inner germinal layer that gives rise to protoscoleces, a middle acellular laminated layer and an outer host-tissue derived fibrous layer. As life cycle depends on carnivores eating infected intermediate hosts, humans are usually a dead end for the parasite.

2.1. Clinical presentation of renal echinococcosis

Hydatid cysts are typically slow growing and clinical presentation seldom suggests diagnosis [9]. Renal echinococcosis usually presents between the third and fifth decades of life and accounts for 2%–3% of all cases [10]. Renal involvement can occur by hematogenous route or larval migration through retroperitoneal lymphatics [3]. Due to the slow-growing nature of the cyst, the renal echinococcosis remains asymptomatic for years. Most common symptoms are palpable mass, flank pain, hematuria, malaise, and fever [11]. Secondary infection can cause high-grade fever, rigors, malaise, and pain [12]. The only hallmark sign of genitourinary echinococcosis is the presence of hydaturia (presence of daughter vesicles in urine), but this is found in 10%–20% of the cases [13]. Reports suggest that left renal involvement is more common than right probably due to the smaller renal artery [4]. Renal lesions are usually found in the cortex and can be uni- or multilocular [9].

2.2. Clinical presentation of adrenal echinococcosis

Adrenal involvement is rare and accounts for less than 1% of the cases [14]. It accounts for 6%–7% of all adrenal cysts [15, 16]. Mostly they are diagnosed incidentally, however, patients may present with vague non-specific dull aching pain in flank. Adrenal hydatid may cause hypertension, known as Goldblatt phenomenon, due to irritation of the functional tissue of the adrenal by the growing cyst [17]. Many authors believe that adrenal involvement is usually secondary and part of a generalized echinococcosis [14, 18].

2.3. Clinical presentation of pelvic echinococcosis

Primary pelvic hydatid cyst is rare with an incidence of 0.2%–2.25% [19]. Among the pelvic organs, ovaries are most commonly involved [20]. Symptomatology of pelvic echinococcosis is non-specific and can include abdominal pain, menstruation irregularities, infertility, and urinary disturbances [21]. Ovarian echinococcosis can mimic polycystic disease or malignancy [22]. Ovarian echinococcosis can also mimic endometriosis [23]. Although ovarian cysts are usually uni-locular, multilocular cysts have also been described [24]. Uterine echinococcosis can present with menorrhagia, and may be misdiagnosed as molar pregnancy [25]. Due to their large size, they can cause prolonged and obstructed labour requiring caesarean section [26]. Primary hydatid cyst of the broad ligament is extremely rare and may be misdiagnosed as pedunculated fibroid or a paraovarian cyst [27]. In one study of echinococcosis in an endemic region, the incidence of broad ligament echinococcosis was 0.37% among all cases of hydatid cyst [28].

Bladder hydatid cysts are characterized by clinical latency. Acute urinary retention is a commonly reported symptom [29] apart from frequency, urgency, and nocturia. Hydaturia, although specific, is uncommonly reported. Pelvic retrovesicle hydatidosis occurs by peritoneal dissemination, hematogenous or lymphatic seeding or spread from rectal mucosa to the perivesicle and pelvic venous plexus [30]. This site is unusual, even in endemic regions [31], accounting for 2% of all genitourinary echinococcosis [32]. They may present with pelvic pain, dysuria, membranuria, lower urinary tract symptoms, and hematospermia or may mimic ovarian cysts in females [32, 33]. Larger cysts may lead to urinary retention, ureteric compression with renal atrophy [34], renal failure, constipation. and even obstructed labour [35] or may develop fistulous communication with the rectum and bladder [36].

Prostatic cysts can be classified in to six categories: 1) isolated medial cysts; 2) cysts of the ejaculatory duct; 3) simple or multiple cysts of the parenchyma; 4) complicated infectious or hemorrhagic cysts; 5) cystic tumors; and 6) cysts secondary to a parasitic disease. Hydatid cyst of the prostate is a rare differential diagnosis of prostatic cyst [37]. Prostatic involvement occurs by hematogenous dissemination with cyst development within the prostatic stroma. They can clinically present as intraprostatic cystic mass. Growing cyst may rupture into the urethra causing hydaturia. Intracystic stone formation can occur due to urinary stagnation.

2.4. Other genitourinary sites of involvement

Rare case reports of scrotal, testicular, epididymal, and seminal vesicle hydatid cysts exist in literature [38-41]. Blood-testis barrier may account for testicular resistance to echinococcosis [42]. It mimics testicular mass, with diagnosis being proven on final histopathology of orchidectomy specimen. Testicular infestation can be primary or secondary to rupture of an intra-abdominal hydatid cyst [43]. Testicular echinococcosis, although rare, should be remembered as a differential diagnosis of testicular mass. Seminal vesicle hydatid cysts may present with lower urinary tract symptoms [44].

3. Diagnostic investigation

Imaging plays a central role in the diagnosis of echinococcosis. Various serological tests have evolved over time and contribute to diagnosis making, although they have low sensitivity [45]. Insensitive and nonspecific tests such as Casoni intradermal test, complement fixation test, indirect hemagglutination, and latex agglutination tests are now replaced by ELISA, immunoelectrophoresis, indirect immunofluorescence antibody test, and immunoblotting in routine laboratory testing [46, 47]. ELISA has positive titers in up to 80% of the cases [9]. Dipstick assays have been developed with nearly 100% sensitivity and approximately 91% specificity [48]. Newer immunodiagnostic tests are based on detection of echinococcal antigens in hydatid fluid fraction. These include *E.granulosus* antigen B (AgB), *E. granulosus* antigen 5 and EpC1. AgB8/2 antigen has provided the highest diagnostic sensitivity (84%–93.1%) and specificity (98%–99.5%) [49, 50]. Serology has a definite role in the follow up of cases, as the titer should fall after definitive treatment [51]. Eosinophilia occurs in 20%–50% of the cases [12].

Ultrasound is the key imaging tool to clinch the diagnosis. It demonstrates the floating membranes, daughter cysts, and hydatid sand apart from demonstrating the site, size, and number of cysts. The WHO/IWG-E classification for diagnosis and treatment is based on ultrasound imaging characteristics. It classifies the cyst into six subtypes (CL, CE1 to CE5) and three relevant groups: active (CE1 and 2), transitional (CE3), and inactive (CE4 and 5) [4]. "CL" is a univesicular, cystic lesion with uniform echoes, clear boundary, and thin visible wall. If it is a hydatid cyst, it is active. "CE1" is a univesicular anechoic cyst with presence of hydatid sand, double wall, and snowflake sign. The disease is active. "CE2" includes multi-vesicular, multi-septated cysts. Cyst septations produce "wheel-like" structures, and the presence of daughter cysts is indicated by "rosette-like" structure. "CE3a" is the detachment of laminated membrane from the cyst wall, visible as a "big snake sign" or as a "water-lily sign". The disease status is transitional. "CE3b" shows an intracystic shadow of the daughter vesicles and solid septation, manifested as complex cyst shadow. The parasite is dying. "CE4" has heterogenous, hypoechoic, or hyperechoic contents in the cyst. "CE5" is intracystic solid degeneration and calcification of the cystic wall. The parasite is inactive. Transrectal ultrasound is helpful in evaluating pelvic cystic lesions.

On CT scan, unilocular or multilocular cystic lesions are identified with frequently calcified walls, debris, small daughter cysts, and increased tissue density of hydatid membrane that enhances on intravenous contrast administration [7]. CT scan provides information regarding the number of cysts, the organ of origin, residual parenchyma in the affected organ, and relationship of the cyst with the adjacent structures [Figure 1–4]. This preoperative assessment is essential for planning the approach and type of surgery. Retrograde pyelography may not demonstrate communication with the pelvicalyceal system because of high intracystic pressures [52]. Communication may be demonstrated soon after cyst decompression. CT-guided diagnostic needle aspiration is not indicated when echinococcal cyst is suspected due to risk of dissemination and anaphylactic reaction. Magnetic resonance imaging provides better tissue delineation especially in cases of pelvic hydatid cysts. In one study, the preoperative diagnostic accuracy for serological test was 73.3%, while it was 74% and 87.5% for ultrasound and CT scan respectively [4].

Hydatid cysts should be considered in the differential diagnosis of cystic masses of the genitourinary tract as they can radiologically and clinically mimic tumors, benign and malignant, and other cystic lesions of genitourinary tract.

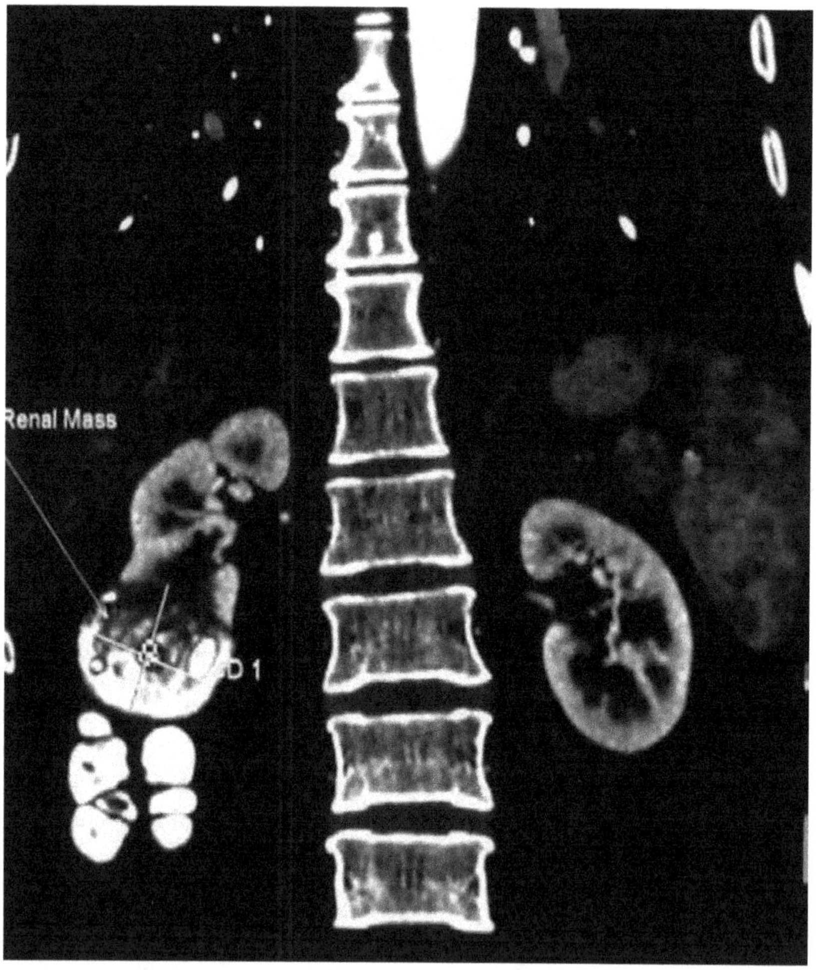

Legend: Contrast-enhanced CT scan of the abdomen (coronal view) showing a multiloculated, exophytic, cystic lesion arising from lower pole of the right kidney with calcification of the cyst wall *(Courtesy: Kumar et al. J Endourol. 2008;22:1709–1713.)*

Figure 1. CT imaging of Renal Hydatid.

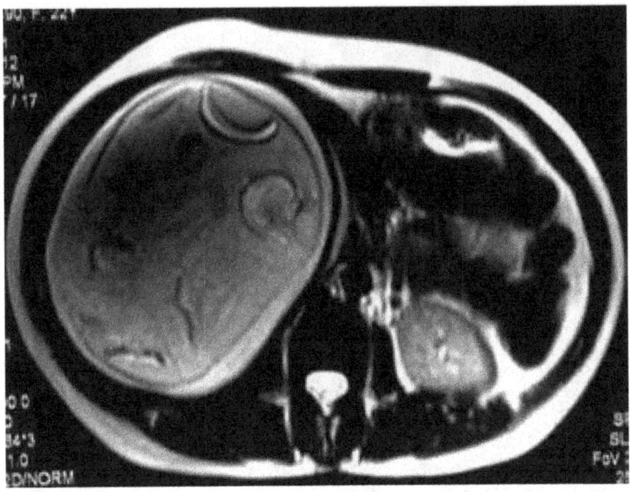

Legend: Abdominal MRI revealing a multiloculated hydatid cyst of a kidney with a cyst-in-cyst appearance. *(Courtsey: Kumar et al. Asian J Endosc Surg. 2013;6:342–345.)*

Figure 2. MRI of renal hydatid cyst.

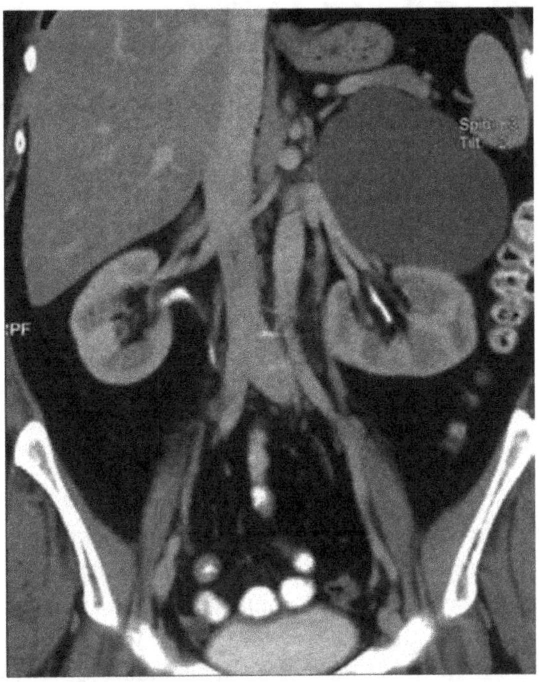

Legend: Contrast-enhanced computed tomography scan showing a cystic lesion involving the left adrenal gland without sepatations or daughter cyst. *(Courtesy: Kumar et al. Korean J Urol. 2014;55:493–495.)*

Figure 3. CT scan of adrenal hydatid cyst.

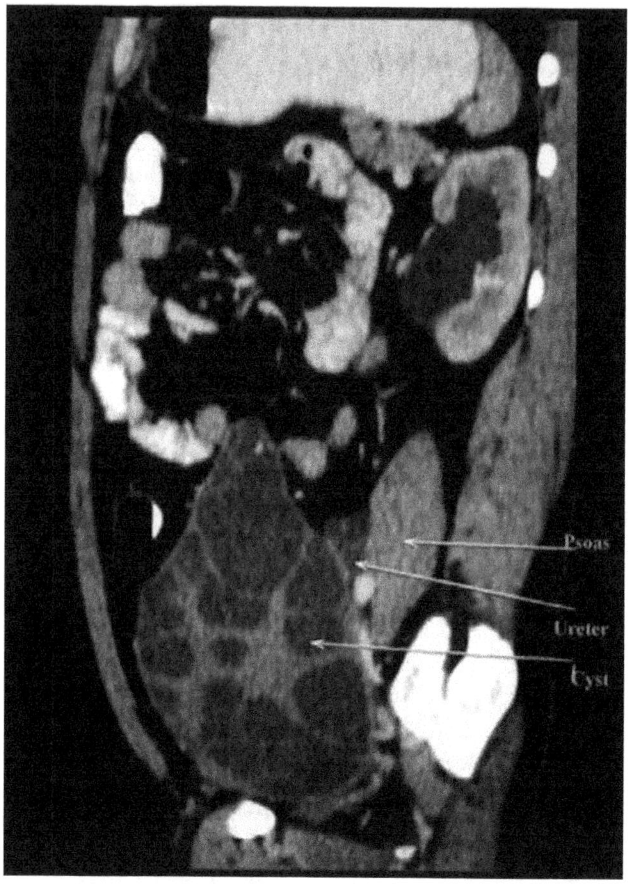

Legend: Contrast-enhanced CT of the abdomen (sagittal view) showing a retrovesical cyst with left hydroureteronephrosis. *(Courtesy: Kumar et al. J Endourol. 2008;22:1709–1713.)*

Figure 4. CT scan of retrovesicle hydatid cyst.

4. Management

Treatment depends on disease activity and symptom status. Actively growing or symptomatic cysts need to be treated. Treatment modalities include medical therapy, percutaneous intervention, and open and minimally invasive surgery. Surgical excision provides the best chance of cure. Medical therapy is used either as an adjunct to surgical excision or as a primary mode of treatment in poor surgical candidates, cases of disseminated hydatidosis, or cases of brain or bony hydatidosis [7]. Preoperative therapy with albendazole (10–15 mg/kg per day) with or without praziquantel (50 mg/kg) for 4 weeks before surgery may kill the scolices, decrease cyst material antigenicity, make the cyst inactive, reduce cyst wall tension thereby reducing risk of spillage [15]. In a study by Arif et al. on liver echinococcosis, patients who received preoperative Albendazole had a recurrence rate of 4.16%, while it was 18.75% in those who did not receive Albendazole [53]. One of the limitations of medical therapy is the serious drug-related adverse effect such as hepatotoxicity, leukopenia, allergic reactions, and alopecia [54] and the limited amount of literature available on its use in genito-urinary echinococcosis.

Percutaneous puncture, aspiration, instillation of scolicidal agent, and re-aspiration techniques (PAIR) under ultrasound guidance have been devised in an attempt to reduce the morbidity associated with open surgical procedures in cases of unilocular cysts not communicating with the pelvicalyceal system. However, it carries the risk of dissemination of daughter cysts and lethal anaphylaxis has been reported in 0.03%–0.04% of percutaneous procedures [55].

The surgical treatment planning for renal hydatid is based on residual renal function, hydatid cyst size, location, number, and degree of renal involvement. With the advent of minimally invasive surgery, the morbidity associated with open surgery has reduced. Smaller incisions result in reduced wound-related complications, early ambulation, and early return to work. Surgical treatment options for renal echinococcosis include cysto-pericystectomy, cyst de-roofing with endocyst evacuation, and partial or total nephrectomy. Laparoscopic management of renal hydatid cyst dates back to 1991 and includes laparoscopic cystopericystectomy, laparoscopic partial nephrectomy, laparoscopic aspiration, instillation of scolicidal agent, and suction [52]. Superficial hydatid cysts involving little renal parenchyma can be managed by pericystectomy while larger, deep seated cysts may require partial cystectomy or de-roofing with omentopexy, partial or total nephrectomy. In most cases, nephrectomy can be avoided and kidney can be preserved considering the benign nature of the disease and the fact that in hydatid cyst, the renal parenchyma is compressed and not invaded. Ex-vivo surgery with orthotopic replantation of the kidney for a centrally located hydatid cyst has been performed with good short-term outcome [56]. Partial nephrectomy may be necessary for thickened or calcified cysts with doubtful diagnosis [7]. Nephron-sparing surgeries are possible in 75% of the cases [57]. Nephrectomy may be needed in cases where the entire kidney is replaced by a hydatid cyst or in cases of poorly functioning kidney, cyst hemorrhage, cyst infection, or communicating cyst [7]. Techniques of controlled evacuation are used to prevent spillage and dissemination of daughter cysts. In controlled evacuation, one third of the cyst content is aspirated, followed by instillation of scolicidal agents such as 30% sodium chloride, 10% povidone iodine, 0.5% silver nitrate, or 95% ethanol [12, 15]. Moreover, during surgery, the cysts should be packed on all sides with gauze soaked in scolicidal solutions including 20% normal saline solution, 1% iodine, 10% cetrimide, 10% povidone-iodine, or 0.5% silver nitrate [58].

The laparoscopic approach for hydatid cyst management is safe and feasible with better postoperative recovery. The smaller incision, as compared to conventional open surgery leads to less postoperative pain, and wound-related complications. During surgery for hydatid cyst, the anesthetist should be ready with epinephrine injections, should severe anaphylactic reaction occur [58]. Both transperitoneal and retroperitoneal laparoscopic approaches have been described [59]. Transperitoneal approach provides a larger working space outside the Gerota fascia and prevents inadvertent cyst rupture [60]. Two of the main challenges in minimal invasive surgery for hydatid disease are the risk of intraperitoneal spillage and the difficult evacuation of particulate cyst contents including the daughter cyst and laminated membranes. However, even giant multilocular renal hydatid cysts have been successfully treated by percutaneous nephroscopic aspiration, instillation, and re-aspiration through single-incision laparoscopic approach—the Santosh-PGI technique (Figure 5) [52]. In this technique following pneumoperitoneum, three conventional laparoscopic trocars with cannula (one 10 mm and two 5 mm) are inserted through a single periumbilical incision. After medial mobilization of the colon, the cyst is punctured with a 18-gauge 20 cm puncture needle introduced through the right lumbar region. 10% povidone-iodine solution is instilled for 10 minutes, followed by the passage of a 0.8128 mm Terumo guidewire through the puncture needle. The tract is dilated with Amplatz dilators to accommodate 30 French instruments. Two separate camera monitors are used: one for laparoscopy and the other for hydatid cystoscopy. A suction catheter is placed through the 5-Fr periumbilical port to help suck out small amount of fluid that may spill during the process of tract dilatation. Following dilatation of tract with Amplatz dilator, a 24-French caliber 25-degree nephroscope is introduced into the cyst and the contents are aspirated under vision followed by the removal of the laminated membrane with grasping forceps. This is an attractive technique because of its acceptable success rate and reduced morbidity. It highlights the feasibility of successful laparoscopic treatment even in cases of a giant hydatid cyst. Laparoscopic guidance for cysts puncture avoids inadvertent colonic injury. The use of conventional laparoscopic instruments through a single periumbilical incision not only reduces operative costs but also provides excellent cosmesis.

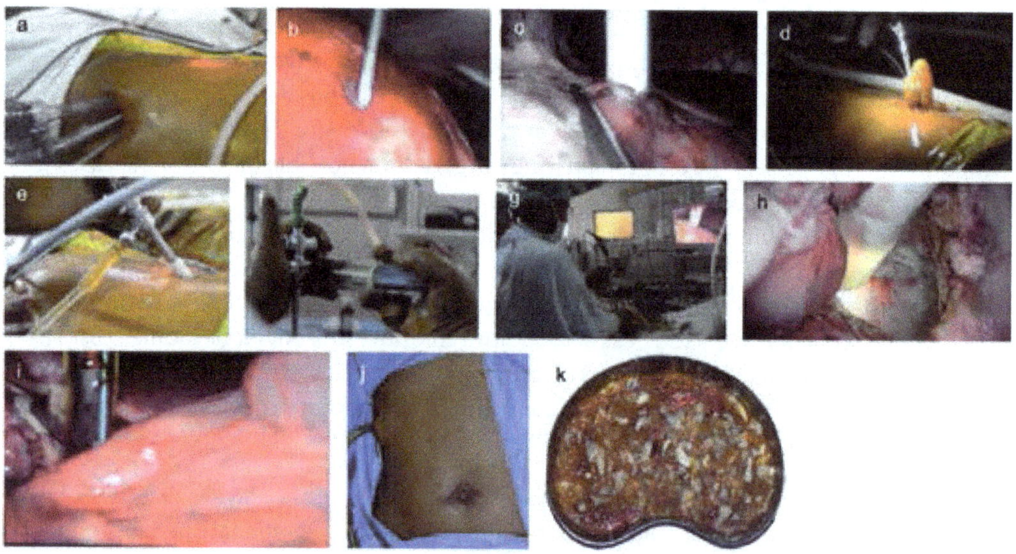

Legend: Surgical procedure. (a) Three conventional laparoscopic trocars, one 10 mm and two 5 mm, were inserted through the umbilical incision. (b) Laparoscopic guidance was used to puncture the cyst. (c) Tract dilatation with Amplatz dilators. (d,e) With the help of a nephroscope, all the cyst contents were aspirated until the clear cyst wall could be seen all around. (f) Injection of 10% povidone-iodine solution. (g) Cyst removal with grasping forceps through the nephroscope. (h) Deroofing the cyst. (i) Placement of the Portex drain into cyst cavity. (j) Closed port site. (k) Removed cyst contents. *(Courtesy: Kumar et al. Asian J Endosc Surg. 2013;6:342–345.)*

Figure 5. Percutaneous nephroscopic management of an isolated giant renal hydatid cyst guided by single-incision laparoscopy using conventional instruments: The Santosh-PGI technique.

The Palanivelu Hydatid System (PHS) helps in the controlled evacuation of the cyst contents, laparoscopically minimizing the fear of intraperitoneal spillage [61]. It consists of a 12 mm trocar and cannula assembly along with 5 mm and 8 mm reducers. The pyramidal tip of the trocar has fenestrations and the shaft is hollow to accommodate suction cannula. The 26 cm long cannula has 12 mm inner diameter with suction and irrigation channels [Figure 6]. This unique architecture of trocar and cannula allows for easy suction of scolices, as well as avoids spillage of contents. Following aspiration, the same cannula can be used for visualization of intracystic architecture and rule out its communication with the collecting system. Following the aspiration of the scolicidal agent after 10 minutes of contact time, the residual cyst can be marsupialized or excised depending on the location. The specimen is retrieved through a specimen retrieval bag.

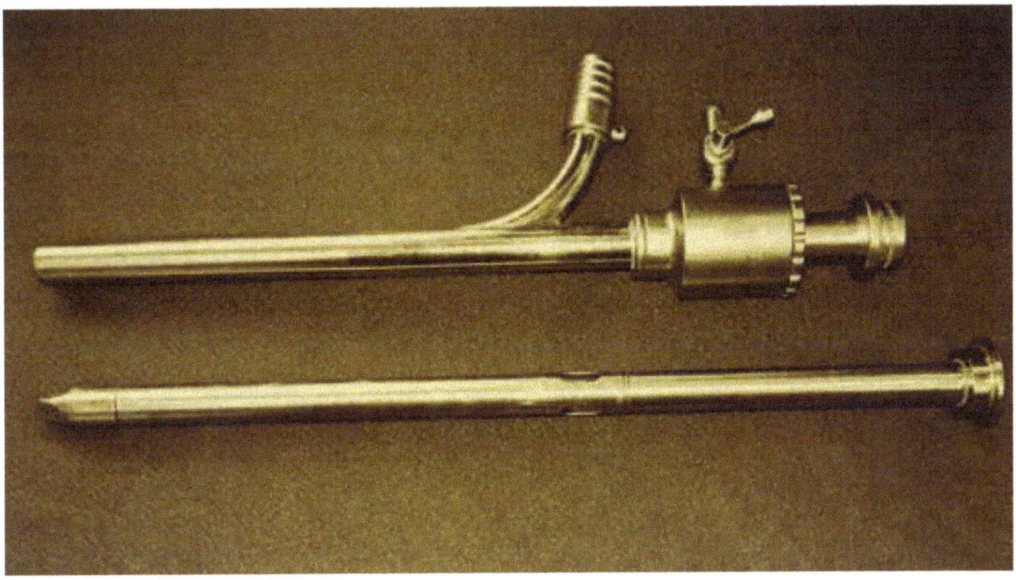

Legend: Palanivelu hydatid system showing the long trocar and cannula with two side channels for suction and irrigation.

Figure 6. The Palanivelu Hydatid System (PHS).

Retroperitoneoscopic approach further minimizes the risk of intraperitoneal spillage of cyst contents. With the increasing experience in retroperitoneoscopy, reports of retroperitoneoscopic hydatid cyst excision are emerging [62]. The technique involves standard three-port (5 mm, 10 mm, 10 mm) retroperitoneal access under the vision of a 30-degree telescope at 90-degree flank position, with the help of balloon dilatation. The cyst wall is packed with gauze soaked in scolicidal agent. In the technique described by Ozden and colleagues, a purse-string suture was placed on the cyst wall followed by cyst perforation with hook dissector. The fluid content was aspirated, followed by the instillation of scolicidal agent. Cystopericystectomy was performed and the intact cyst could be removed. The authors emphasize the technical feasibility of this approach, along with the advantage of limited risk of intraperitoneal spillage.

Surgical management of adrenal hydatid cyst involves partial or complete excision of the cyst by laparoscopic or open techniques. In a series of nine cases by Ackay and colleagues, adrenalectomy was performed in all cases with no recurrence at a median follow-up of 16 months (range: 6–64 months)[14]. Due to the limited amount of available data, it is difficult to say whether complete excision of adrenal is mandatory. Kumar and colleagues did transperitoneal laparoscopic aspiration with instillation of scolicidal agent with partial cystectomy for adrenal hydatid cyst. The area around the cyst was packed with Betadine-soaked gauze pieces. The cyst was aspirated during the procedure followed by the instillation of the scolicidal agent and maintained for 10 minutes. An appropriate plane between the cyst and adrenal gland could not be made. A 10 mm trocar was introduced inside the cyst and the cyst contents were sucked out, including the germinal layer. Partial excision of the cyst wall was done as it was adherent to renal vessels. Patient had no recurrence at sixth-month follow up. Total adrenalectomy may not be essential and may be required only when there is complete destruction of the gland [63]. Complete evacuation of the cyst contents, along with the prevention of intraperitoneal spillage of viable scolices, is the key principle in managing the adrenal hydatid cyst.

Retrovesicle hydatid cyst contains small bowel, sigmoid colon, rectum, ureter, urinary bladder, pelvic vessels, or internal genitelia of females as part of the pericyst. Although complete cyst excision has been described in few reports [64], it carries a high risk of inadvertent pelvic visceral injury. The narrow pelvic space along with dense adhesions to the surrounding structures may render difficulties in complete excision of pelvic hydatid cysts. Few case reports exist in literature regarding their management. In cases of pelvic or peri-vesical hydatid, where the cyst is large and adherent to adjacent vital organs, partial excision of hydatid cyst with adequate drainage is an acceptable alternative [7]. Laparoscopic cyst aspiration with instillation of scolicidal agent (LAIS) and suction has been successfully employed in the perivesical hydatid cyst (Figure 7) [7]. In this technique, pneumoperitoneum is created using Verres' needle in the epigastrium. Four ports are placed: a 12 mm camera port in the midline above the umbilicus; two 12 mm lateral working ports in the lower abdomen at lateral border of rectus; and an additional 5 mm port can be placed in the iliac fossa to help in retraction. Laparoscopy guided percutaneous puncture of the cyst with an 18 G needle is performed, followed by aspiration with instillation of scolicidal agent. The procedure is repeated to ensure the instillation of the scolicidal agent into the entire cyst. The ectocyst is opened and the lateral port is negotiated into the cyst for complete cyst evacuation using a wide-bore suction cannula followed by visual inspection of the cyst lumen to ensure the complete removal of scolices. Complete ectocyst excision is difficult with associated risk of inadvertent bladder-bowel injury. However, even in cases with partial or no excision of ectocyst, complete evacuation of daughter cysts, germinal layer, and lamellated membrane combined with medical therapy results in an acceptable short-term outcome. Even partial cystectomy can be difficult and may lead to inadvertent adjacent visceral injury [7]. However, on table recognition of such complication and primary repair reduces post-operative morbidity. With the advances in laparoscopic techniques, such visceral injuries can be managed laparoscopically.

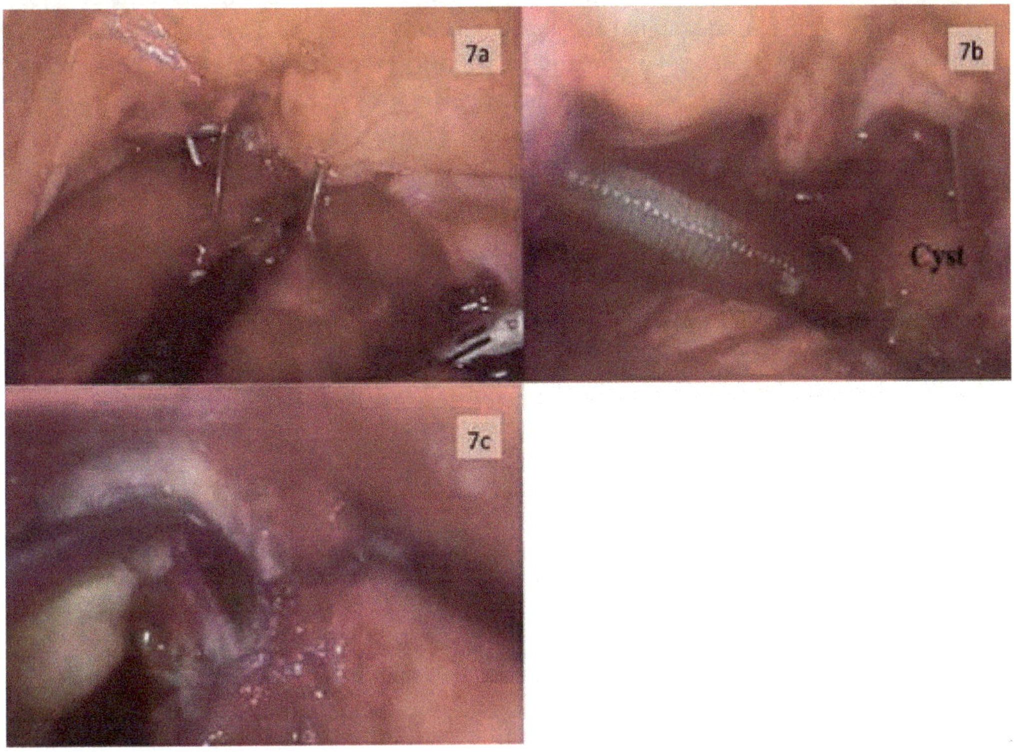

Legend: (a) Laparoscopic-guided percutaneous cyst puncture, aspiration, and instillation of 10% povidone iodine solution. (b) Cyst contents and laminated membrane being sucked out through the port using a wide-bore suction cannula. (c) Excision of part of the ectocyst led to iatrogenic bladder injury, which was repaired by intra-corporeal suturing. *(Courtesy: Kumar et al. J Endourol. 2008;22:1709–1713.)*

Figure 7. LAIS for retrovesicle hydatid cyst.

The PHS system has also been successfully used for managing pelvic echinococcal cysts [65]. Ports include a 12 mm midline supra-umbilical port, two para-rectal lower abdominal ports (12 mm and 5 mm) and an accessory port in iliac fossa. After dissecting the ectocyst from adjacent viscera, Betadine-soaked gauzes are placed around the cyst. The puncture and aspiration technique is similar to the one described for renal echinococcosis. Complex retrovesicle echinococcal cysts may communicate with the bladder or rectum [36]. Their management is a challenge. Retrovesicle cysts communicating with the bladder have been managed with intravesicle instillation of scolicidal agents with good outcome [66]. Pelvic retroperitoneal cysts can also be evacuated by transvaginal route [67].

Nowadays even robot-assissted surgical excision of the pelvic hydatid cyst has been performed [68]. Patient position is same as for robotic radical prostatectomy. Superior magnification, 3D vision, and endowrist technology help in the accurate dissection with minimal collateral damage thereby, helping in complete cyst excision. Robot assisted laparoscopic surgery is a safe and feasible option in the management of pelvic hydatid cyst.

Prostatic hydatid cysts are rarely reported with only few case reports discussing their management. Sallami et al. described endoscopic management of prostatic hydatid cyst [69]. Surgery was performed under spinal anesthesia. Cystoscopy revealed a bulge in the posterior urethral wall. The posterior wall of the urethra was incised with a cold knife, taking care not to injure the bladder neck and verumontanum. Scolicidal agent was injected, followed by the aspiration of the cyst fluid. The cyst wall was opened, followed by the immediate suction of the cyst contents including the daughter cyst. The germinal layer was completely removed, followed by the re-instillation of the scolicidal agent. Post-procedure, a Foley catheter was placed for four days. Laparoscopic excision of the prostatic hydatid cyst is also safe and feasible [70]. Therapeutic principles are the same.

Preoperative diagnosis of testicular echinococcosis is difficult. In the cases reported, diagnosis was made based on histopathological examination of the orchidectomy specimen. The indications for orchidectomy were either suspicion of testicular malignancy or tuberculosis [39]. Ovarian echinococcal cysts have been rarely reported [22]. Although ovarian cystectomy shall be the ideal treatment, cyst marsupialization with evacuation of daughter cysts also has acceptable results [22].

5. Outcome

Majority of the literature available on genitourinary echinococcosis include case series and case reports. Many of the therapeutic principles are extrapolation of the experience with the hepatic hydatid cyst. Given the rarity of the disease, no randomized control trial comparing the treatment modalities for genitourinary hydatid exist. Moreover, long-term follow up in many cases is unavailable. Overall, the incidence of local and systemic recurrence is low. In a series of 30 cases of renal echinococcosis, only one patient had local recurrence, while extrarenal recurrence occurred in three more cases [4]. Risk factors for recurrence includes spillage of viable daughter cysts and scolices, incomplete removal of germinal layer, undetected cyst at other location, and return to endemic area.

6. Conclusion

Genitourinary echinococcosis is an uncommon disease. Preoperative diagnosis requires a high index of suspicion. It should be considered in differential diagnosis of cystic mass of genitourinary tract, especially in endemic regions. Computed tomography, ultrasonography, and antibody testing aid in diagnosing and classifying the stage of the cyst. Although a number of operative techniques have been described, complete removal of germinal layer with daughter cysts without spillage of viable cyst contents with perioperative medical therapy provide an optimum chance of cure with minimal morbidity. Considering the benign nature of the disease, organ preservation is feasible in majority of the cases. The conventional open surgical treatment has evolved into minimally invasive laparoscopic, endoscopic, and even robotic techniques with concomitant improvement in wound-related morbidity and cosmetic outcome.

Author details

Santosh Kumar* and Shivanshu Singh

*Address all correspondence to: santoshsp1967jaimatadi@yahoo.co.in ; santoshsp1967@yahoo.co.in

Advanced Urology Center, Department of Urology, Postgraduate Institute of Medical Education and Research. Chandigarh, India

References

[1] Strohmaier WL, Bichler KH, Wilbert DM, Seitz HM. Alveolar echinococcosis with involvement of the ureter and testis. J Urol. 1990;144:733–734.

[2] Kern P, Bardonnet K, Renner E, Auer H, Pawlowski Z, Ammann RW, et al. European echinococcosis registry: Human alveolar echinococcosis, Europe, 1982-2000. Emerg Infect Dis. 2003;9:343–349.

[3] Choi H, Park JY, Kim JH, Moon DG, Lee JG, Bae JH. Primary renal hydatid cyst: Mis-Interpretation as a renal malignancy. Korean J Parasitol. 2014;52:295–298.

[4] Rexiati M, Mutalifu A, Azhati B, Wang W, Yang H, Sheyhedin I, et al. Diagnosis and surgical treatment of renal hydatid disease: A retrospective analysis of 30 cases. PLoS ONE 2014;9:e96602. DOI:10.1371/journal.pone.0096602.

[5] Brunetti E, Garcia HH, Junghanss T. Cystic echinococcosis: Chronic, complex, and still neglected. PLoS Negl Trop Dis. 2011;5:e1146. DOI:10.1371/journal.pntd.0001146.

[6] McManus DP, Zhang W, Li J, Bartley PB. Echinococcosis. Lancet. 2003;18:1295–1304.

[7] Kumar S, Pandya S, Agarwal S, Lal A. Laparoscopic management of genitourinary hydatid cyst disease. J Endourol. 2008;22:1709–1713.

[8] Zhang W, Li J, McManus DP. Concepts in immunology and diagnosis of hydatid disease. Clin. Microbiol. Rev. 2003;16:18. DOI:10.1128/CMR.16.1.18-36.2003.

[9] Karabekios S, Gouliamos A, Kalovidouris A, Vlahos L, Papavasiliou C, Sakkas J. Features of computed tomography in hydatid cysts of the urinary tract. Br J Urol. 1989;64:575–578.

[10] Shetty SD, Al-saigh A, Ibrahim AI, Patil KP, Bhattachan CL. Management of hydatid cysts of the urinary tract. Br J Urol. 1992;70:258–261.

[11] Horchani A, Nouira Y, Kbaier I. Hydatid cyst of the kidney: A report of 147 controlled cases. Eur Urol. 2000;38:461–467.

[12] Gogus O, Beduk Y, Topukcu Z. Renal hydatid disease. Br J Urol 1991;68:466.

[13] Shukla S, Singh SK, Pujani M. Multiple disseminated abdominal hydatidosis presenting with gross hydatiduria: A rare case report. Indian J Pathol Microbiol. 2009;52:213–214.

[14] Akcay MN, Akcay G, Balik AA, Boyuk A. Hydatid cysts of the adrenal gland: Review of nine patients. World J Surg 2004;28:97–99. DOI:10.4111/kju.2014.55.7.493.

[15] Goel MC, Agarwal MR, Misra A. Percutaneous drainage of renal hydatid cyst: Early results and follow-up. Br J Urol. 1995;75:724–728.

[16] Foster DG. Adrenal cysts: Review of literature and report of case. Arch Surg. 1966;92:131–143.

[17] Yeniyol CO, Minareci S, Ayder AR. Primary cyst hydatid of adrenal: A case report. Int Urol Nephrol. Int Urol Nephrol. 2000;32:227–229.

[18] Schoretsanitis G, de Bree E, Melissas J, Tsiftsis D. Primary hydatid cyst of the adrenal gland. Scand J Urol Nephrol. 1998;32:51–53.

[19] Tampakoudis P, Assimakopoulos E, Zafrakas M, Tzevelekis P, Kostopoulou E, Bontis J. Pelvic echinococcus mimicking multicystic ovary. Ultrasound Obstet Gynecol. 2003;22:196–198.

[20] Diaz-Recasens J, Garcia-Enguidanos A, Munoz I, Sainz de la Cuesta R. Ultrasonographic appearance of an echinococcus ovarian cyst. Obstet Gynecol. 1998;91:841–842.

[21] Dede S, Dede H, Caliskan E, Demir B. Recurrent pelvic hydatid cyst obstructing labor, with a concomitant hepatic primary: A case report. J Reprod Med. 2002;47:164–166.

[22] Cattorini L, Trastulli S, Milani D, Cirocchi R, Giovannelli G, Avenia N, et al. Ovarian hydatid cyst: A case report. International Journal of Surgery Case Reports. 2011;2:100–102. DOI:10.1016/j.ijscr.2010.12.005.

[23] Bozkurt M, Bozkurt DK, CIL AS, Karaman M. Primary Ovarian and Pararectal Hydatid Cysts Mimicking Pelvic Endometriosis. Acta Medica Iranica. 2012;50:839–842.

[24] Kaya A, Yildiz S, Ozaras R, Mert A. A primary giant hydatid cyst of ovary. Iran J Radiol. 2012;9:165–166. DOI:10.5812/iranjradi-ol.7955.

[25] Rashid SQ. Primary and solitary uterine hydatid cyst: A most unusual site. Journal of Medical Ultrasound. 2011;19:57–60.

[26] Thakare PY. Hydatid cysts in a pregnant uterus. The Journal of Obstetrics and Gynecology of India. 2014;64:215–217.

[27] Bhattacharya A, Saha R, Mitra S, Nayak P. Primary hydatid cyst of broad ligament. Tropical Parasitology. 2013;3:155–157. DOI:10.4103/2229-5070.122148.

[28] Bickers WM. Hydatid disease of the female pelvis. Am J Obstet Gynecol. 1970;107:477–483.

[29] Deodhar SD, Patel VC, Kirloskar MS. Hydatid disease of urinary bladder (a case report). J Postgrad Med. 1986;32:46B–48B.

[30] Angulo JC, Escribano J, Diego A, Sanchez-Chapado M. Isolated retrovesical and extra-renal retroperitoneal hydatidosis: Clinical study of 10 cases and literature review. J Urol. 1998;159:76–82.

[31] Horchani A, Nouira Y, Chtourou M, Kacem M, Ben Safta Z. Retrovesical hydatid disease: A clinical study of 27 cases. Eur Urol. 2001;40:655–660.

[32] Nasr R, Saad GA, Shahait M, Khater N. Retrovesical hydatid cyst presenting with urinary retention and left kidney atrophy. Urol Ann. 2014;6:68–70.

[33] Kumar S, Sarkar D, Prasad S, Gupta V, Ghosala P, Kaman L, et al. Large pelvic masses of obscure origin: Urologist's perspective. Urologia Internationalis. 2012;88:215–224.

[34] Srinivasan S. Retrovesical hydatid cyst presenting with urinary retention and left kidney atrophy. Urol Ann. 2014;6:70–71.

[35] Parray FQ, Wani SN, Bazaz S, Khan SR, Malik NS. Primary pelvic hydatid cyst: A case report. case reports in surgery. Vol. 2011, Article ID 809387, 3 pages. 2011. DOI: 10.1155/2011/809387.

[36] Kumar S, Naveen A, Mandal A, Singh SK. Case report unusual presentation of retrovesical hydatid cyst: Report of three cases. African Journal of Urology. 2007;14:155–157.

[37] Nouira Y, Binous MY, Nouira K, Mekni A, Kallel Y, Fitouri Z, et al. Intraprostatic hydatid cyst: An unusual presentation. Scientific World Journal. 2006;6:2315–2318.

[38] Bouchikhi AA, Lamrani YA, Tazi MF, Mellas S, Elammmari J, Khallouk A, et al. Unilateral primitive hydatid cyst with surgical resection of the scrotum: A case report. Journal of medical case reports. 2013;7:109. DOI:10.1186/1752-1947-7-109

[39] Singh B, Wani AA, Ganai AA, Singh M, Baba K. Hydatid cyst of testis: An unusual presentation of hydatid disease - Case report and review of literature. Indian J Urol. 2001;18:94–96.

[40] Kumar PVN, Jahanshahi SH. Hydatid cyst of testis: A case report. J Urol. 1987;137:511–512.

[41] Sağlam M, Taşar M, Bulakbaşi N, Tayfun C, Somuncu I. TRUS, CT and MRI findings of hydatid disease of seminal vesicles. Eur Radiol. 1998;8:933–935.

[42] Ahmadnia H, Kalantari MR, Ghanbarizadeh SR. Why testes are resistant to hydatidosis: Is blood-testis-barrier responsible for this resistance? Nigerian Journal of Parasitology. 2008;29:84-87.

[43] Khan RA, Wahab S, Chana RS, Fareed R. Isolated retroperitoneal hydatid cyst in a child: A rare cause of acute scrotal swelling? J Pediatr Surg. 2010;45:1717–1719. DOI: 10.1016/j.jpedsurg.2010.04.019

[44] Mushtaque M, Mir MF, Nazir P, Khan PS. Primary isolated echinococcal cyst of the seminal vesicle: A rare case. Urology Annals. 2012;4:122–125. DOI: 10.4103/0974-7796.95571

[45] Stojkovic M, Rosenberger K, Kauczor HU. Diagnosing and staging of cystic echinococcosis: How do CT and MRI perform in comparison to ultrasound? PLoS Negl Trop Dis. 2012;6:e1880.

[46] Lightowlers, MW, Gottstein B. Echinococcosis/hydatidosis: Antigens, immunological, and molecular diagnosis. Wallingford, Oxon, UK: CAB International. 1995.

[47] Nasrieh MA, Abdel-Hafez SK. Echinococcus granulosus in Jordan: Assessment of various antigenic preparations for use in the serodiagnosis of surgically confirmed cases using enzyme immuno assays and the indirect haemagglutination test. Diagn Microbiol Infect Dis. 2004;48:117-123.

[48] Al-Sherbiny MM, Farrag AA, Fayad MH, Makled MK, Tawfeek GM, Ali NM. Application and assessment of a dipstick assay in the diagnosis of hydatidosis and trichinosis. Parasitol Res. 2004;93:87–95.

[49] Rott MB, Fernandez V, Farias S, Ceni J, Ferreira HB, Haag KL, et al. Comparative analysis of two different subunits of antigen B from Echinococcus granulosus: Gene sequences, expression in Escherichia coli and serological evaluation. Acta Trop. 2000;75:331–340.

[50] Virginio VG, Hernandez A, Rott MB, Monteiro KM, Zandonai AF, Nieto A, et al. A set of recombinant antigens from Echinococcus granulosus with potential for use in the immunodiagnosis of human cystic hydatid disease. Clin Exp Immunol. 2003;132(2):309–315.

[51] Feki W, Ghozzi S, Khiari R, Ghorbel J, Elarbi H, Khouni H, et al. Multiple unusual locations of hydatid cysts including bladder, psoas muscle, and liver. Parasitology International. 2008;57:83–86.

[52] Kumar S, Choudhary GR, Pushkarna A, Najjapa B, Vatasla Ht. Percutaneous nephroscopic management of an isolated giant renal hydatid cyst guided by single-incision laparoscopy using conventional instruments: The Santosh-PGI technique. Asian J Endosc Surg. 2013;6:342–345. DOI:10.1111/ases.12050.

[53] Arif SH, Shams Ul B, Wani NA, Zargar SA, Wani MA, Tabassum R, et al. Albendazole as an adjuvant to the standard surgical management of hydatid cyst liver. Int J Surg. 2008;6:448–451.

[54] Von Sinner WN, Hellstorm M, Kavegi I, Norlen BJ. Hydatid disease of urinary tract. J Urol. 1993;149:577–580.

[55] Neumayr A, Troia G, de Bernardis C, Tamarozzi F, Goblirsch S, Piccoli L, et al. Justified concern or exaggerated fear: The risk of anaphylaxis in percutaneous treatment of cystic echinococcosis-a systematic literature review. PLoS Negl Trop Dis. 2011;5:e1154.

[56] Tscholl R, Ausfeld R. Renal replantation (orthotopic autotransplantation) for echinococcosis of the kidney. J Urol. 1985;133:456457.

[57] Zmerli S, Ayed M, Horchani A, Chami I, El Ouakdi M, Ben Slama MR. Hydatid cyst of the kidney: Diagnosis and treatment. World J Surg. 2001;25:68–74.

[58] Afsar H, Yagci F, Aybasti N, Meto S. Hydatid disease of the kidney. Br J Urol. 1994;73:17–22.

[59] Aggarwal S, Bansal A. Laparoscopic Management of Renal Hydatid Cyst. JSLS. 2014;18:361–366. DOI:10.4293/108680813X13753907291396.

[60] Shah KJ, Ganpule AP, Desai MR. Isolated renal hydatid cyst managed by laparoscopic transperitoneal nephrectomy. Indian J Urol. 2009;25:531–533.

[61] Chipde SS, Yadav A, Ranjan P, Prakash A, Kapoor R. Total laparoscopic management of a large renal hydatid cyst by using hydatid trocar cannula system. Journal of Surgical Technique and Case Report. 2012;4:32–35. DOI:10.4103/2006-8808.100351

[62] Ozden E, Bostanci Y, Mercimek MN, Yakupoglu YK, Yilmaz AF, Sarıkaya S. Renal hydatid cyst treatment: Retroperitoneoscopic "closed cyst" pericystectomy. International Journal of Urology. 2011;18:237–239. DOI: 10.1111/j.1442-2042.2010.02703.x

[63] Kumar S, Nanjappa B, Gowda KK. Laparoscopic management of a hydatid cyst of the adrenal gland. Korean J Urol. 2014;55:493–495.

[64] Turan T, Tuncay L, Kayik S, Atahan O, Aybek Z. Retrovesical hydatid cyst. J Urol. 1998;159:2085–2086.

[65] Subramaniam B, Abrol N, Kumar R. Laparoscopic Palanivelu-hydatid-system aided management of retrovesical hydatid cyst. Indian Journal of Urology: IJU: Journal of the Urological Society of India. 2013;29:59–60. DOI:10.4103/0970-1591.109987.

[66] Vaidyanathan S, Rao MS, Sharma SK, Rajendran LJ, Subudhi CL, Rao KM, et al. Non-operative management of a pelvic hydatid cyst communicating with the bladder. J Urol. 1979;121:245–247.

[67] Görgen H, Api M, Çetin A. Primary adnexial hydatid cyst mimicking ovarian tumor. Journal of the Turkish German Gynecological Association. 2009;10:232–234.

[68] Dogra P, Javeli T, Saini A, Sharma S, Gupta N. Isolated retrovesical hydatid cyst [Internet]. 2010. Available from: http://www.bjui.org/ContentFullItem.aspx?id=546.

[69] Sallami S, Nouira Y, Rhouma SB, Tanguour M, Cherif K, Rebai S, et al. Endoscopic treatment of a primary prostatic hydatid cyst: A mini-invasive therapeutic approach. Urol J. 2010;7:270-274.

[70] El-Kappany HA, El-Nahas AR, El-Nahas HA. Laparoscopic excision of prostatic hydatid cyst: Case report and review of literature. Journal of Endourology. April 2005:19:3:290–294. DOI:10.1089/end.2005.19.290.

Section 3

Treatment and Prevention

10

Hydatidosis and Intervention Strategies

YuRong Yang

Abstract

Human echinococcosis is a zoonotic infection caused by larval forms (metacestodes) of tapeworms of the genus *Echinococcus*. Among the recognised species, *Echinococcus granulosus* and *E. multilocularis* are of considerable medical importance, causing cystic and alveolar echinococcosis (AE and CE), respectively. The factors of immunology, host-genetic inherits, and Echinococcus genetic-diversity and adaption clearly influence infectious establishment and disease progression. However, subtle mechanisms between host and parasite interactions/relationships are still open to study for answers. Despite the global burden, echinococcosis remains a neglected zoonosis. The importance of environmental factors influencing the transmission intensity and distribution of *Echinococcus* species is increasingly being recognised. The intervention strategies for this public health threat have integrated host immune-genetic research, parasite adaptation, and genetic diversity analysis, as well as the transmission dynamic investigations; the limitations of current control programmes are clearly presented in this study that hampers the elimination of *Echinococcus* species worldwide. Continuous efforts by multidiscipline researches are needed.

Keywords: *Echinococcus* species, host immunology and genetics, *Echinococcus* genetic diversity and adaptation, intervention strategies

1. Introduction

The zoonotic disease of echinococcosis (hydatidosis) is one of the most important parasitic helminth diseases, with over three million people infected worldwide. The two major species infecting man are *Echinococcus multilocularis* that causes alveolar echinococcosis (AE) and

Echinococcus granulosus that causes cystic echinococcosis (CE). Both CE and AE are life threatening and are associated with severe morbidity. The global burden of human CE exceeds one million disability-adjusted life years (DALYs), resulting in a loss of at least US$760 million per annum. Case series and clinical trials show a mortality rate of 2%–4% for CE, but this increase is marked with poor treatment and care. CE also impacts upon agriculture as *E. granulosus* infects domestic livestock, further adding to economic loss. There are 0.4 million cases of human AE, and survival analysis has shown that, if untreated or if limited treatment is provided, mortality exceeds 90%, 10–15 years post-diagnosis. There are approximately 18,000 new cases of AE annually, with a total annual burden of 666,434 DALYs.

2. Transmission of *Echinococcus* species

All *Echinococcus* species are transmitted to intermediate hosts via the ingestion of eggs and are transmitted to definitive hosts by means of eating infected cyst/lesion containing organs. The life cycle of *E. multiclocularis* involves carnivorous definitive hosts (foxes and dogs) and intermediate hosts (predominantly microtine rodents).

For *E. granulosus,* dogs are the major definitive hosts and sheep and other livestock are typical intermediate hosts. In Australia, however, the definitive hosts for *E. granulosus* also include wild dogs and dingoes, while sheep, kangaroos, and wallabies are common intermediate hosts.

Human echinococcosis occurs through the ingestion of *Echinococcus* eggs from environments that have been contaminated by the faeces of infected dogs or foxes. Mostly, following close contact with infected canines carrying *Echinococcus* eggs on their fur; by ingestion of egg-contaminated water or food; or by coprophagic flies serving as mechanical vectors for transmission. Once inside the body, the eggs release oncospheres in the intestine that then migrate through the circulatory system to various organs of the host, notably the liver and lungs. Generally, echinococcosis is associated with poverty, which impacts on sanitation and hygiene, and access to health services, particularly in livestock-raising communities.

3. Epidemiology in Australia and China

Cosmopolite distribution of *E. granulosus* in a few of countries is completely free from this parasite contamination, while *E. multilocularis* mainly occurs in the northern hemisphere; but it will be an emerging or re-emerging disease in certain countries as a result of ecological alternatives in modern life (Figure 1). AE and CE are of considerable public health concern, particularly in parts of Central and Eastern Europe, and especially Northwest China. While the annual incidence of AE may appear low in many endemic areas (0.03–1.2 per 100,000 inhabitants), it is estimated that many cases are undiagnosed. Human CE is endemic in many pastoral communities. The mortality rate from CE is lower than that from AE (about 2%–4%), but increases considerably if medical treatment is unavailable or inadequate.

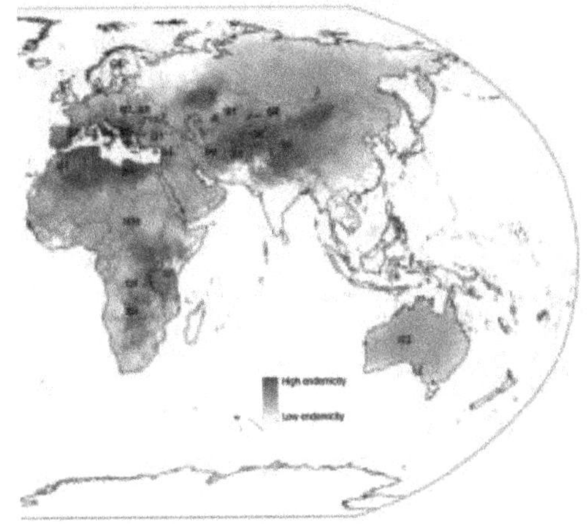

Figure 1. The distribution of *Echinococcus* spp. in Eastern parts of world (Asian and Australia).

3.1. In Australia

E. granulosus occurs in Australia and is prevalent in wildlife. The true extent of human CE in Australia is not accurately known. It is estimated that 80–100 new cases of CE are diagnosed annually; however, CE is not a notifiable disease in Australia and has notoriously been under-reported so the true prevalence of CE is likely to be considerably higher than described. Of few data that are available for rural Australian communities, it is apparent that some have an infection index as high as 23.5/100,000. Other data from Western Australia have shown that the incidence in Aboriginal people was 12.2 times higher than in the equivalent non-Aboriginal rural population.

3.2. In China

There are approximately 1.3 million people with echinococcosis in China, where the disease burden is greater than that of any other country. Of the 33 provinces, autonomous regions, and municipalities in China, at least 20 are considered to be endemic for *E. granulosus* and at least five for *E. multilocularis*. The provinces and autonomous regions with the highest risk of echinococcosis include Xinjiang, Qinghai, Sichuan, Gansu, and Ningxia Hui Autonomous Region (NHAR). These provinces/regions are co-endemic for both human CE and AE, with common cases of co-infections. In addition, significant numbers of CE cases occur in Tibet, Shaanxi, as well as Inner Mongolia, Heilongjiang Province. There are now 66 million people at risk of infection.

4. Pathogenesis of human echinococcosis

The initial phase of a primary infection is always asymptomatic for both AE and CE in humans and may remain so for a matter of months up to many (typically more than 10) years.

The metacestodes of *E. multilocularis* develop almost exclusively in the liver as a tumour-like, infiltrative growth. The rapidly growing cysts can grow up to 20 cm or more in diameter, often with a central necrotic cavity. A primary infection of *E. multilocularis* outside of the liver is rare, but the spread of parasitic larvae from the primary site in the liver to other organs by metastatic infiltration is not uncommon. AE is typically identified following the investigation of symptoms such as fatigue and weight loss, hepatomegaly and abnormal US, or through routine laboratory examination.

In CE, *E. granulosus* metacestodes may develop in almost any organ. For the majority of patients, however, a single-organ infection site is generally observed with a solitary cyst localized to the liver or to the lungs. Ultrasound surveys have shown that, while some cysts may grow up to 50 mm per year, others may persist without change for many years. Liver cysts also appear to grow at a lower rate than lung cysts. Most CE cases remain asymptomatic until the cyst compresses or ruptures into neighbouring structures and organs by which time the disease is already advanced.

5. Disease diagnosis and severity

Patients with AE and CE are diagnosed based on clinical parameters including assessment of hepatomegaly, jaundice and upper abdominal complaints, as well as by imaging techniques such as ultrasound (US), computed tomography (CT) scans and magnetic resonance imaging (MR). ELISA-based detection of serum *Echinococcus* specific-antibodies and histological examination are also used to confirm diagnosis.

To assess the degree of hepatic involvement of the parasite mass, AE patients are classified according to PNM (P: hepatic localization of parasite; N: extrahepatic involvement of neighbouring organs; M: absence or presence of distant metastases) and staged as P1, P2, P3, or P4 as recommended by WHO guidelines and the European Network for concerted surveillance of alveolar echinococcosis classification. For CE patients, classification of disease is based on liver lesion type (CE1, CE2, CE3, CE4 and CE5) at initial diagnosis, as proposed by the WHO Informal Group on Echinococcosis.

6. Susceptibility of human echinococcosis

Despite its public health significance, the susceptibility of human echinococcosis is poorly understood. The general factors that may render an individual more susceptible include malnutrition, co-infection, and immuno-suppression caused by other diseases or through the use of immuno-suppressive drugs. Several reports of children with cystic echinococcosis were predominantly located in the lungs. The reason for lung hydatidosis in children may be explained by either the weaker immune capability in their respiratory system or the faster cyst growth rate (or both) in young ages than that in adults. Pregnancy has also been thought to increase risk of infection or aggravate the disease due to the impaired cellular immunity frequently observed in pregnant women.

6.1. Host immunology

Immuno-suppression is frequently observed in patients with severe AE or CE. High levels of circulating *Echinococcus* antigens can contribute to immune-suppression through polyclonal over-stimulation. The chronicity of *Echinococcus* infection results from persistent antigenic stimulation, polarization of T cell-subset populations and humoral immune responses. Whilst increased Th1 cell activity has been associated with degeneration of CE and AE lesions and successful chemotherapy, high Th2 cell activity is typically associated with active disease and a poor response to chemotherapy. In animals, CE induces local immune-suppression associated with increased IL-10 and TGFβ production. Similarly, in humans, IL-10 production plays a key role in the immune response against *E. multilocularis*. Other studies show, however, a clear immunopathology-associated Th2 polarization in patients with progressive disease related to increased levels of IL-4 and IL-13. Th1/Th2 cytokines have shown association with susceptibility or resistance to both *Em* and *Eg* infection in *in vitro* studies. Immunological markers have proved useful for monitoring the natural course of echinococcosis. High IgG4/IgE levels are associated with active disease whereas IgG1, IgG2 and IgG3 responses occur when cysts became infiltrated and are destroyed by the host. This highlights the importance of measuring IgG subclasses individually for a more sensitive index of disease activity than total IgG levels. Measurement of both cytokine and antibody levels can provide a more sensitive diagnostic tool for studying the immunological mechanisms involved in echinococcosis.

6.2. Host genetics

Despite the high morbidity and mortality associated with echinococcosis, relatively few studies to date have investigated the genetics underlying human susceptibility to the disease.

The case-control studies of candidate genes that have been previously undertaken have identified a number of associations with susceptibility to human echinococcosis in the HLA region for both AE and CE. Of these, however, many have not been replicated, likely reflecting the complexities and diversities of host susceptibility in different ethnic populations, different environmental conditions, and exposure to different *Echinococcus* genotypes or strains. The majority of candidate gene studies have used small cohorts. Only two genes outside of the HLA loci have been investigated in terms of AE and CE susceptibility. These genes, *TAP1* and *TAP2*, belong to the MDR/TAP subfamily and have been previously implicated in autoimmune diseases such as ankylosing spondylitis, type 1 diabetes, and coeliac disease. As with other complex diseases, it is anticipated that host genetic influences on echinococcosis susceptibility are likely to comprise multiple additive loci. Indeed, a recent study has demonstrated that multiple loci exist that contribute to the susceptibility to echinococcosis in mice. This has been supported by recent evidence that implicated a large number of differentially expressed genes in murine AE. However, the relevant genes that determine susceptibility to human echinococcosis and the clinical outcome from this severe disease remain largely unknown. It is clear that any gene variations that interfere with these interactions may alter the etiopathogenesis of disease. Given the highly diverse allelic variation within the MHC region observed between different geographic populations and racial groups, it is plausible that the race and origin of an individual can greatly affect their phenotype and the subsequent outcome of infection.

7. *Echinococcus* adaptation/genetics

Echinococcus species have developed their signalling systems for the microenvironment, encompassing the host insulin acting as a stimulant for larval *E. multilocularis* development and revealed an important factor in the pathology of alveolar echinococcosis predominantly in the host liver.

The extensive genetic variation of *E. granulises* comprises a number of strains (G1–G10) that differ in biological features of intermediate host specificity, with diverse viscera involvements, anitgenicity, transmission dynamics, and infectivity to humans. An abundant AgB in HCF is involved in the evasion of the immune response of the host due to its ability to inhibit elastase activity and neutrophils recruitment and to elicit an immunopathology-associated Th2 cell response. The significantly different expression levels of 14-3-3 proteins in larval *E.multilocularis* and *E.granulosus* provide different growth behaviours of AE and CE in the intermediate hosts, respectively.

8. Public health threat

To date, over five species are recognized in the genus and four species are already revealed to be involved in human diseases. The most common forms are *E. granulosis* and *E. multilocularis* responsible for CE and AE, respectively. Two other forms, namely *E. oligarthrus* and *E. vogeli* cause polycystic echinococcosis; two new species, *E. felidis* and *E. shiquicus* may also contribute to human infection, though little is known.

However, human behavioural changes with economic, technological development, and the spatial expansion of agriculture promoted encroachment into wildlife habits, driven by increasing human population, leading to ecosystem changes and bringing human, domestic animals into closer proximity to wildlife. Many recently emerged zoonoses originated in wildlife have been reported.

9. Intervention strategies

9.1. Immunological/genetic research

Many studies of echinococcosis have provided significant information on risk factors of infection, as well as on socio-economic influences and ecological determinants of parasite transmission. The new immunological/genetic research components for new therapeutic targets, in combination with standard imaging techniques, will enable rapid and efficient evaluation of echinococcosis patients. This will not only greatly assist in monitoring disease progression and treatment efficacy, but also in the development and deployment of new control strategies and disease surveillance fundamental to reducing morbidity caused by long-term chronic infection and at a low cost to the health care systems of areas where echinococcosis is endemic. Further, the genetic study aims that identification of the genes involved in disease susceptibility can provide valuable insight into the protective and pathogenic mechanisms involved in the different clinical outcomes of echinococcosis. Understanding these processes can provide novel therapeutic targets that are essential for the long-term control of the disease worldwide. A significant, but essential challenge will be to develop strategies for translating knowledge of novel susceptibility genes into improved patient outcomes from both AE and CE. Given the considerable inter-individual variation observed in susceptibility to the different clinical phenotypes and their associated clinical outcomes, it is anticipated that subtle manipulation of the host immune response will translate into clinical benefits. Genomics offers a powerful approach to dissect the relevant pathways and may offer novel therapeutic targets for new drugs against both AE and CE, which are urgently needed as the current albendazole treatment is far from satisfactory. Definition of the molecules and pathways that are important in individual patients may eventually lead to a personalised approach to care, with therapy tailored on the basis of an individual's genetic background.

9.2. Animal host intervention

Various methods for animal host interventions have been employed in echinococcosis endemic regions, for example, the culling of dogs/foxes for CE/AE, culling of rodents for AE, and the anthelminthic treatment (with praziquantel (PZQ)) of dog/foxes for CE/AE. Vaccine development has been ongoing and whilst a vaccine targeting the definitive dog/fox hosts could be a "magic bullet", all current candidates have low efficacy. A highly efficacious sheep vaccine for *E. granulosus* (Eg95) is currently under investigation but the evidence base, though growing, is not yet established for its incorporation into control programmes to date.

9.3. Comprehensive intervention and limitation

The use of geographic information system (GIS) have become more common as a tool for public health investigations due to the increase in number and quality of satellites used for terrestrial observation. These systems integrate the use of geographic positions sensors (GPS) tool for infectious disease studies, including *Echinococcus*. Spatial analysis provides an improvement in epidemiological analysis and prediction of future events. Using remote sensors for monitoring *Echinococcus* transmission, particularly *E. multilocularis*, have produced information that has showed much importance in designing a control programme. Apart from the detection of animal host assembling linking transmission dynamics due to prey-predatory relations, in terms of geological and ecological environments, prediction mapping provides geographical identification of *Echinococcus* spp. risk areas, allowing for the allocation of resources in reasonable ways/location. Linking with a mathematical model has been done in many other parasitic disease controls. It is believed to be also useful for the determination of the optimal strategies for control and/or elimination of echinococcosis in specific locations. The optimal intervention strategies can be translated into policy and practice reducing the burden of this disease, leading to improved direct health outcomes. Modelling can also be used for future economic assessments of interventions that reduce the financial impact of the disease.

To date, only five islands (Iceland, New Zealand, Tasmania, Falkland Islands, and Cyprus) have been able to successfully control echinococcosis. Control programmes were predominantly based on health education and control or elimination of home slaughter of sheep, with behaviour change, is central to their success.

Despite the range of intervention strategies, control in endemic regions of the world (especially the poor rural areas) has proved difficult, as demonstrated by the increasing number of cases over the last decade. This failure to effectively control echinococcosis can be attributed to a number of causes: 1) culling of animals has ethical challenges (e.g., use of rodenticides in NHAR resulted in the poisoning of domestic dogs); 2) PZQ is effective in killing adult *E. granulosus* and *E multilocularis* in definitive hosts, but it does not prevent reinfection in the definitive hosts; 3) existing health promotion materials are passive and may not be sufficiently engaging to bring about behaviour change at the population level; and 4) the lack of significant governmental support for control programmes.

10. Conclusion

Hydatid disease is a major cause of morbidity and mortality in many parts of the world. Although immunological research has provided important insight into the mechanisms of immunity in CE and AE, the genetic variants within the host-participating genes may be too subtle or too few to cause much effect on individual risk. The genotypic variation of *Echinococcus* species reflects phenotypic differences with important consequences in terms of increased host infectivity by local *Echinococcus* strains. Such adaptations may also result in different sensitivity to drugs or increased virulence for hosts that will impede controls efforts and even affect vaccination strategies against *Echinococcus*. The environmental factors have been correlated with transmission to humans through changes in animal population, dynamics spatial overlap of competent hosts, and the creation of improved conditions for egg survival. Therefore, echinococcosis is a complex zoonosis with sparse evidence on the effectiveness of control strategies in diverse settings despite many efforts worldwide for decades. Identifying the environmental determinants of the transmission risk to humans will be vital for the design of accurate predictive models to guide preventative public health action against echinococcosis. Mathematic modelling is a useful tool for simulating control packages under locally specific transmission conditions to inform optimal timing and frequency of phased interventions for cost-effective control of echinococcosis.

Acknowledgements

Fund support from the National Health Medical Research Councils (NHMRCs, APP1009539), Australia, and National Nature Science Foundation of China (NNSFC, 30960339).

Author details

YuRong Yang[1,2]

Address all correspondence to: yangyurong@hotmail.com

1 Ningxia Medical University, Yinchuan, Ningxia Hui Autonomous Region, P.R. of China

2 Molecular Parasitology Laboratory, QIMR Berghofer Medical Research Institute, Brisbane, Australia

References

[1] Zhang W, Ross AG, McManus DP: Mechanisms of immunity in hydatid disease: Implications for vaccine development. *Journal of immunology* 2008, 181(10):6679–6685.

[2] McManus DP, Zhang W, Li J, Bartley PB: Echinococcosis. *Lancet* 2003, 362(9392):1295–1304.

[3] Budke CM, Deplazes P, Torgerson PR: Global socioeconomic impact of cystic echinococcosis. *Emerging infectious diseases* 2006, 12(2):296–303.

[4] Brunetti E, Kern P, Vuitton DA, Writing Panel for the W-I: Expert consensus for the diagnosis and treatment of cystic and alveolar echinococcosis in humans. *Acta tropica* 2010, 114(1):1–16.

[5] Brunetti E, Junghanss T: Update on cystic hydatid disease. *Current opinion in infectious diseases* 2009, 22(5):497–502.

[6] Torgerson PR, Schweiger A, Deplazes P, Pohar M, Reichen J, Ammann RW, Tarr PE, Halkik N, Mullhaupt B: Alveolar echinococcosis: From a deadly disease to a well-controlled infection. Relative survival and economic analysis in Switzerland over the last 35 years. *Journal of hepatology* 2008, 49(1):72–77.

[7] Torgerson PR, Keller K, Magnotta M, Ragland N: The global burden of alveolar echinococcosis. *PLoS neglected tropical diseases* 2010, 4(6):e722.

[8] D'Alessandro A, Rausch RL: New aspects of neotropical polycystic (*Echinococcus vogeli*) and unicystic (*Echinococcus oligarthrus*) echinococcosis. *Clin Microbiol Rev* 2008, 21(2):380–401.

[9] Kern P: Clinical features and treatment of alveolar echinococcosis. *Curr Opin Infect Dis* 2010, 23(5):505–512.

[10] Barnes TS, Hinds LA, Jenkins DJ, Coleman GT, Colebrook AL, Kyngdon CT, Gauci CG, Lightowlers MW: Efficacy of the EG95 hydatid vaccine in a macropodid host, the tammar wallaby. *Parasitology* 2009, 136(4):461–468.

[11] Jenkins DJ, Allen L, Goullet M: Encroachment of *Echinococcus granulosus* into urban areas in eastern Queensland, Australia. *Aust Vet J* 2008, 86(8):294–300.

[12] Jenkins DJ: *Echinococcus granulosus* in Australia, widespread and doing well! *Parasitol Int* 2006, 55 Suppl:S203–206.

[13] Gottstein B: [Epidemiology and systematics of cystic and alveolar hydatid disease]. *Chirurg* 2000, 71(1):1–8.

[14] Yang YR, McManus DP, Huang Y, Heath DD: *Echinococcus granulosus* infection and options for control of cystic echinococcosis in Tibetan communities of Western Sichuan Province, China. *PLoS neglected tropical diseases* 2009, 3(4):e426.

[15] Vuitton DA, Zhou H, Bresson-Hadni S, Wang Q, Piarroux M, Raoul F, Giraudoux P: Epidemiology of alveolar echinococcosis with particular reference to China and Europe. *Parasitology* 2003, 127 Suppl:S87–107.

[16] Jimenez S, Perez A, Gil H, Schantz P, Ramalle E, Juste R: Progress in control of cystic echinococcosis in La Rioja, Spain: Decline in infection prevalences in human and animal hosts and economic costs and benefits. *Acta Trop* 2002, 83(3):213–221.

[17] Vuitton DA, Wang Q, Zhou HX, Raoul F, Knapp J, Bresson-Hadni S, Wen H, Giraudoux P: A historical view of alveolar echinococcosis, 160 years after the discovery of the first case in humans: Part 1. What have we learnt on the distribution of the disease and on its parasitic agent? *Chin Med J (Engl)* 2011, 124(18):2943–2953.

[18] Wang YH, Rogan MT, Vuitton DA, Wen H, Bartholomot B, Macpherson CN, Zou PF, Ding ZX, Zhou HX, Zhang XF *et al.*: Cystic echinococcosis in semi-nomadic pastoral communities in north-west China. *Trans R Soc Trop Med Hyg* 2001, 95(2):153–158.

[19] Barnes TS, Goldizen AW, Morton JM, Coleman GT: Cystic echinococcosis in a wild population of the brush-tailed rock-wallaby (Petrogale penicillata), a threatened macropodid. *Parasitology* 2008, 135(6):715–723.

[20] Jenkins DJ, Romig T, Thompson RC: Emergence/re-emergence of *Echinococcus* spp.—A global update. *Int J Parasitol* 2005, 35(11-12):1205–1219.

[21] Jenkins DJ: Cystic Echinococcosis in Australia: The current situation. *Southeast Asian J Trop Med Public Health* 2004, 35(1).

[22] Budke CM, Jiamin Q, Qian W, Torgerson PR: Economic effects of echinococcosis in a disease-endemic region of the Tibetan Plateau. *The American journal of tropical medicine and hygiene* 2005, 73(1):2–10.

[23] Yang YR, Craig PS, Sun T, Vuitton DA, Giraudoux P, Jones MK, Williams GM, McManus DP: Echinococcosis in Ningxia Hui Autonomous Region, northwest China. *Transactions of the Royal Society of Tropical Medicine and Hygiene* 2008, 102(4):319–328.

[24] Li T, Chen X, Zhen R, Qiu J, Qiu D, Xiao N, Ito A, Wang H, Giraudoux P, Sako Y *et al.*: Widespread co-endemicity of human cystic and alveolar echinococcosis on the

eastern Tibetan Plateau, northwest Sichuan/southeast Qinghai, China. *Acta tropica* 2010, 113(3):248–256.

[25] Craig PS, Li T, Qiu J, Zhen R, Wang Q, Giraudoux P, Ito A, Heath D, Warnock B, Schantz P *et al.*: Echinococcosis and Tibetan communities. *Emerging infectious diseases* 2008, 14(10):1674–1675.

[26] Yang YR, Liu XZ, Vuitton DA, Bartholomot B, Wang YH, Ito A, Craig PS, McManus DP: Simultaneous alveolar and cystic echinococcosis of the liver. *Transactions of the Royal Society of Tropical Medicine and Hygiene* 2006, 100(6):597–600.

[27] Zhang T, Yang D, Zeng Z, Zhao W, Liu A, Piao D, Jiang T, Cao J, Shen Y, Liu H *et al.*: Genetic characterization of human-derived hydatid cysts of *Echinococcus granulosus* sensu lato in Heilongjiang Province and the first report of G7 genotype of *E. canadensis* in humans in China. *PloS one* 2014, 9(10):e109059.

[28] Zheng Q, Vanderslott S, Jiang B, Xu LL, Liu CS, Huo LL, Duan LP, Wu NB, Li SZ, Xia ZG *et al.*: Research gaps for three main tropical diseases in the People's Republic of China. *Infectious diseases of poverty* 2013, 2(1):15.

[29] Moro P, Schantz PM: Echinococcosis: A review. *International journal of infectious diseases : IJID : official publication of the International Society for Infectious Diseases* 2009, 13(2):125–133.

[30] De U: Rare primary extrahepatic intra-abdominal hydatid cysts. *Tropical doctor* 2009, 39(3):172–175.

[31] McManus DP, Li Z, Yang S, Gray DJ, Yang YR: Case studies emphasising the difficulties in the diagnosis and management of alveolar echinococcosis in rural China. *Parasites & vectors* 2011, 4:196.

[32] Yang YR, Cheng L, Yang SK, Pan X, Sun T, Li X, Hu S, Zhao R, Craig PS, Vuitton DA *et al.*: A hospital-based retrospective survey of human cystic and alveolar echinococcosis in Ningxia Hui Autonomous Region, PR China. *Acta tropica* 2006, 97(3):284–291.

[33] Macpherson CN, Bartholomot B, Frider B: Application of ultrasound in diagnosis, treatment, epidemiology, public health and control of *Echinococcus granulosus* and *E. multilocularis*. *Parasitology* 2003, 127 Suppl:S21–35.

[34] Kern P, Wen H, Sato N, Vuitton DA, Gruener B, Shao Y, Delabrousse E, Kratzer W, Bresson-Hadni S: WHO classification of alveolar echinococcosis: principles and application. *Parasitology international* 2006, 55 Suppl:S283–287.

[35] Powanda MC, Beisel WR: Hypothesis: leukocyte endogenous mediator/endogenous pyrogen/lymphocyte-activating factor modulates the development of nonspecific and specific immunity and affects nutritional status. *The American journal of clinical nutrition* 1982, 35(4):762–768.

[36] Sailer M, Soelder B, Allerberger F, Zaknun D, Feichtinger H, Gottstein B: Alveolar echinococcosis of the liver in a six-year-old girl with acquired immunodeficiency syndrome. *The Journal of pediatrics* 1997, 130(2):320–323.

[37] Yang YR, Gray DJ, Ellis MK, Yang SK, Craig PS, McManus DP: Human cases of simultaneous echinococcosis and tuberculosis—Significance and extent in China. *Parasites & vectors* 2009, 2(1):53.

[38] Kern P, Bardonnet K, Renner E, Auer H, Pawlowski Z, Ammann RW, Vuitton DA, Kern P, European Echinococcosis R: European echinococcosis registry: Human alveolar echinococcosis, Europe, 1982-2000. *Emerging infectious diseases* 2003, 9(3):343–349.

[39] Matsaniotis N, Karpathios T, Koutoyzis J, Nicolaidou P, Fretzayas A, Papadellis F, Thomaidis T: Hydatid disease in Greek children. *The American journal of tropical medicine and hygiene* 1983, 32(5):1075–1078.

[40] Romig T, Zeyhle E, Macpherson CN, Rees PH, Were JB: Cyst growth and spontaneous cure in hydatid disease. *Lancet* 1986, 1(8485):861.

[41] Srour SF, Sayfan J: Echinococcosis of the spleen during pregnancy. *The Israel Medical Association journal : IMAJ* 2001, 3(4):290–291.

[42] Vuitton DA, Zhang SL, Yang Y, Godot V, Beurton I, Mantion G, Bresson-Hadni S: Survival strategy of *Echinococcus multilocularis* in the human host. *Parasitology international* 2006, 55 Suppl:S51–55.

[43] Kacprzak E, Stefaniak J: Evaluating the activity of liver cystic echinococcosis using the delayed-hypersensitivity skin reaction to common antigens. *Annals of tropical medicine and parasitology* 1995, 89(1):25–29.

[44] Kolligs FT, Gerbes AL, Durr EM, Schauer R, Kessler M, Jelinek T, Loscher T, Bilzer M: [52-year-old patient with subcutaneous space-occupying lesion in immunosuppression]. *Der Internist* 2003, 44(6):740–745.

[45] Bonifacino R, Carter SD, Craig PS, Almeida I, Da Rosa D: Assessment of the immunological surveillance value of humoral and lymphocyte assays in severe human cystic echinococcosis. *Transactions of the Royal Society of Tropical Medicine and Hygiene* 2000, 94(1):97–102.

[46] Rigano R, Profumo E, Ioppolo S, Notargiacomo S, Teggi A, Siracusano A: Cytokine patterns in seropositive and seronegative patients with *Echinococcus granulosus* infection. *Immunology letters* 1998, 64(1):5–8.

[47] Ortona E, Margutti P, Delunardo F, Nobili V, Profumo E, Rigano R, Buttari B, Carulli G, Azzara A, Teggi A *et al.*: Screening of an *Echinococcus granulosus* cDNA library with IgG4 from patients with cystic echinococcosis identifies a new tegumental protein involved in the immune escape. *Clinical and experimental immunology* 2005, 142(3): 528–538.

[48] Rigano R, Buttari B, De Falco E, Profumo E, Ortona E, Margutti P, Scotta C, Teggi A, Siracusano A: *Echinococcus granulosus*-specific T-cell lines derived from patients at various clinical stages of cystic echinococcosis. *Parasite immunology* 2004, 26(1):45–52.

[49] Rigano R, Ioppolo S, Ortona E, Margutti P, Profumo E, Ali MD, Di Vico B, Teggi A, Siracusano A: Long-term serological evaluation of patients with cystic echinococcosis treated with benzimidazole carbamates. *Clinical and experimental immunology* 2002, 129(3):485–492.

[50] Bresson-Hadni S, Vuitton DA, Bartholomot B, Heyd B, Godart D, Meyer JP, Hrusovsky S, Becker MC, Mantion G, Lenys D *et al.*: A twenty-year history of alveolar echinococcosis: analysis of a series of 117 patients from eastern France. *European journal of gastroenterology & hepatology* 2000, 12(3):327–336.

[51] Mondragon-de-la-Pena C, Ramos-Solis S, Barbosa-Cisneros O, Rodriguez-Padilla C, Tavizon-Garcia P, Herrera-Esparza R: *Echinococcus granulosus* down regulates the hepatic expression of inflammatory cytokines IL-6 and TNF alpha in BALB/c mice. *Parasite* 2002, 9(4):351–356.

[52] Harraga S, Godot V, Bresson-Hadni S, Mantion G, Vuitton DA: Profile of cytokine production within the periparasitic granuloma in human alveolar echinococcosis. *Acta tropica* 2003, 85(2):231–236.

[53] Rigano R, Profumo E, Bruschi F, Carulli G, Azzara A, Ioppolo S, Buttari B, Ortona E, Margutti P, Teggi A *et al.*: Modulation of human immune response by *Echinococcus granulosus* antigen B and its possible role in evading host defenses. *Infection and immunity* 2001, 69(1):288–296.

[54] Godot V, Harraga S, Beurton I, Deschaseaux M, Sarciron E, Gottstein B, Vuitton DA: Resistance/susceptibility to *Echinococcus multilocularis* infection and cytokine profile in humans. I. Comparison of patients with progressive and abortive lesions. *Clinical and experimental immunology* 2000, 121(3):484–490.

[55] Rigano R, Profumo E, Ioppolo S, Notargiacomo S, Ortona E, Teggi A, Siracusano A: Immunological markers indicating the effectiveness of pharmacological treatment in human hydatid disease. *Clinical and experimental immunology* 1995, 102(2):281–285.

[56] Daeki AO, Craig PS, Shambesh MK: IgG-subclass antibody responses and the natural history of hepatic cystic echinococcosis in asymptomatic patients. *Annals of tropical medicine and parasitology* 2000, 94(4):319–328.

[57] Dreweck CM, Luder CG, Soboslay PT, Kern P: Subclass-specific serological reactivity and IgG4-specific antigen recognition in human echinococcosis. *Tropical medicine & international health: TM & IH* 1997, 2(8):779–787.

[58] Dixon JB: Echinococcosis. *Comparative immunology, microbiology and infectious diseases* 1997, 20(1):87–94.

[59] Al-Ghoury AB, El-Hamshary EM, Azazy AA, Hussein EM, Rayan HZ: HLA class II alleles: susceptibility or resistance to cystic echinococcosis in Yemeni patients. *Parasitol Res* 2010, 107(2):355–361.

[60] Aydinli B, Pirim I, Polat KY, Gursan N, Atamanalp SS, Ezer M, Donmez R: Association between hepatic alveolar echinococcosis and frequency of human leukocyte antigen class I and II alleles in Turkish patients. *Hepatol Res* 2007, 37(10):806–810.

[61] Eiermann TH, Bettens F, Tiberghien P, Schmitz K, Beurton I, Bresson-Hadni S, Ammann RW, Goldmann SF, Vuitton DA, Gottstein B *et al.*: HLA and alveolar echinococcosis. *Tissue Antigens* 1998, 52(2):124–129.

[62] Li F, Shi Y, Shi D, Vuitton DA, Craig PS: HLA-DRB1 allele in 35 patients with alveolar echinococcosis in Gansu Province of China. *Chin Med J (Engl)* 2003, 116(10): 1557-1560.

[63] Li F, Shi Y, Shi D: [Association of HLA-DRB1 allele and the susceptibility to alveolar echinococcosis in the west of China]. *Zhonghua Yi Xue Za Zhi* 2000, 80(6):414–416.

[64] Kiper N, Gerceker F, Utine E, Yalcin E, Pekcan S, Cobanoglu N, Aslan A, Kose M, Dogru D, Ozcelik U *et al.*: TAP1 and TAP2 gene polymorphisms in childhood cystic echinococcosis. *Parasitol Int* 2010, 59(2):283–285.

[65] Zhang S, Penfornis A, Harraga S, Chabod J, Beurton I, Bresson-Hadni S, Tiberghien P, Kern P, Vuitton DA: Polymorphisms of the TAP1 and TAP2 genes in human alveolar echinococcosis. *Eur J Immunogenet* 2003, 30(2):133–139.

[66] Emery I, Leclerc C, Houin R, Vuitton DA, Liance M: Lack of H-2 gene influence on mouse susceptibility to secondary alveolar echinococcosis. *Int J Parasitol* 1997, 27(11): 1433–1436.

[67] Nakao R, Kameda Y, Kouguchi H, Matsumoto J, Dang Z, Simon AY, Torigoe D, Sasaki N, Oku Y, Sugimoto C *et al.*: Identification of genetic loci affecting the establishment and development of *Echinococcus multilocularis* larvae in mice. *Int J Parasitol* 2011, 41(11):1121–1128.

[68] Hemer S, Konrad C, Spiliotis M, Koziol U, Schaack D, Forster S, Gelmedin V, Stadelmann B, Dandekar T, Hemphill A *et al.*: Host insulin stimulates *Echinococcus multilocularis* insulin signalling pathways and larval development. *BMC biology* 2014, 12:5.

[69] McManus DP, Thompson RC: Molecular epidemiology of cystic echinococcosis. *Parasitology* 2003, 127 Suppl:S37-51.

[70] Parkinson J, Wasmuth JD, Salinas G, Bizarro CV, Sanford C, Berriman M, Ferreira HB, Zaha A, Blaxter ML, Maizels RM *et al.*: A transcriptomic analysis of *Echinococcus granulosus* larval stages: implications for parasite biology and host adaptation. *PLoS neglected tropical diseases* 2012, 6(11):e1897.

[71] Siles-Lucas M, Nunes CP, Zaha A: Comparative analysis of the 14-3-3 gene and its expression in *Echinococcus granulosus* and *Echinococcus multilocularis* metacestodes. *Parasitology* 2001, 122(Pt 3):281–287.

[72] Huttner M, Nakao M, Wassermann T, Siefert L, Boomker JD, Dinkel A, Sako Y, Mackenstedt U, Romig T, Ito A: Genetic characterization and phylogenetic position of *Echinococcus felidis* (Cestoda: Taeniidae) from the African lion. *International journal for parasitology* 2008, 38(7):861–868.

[73] Xiao N, Qiu J, Nakao M, Li T, Yang W, Chen X, Schantz PM, Craig PS, Ito A: *Echinococcus shiquicus*, a new species from the Qinghai-Tibet plateau region of China: discovery and epidemiological implications. *Parasitology international* 2006, 55 Suppl:S233–236.

[74] Jones BA, Grace D, Kock R, Alonso S, Rushton J, Said MY, McKeever D, Mutua F, Young J, McDermott J *et al.*: Zoonosis emergence linked to agricultural intensification and environmental change. *Proceedings of the National Academy of Sciences of the United States of America* 2013, 110(21):8399–8404.

[75] McManus DP, Gray DJ, Zhang W, Yang Y: Diagnosis, treatment, and management of echinococcosis. *Bmj* 2012, 344:e3866.

[76] Yang YR, Clements AC, Gray DJ, Atkinson JA, Williams GM, Barnes TS, McManus DP: Impact of anthropogenic and natural environmental changes on *Echinococcus transmission* in Ningxia Hui Autonomous Region, the People's Republic of China. *Parasites & vectors* 2012, 5:146.

[77] Yang Y, Ellis MK, McManus DP: Immunogenetics of human echinococcosis. *Trends in parasitology* 2012, 28(10):447–454.

[78] Zhang W, Zhang Z, Shi B, Li J, You H, Tulson G, Dang X, Song Y, Yimiti T, Wang J *et al.*: Vaccination of dogs against *Echinococcus granulosus*, the cause of cystic hydatid disease in humans. *The Journal of infectious diseases* 2006, 194(7):966–974.

[79] Lightowlers MW: Vaccination against hydatid disease. *Developments in biologicals* 2002, 110:81–87.

[80] Larrieu E, Herrero E, Mujica G, Labanchi JL, Araya D, Grizmado C, Calabro A, Talmon G, Ruesta G, Perez A *et al.*: Pilot field trial of the EG95 vaccine against ovine cystic echinococcosis in Rio Negro, Argentina: early impact and preliminary data. *Acta tropica* 2013, 127(2):143–151.

[81] Heath DD, Robinson C, Lightowlers MW: Maternal antibody parameters of cattle and calves receiving EG95 vaccine to protect against *Echinococcus granulosus*. *Vaccine* 2012, 30(50):7321–7326.

[82] Pleydell DR, Yang YR, Danson FM, Raoul F, Craig PS, McManus DP, Vuitton DA, Wang Q, Giraudoux P: Landscape composition and spatial prediction of alveolar

echinococcosis in southern Ningxia, China. *PLoS neglected tropical diseases* 2008, 2(9):e287.

[83] Graham AJ, Danson FM, Giraudoux P, Craig PS: Ecological epidemiology: landscape metrics and human alveolar echinocossis. *Acta tropica* 2004, 91(3):267–278.

[84] Giraudoux P, Raoul F, Afonso E, Ziadinov I, Yang Y, Li L, Li T, Quere JP, Feng X, Wang Q *et al*: Transmission ecosystems of *Echinococcus multilocularis* in China and Central Asia. *Parasitology* 2013, 140(13):1655–1666.

[85] Atkinson JA, Williams GM, Yakob L, Clements AC, Barnes TS, McManus DP, Yang YR, Gray DJ: Synthesising 30 years of mathematical modelling of *Echinococcus* transmission. *PLoS neglected tropical diseases* 2013, 7(8):e2386.

[86] Atkinson JA, Gray DJ, Clements AC, Barnes TS, McManus DP, Yang YR: Environmental changes impacting *Echinococcus* transmission: research to support predictive surveillance and control. *Global change biology* 2013, 19(3):677–688.

[87] Craig PS, McManus DP, Lightowlers MW, Chabalgoity JA, Garcia HH, Gavidia CM, Gilman RH, Gonzalez AE, Lorca M, Naquira C *et al*.: Prevention and control of cystic echinococcosis. The Lancet Infectious diseases 2007, 7(6):385–394.

[88] Heath D, Yang W, Li T, Xiao Y, Chen X, Huang Y, Yang Y, Wang Q, Qiu J: Control of hydatidosis. Parasitology international 2006, 55 Suppl:S247–252.

11

Immunotherapy Can Enhance Anthelmintic Efficacy in Alveolar Echinococcosis

Emília Dvorožňáková

Abstract

The immune response of the intermediate host with alveolar echinococcosis was investigated on mice intraperitoneally infected with *Echinococcus multilocularis* protoscoleces. The study was focused on cell-mediated immune response (dependent on interactions of T lymphocytes and macrophages), which is considered protective in alveolar echinococcosis. The immune response to *E. multilocularis* is regulated by Th1/Th2 cytokines produced by the CD4+ T lymphocyte subpopulation. Metacestode has been known for its ability to modify immune functions and suppress effective specific cell response to ensure its survival in host organism. The influence of immunomodulatory substances – muramyltripeptide (L-MTP-PE), glucan (Gl), glucan with zinc (GlZn), and transfer factor (TF) – applied alone or combined with anthelmintic albendazole (ABZ) on regulative and effector components of immunity were tested and at the same time, antiparasitic efficacy of immunomodulators was evaluated.

Keywords: *Echinococcus multilocularis*, therapy, muramyltripeptide, glucan, transfer factor

1. Introduction

The larval stage of *Echinococcus multilocularis* causes alveolar echinococcosis, the serious helminthozoonosis with a high mortality in patients with late treatment [1]. The disease is characterized by an infiltrative, tumor-like growth of the *E. multilocularis* larval cysts, affecting the liver of intermediate hosts such small mammals or man [2]. The therapy of this disease represents an important problem. The treatment with available anthelmintics (benzimidazoles, praziquantel a.o.) is long term and relatively little effective. A surgical extirpation of cysts is not always successful owing to their ability to form metastatic foci in secondarily infected organs [3, 4]. The available treatment has only parasitostatic effect and is therefore performed over many years, often through the patient's life [5]. This brings the risk of adverse reactions of drugs, among which gastrointestinal disturbances, reversible alopecia, hepatitis, proteinuria, neurological symptoms are the most frequent [5, 6], apart from a strong teratogenic effect [7]. The disadvantage of benzimidazoles consists also in irresponsiveness to treatment in some patients and recurrence of the disease after intermission of the therapy [8]. There is still no consensus regarding the effective dosage and duration of treatment [9, 10]. Moreover, the immunological status of the host, host susceptibility, and actual stage of infection influence the results of treatment [11]. The generalized immunosuppression induced by *E. multilocularis* may complicate therapy efficacy in alveolar echinococcosis. *E. multilocularis* evades the host immune response by mechanisms that protect the parasite or modify the host immunity to ensure its long-lasting survival in the host organism [12, 13]. Application of immunomodulatory substances could improve host immune status during *E. multilocularis* infection and limit the growth of the parasite. Results of alternative therapeutic strategies with use of immunomodulatory substances seem to be promising and might contribute to higher efficacy of the anti-*Echinococcus* treatment.

E. multilocularis induces parasite-specific cellular and humoral immune response in intermediate host [14]. The infection induces strong cellular immune response and production of all antibody isotypes, which are not effective in killing and elimination of parasites. Cellular immune response, leading to granulomatous infiltration of peri-parasite tissue, plays the dominant role in the fight with echinococcus [15]. Cell-mediated immune response depending on interaction of macrophages and T lymphocytes is regarded as protective against *E. multilocularis* infection [16]. On the contrary, *E. multilocularis* is able to evade host immune response or modify it to ensure its long-lasting survival in the organism of the intermediate host [12, 13]. Different activation of T cells subsets (CD4+, CD8+) and the combined Th1 and Th2 cytokine profile appear crucial for prolonged metacestode growth and survival. Regressive, as well as progressive course of the disease correlates with stadium-specific granuloma cell composition and antigen-specific T cell response [17]. An activation of Th1 CD4 T lymphocytes is connected with the control of the infection [18] and a reversion to Th2 response may contribute to long-lasting manifestation of *E. multilocularis* infection in humans [12, 19]. The *E. multilocularis* metacestode can specifically manipulate the balance between Th1 and Th2 response leading to lowered effectiveness of immune response [20]. Macrophages on the periphery of the periparasitic granuloma can produce proinflammatory cytokines continually serving as mediators of acute phase of protein secretion and fibrogenesis [14]. Granuloma generation and fibrosis can restrict larval growth, but also reduces anthelmintic drug transport to the lesion and thus may be the reason for partial or total ineffectiveness of treatment [20]. Application of immunomodulatory substances could improve the host immune status during *E. multilocularis* infection and limit the growth of the parasite. New therapeutic approaches to alveolar echinococcosis use immunomodulators to overcome patient's immunosuppression (caused by *E. multilocularis* metacestode) that complicates benzimidazole therapy. The application of cytokine IFN-γ or IL-12 together with benzimidazoles stopped the progression of disease or limited the metacestode growth [17, 21], suggesting its usefulness in therapy. However, the use of recombinant cytokines in therapy is technically and financially demanding. Therefore, new ways to support a secretion of endogenous cytokines in patients are sought.

In our study, we focused on the activity of three immunomodulators (liposomized muramyl-tripeptide, glucan with zinc, and transfer factor) in enhancing of the host antiparasite defence and the efficacy of anthelmintic albendazole treatment in alveolar echinococcosis.

2. Materials and methods

Experiments were performed on pathogen-free BALB/c mice, males, weighing 20–25 g. Mice were kept under a 12-h light/dark regime at room temperature (21±3°C) and 50–60% relative humidity on a commercial diet and water. The experimental protocols complied with the current Slovak ethics law.

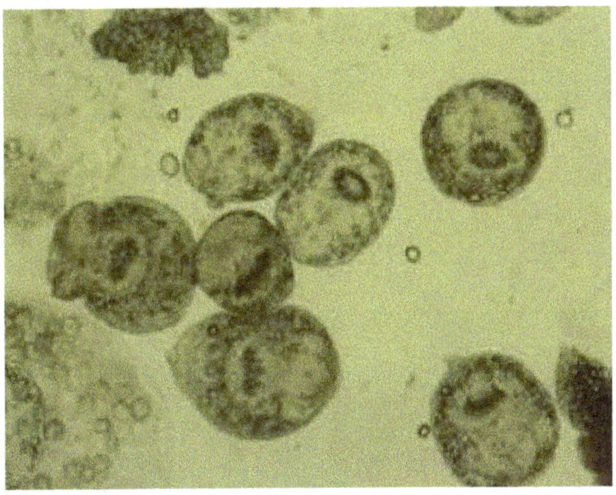

Figure 1. Protoscoleces of *Echinococcus multilocularis*.

2.1. Infection

E. multilocularis metacestode (strain provided by Department of Medical Parasitology, Clinical Institute of Hygiene and Medical Microbiology, Medical University of Vienna, Austria) was passaged in our laboratory by intraperitoneal injection of Mongolian jirds *Meriones unguiculatus*.

Parasite cysts were isolated 4 months post infection (p.i.) and cut into pieces in sterile RPMI 1640 medium (Sigma-Aldrich, Germany) supplemented with antibiotics, 100 U/ml penicillin and 100 μg/ml streptomycin (Sigma-Aldrich, Germany), and passed through a Cell Dissociation Sieve Tissue Grinder Kit using apertures ranging from 380 to 45,7 μm (Sigma-Aldrich, Germany).

Protoscoleces obtained after the last filtration were maintained in RPMI and counted for an infective dose.

2.2. Efficacy of treatment

The antiparasitic efficacy of immunotherapy was evaluated by the cyst development in infected mice. *E. multilocularis* cysts were isolated from sacrificed mice and parasite cysts were weighed and subsequently mean value ± S.D. was determined (n=3 or n=4).

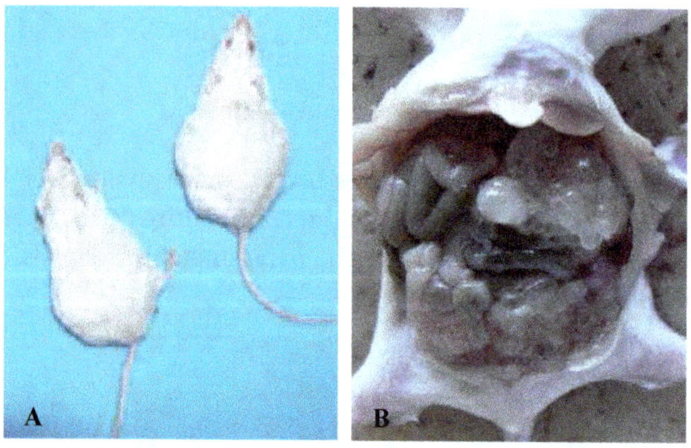

Figure 2. A – Mice infected with *E. multilocularis*. B – Cysts of *E. multilocularis* in the peritoneal cavity of an infected mouse (4th month after the infection).

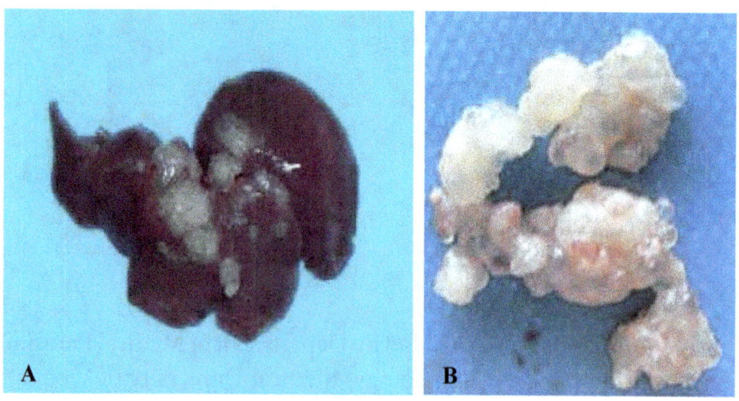

Figure 3. A – The affected liver with *E. multilocularis* cysts. B – Cysts of *E. multilocularis* isolated from the peritoneal cavity of an infected mouse (4th month after the infection).

2.3. T and B lymphocyte proliferation assay

The spleen was aseptically homogenized in phosphate-buffered saline (PBS) (pH 7.2) to obtain cells. Cell suspension was washed twice with PBS and finally with RPMI 1640 medium (Sigma-Aldrich, Germany). Erythrocytes were removed by lysis in hypotonic solution (0.85 % NH_4Cl) and lymphocytes were resuspended to a final concentration of 5×10^6 cells /ml in RPMI 1640 medium. The assay was performed in 96 wells plates (Nunc, Denmark) and cells were incubated in RPMI 1640 medium (100 μl) containing 10 % bovine fetal serum, 100 U/ml penicillin, and 100 μg/ml streptomycin. Mitogens Concanavalin A (Con A) (T cells) and lipopolysaccharide (LPS) (B cells) (Sigma-Aldrich, Germany) were added in a dose 100 μl (concentration 10 μg/ml) to the cell suspensions and incubated at 37 °C in 5 % CO_2 and 85 % humidity for 72 h. Then 20 μl of 3,4-dimethylthiazolyl 2,5-diphenyltetrazolium bromide (Sigma-Aldrich, Germany) (0.1 % solution) was added to the cell suspensions and incubated at 37 °C and 5 % CO_2 for 4 h followed by centrifugation at 800 x *g* for 5 min. Reaction was terminated with dimethylsulfoxide (Sigma-Aldrich, Germany) (100 μl/cell sample) and read on ELISA reader (Multiskan Plus, Labsystem, Finland) at 540 and 630 nm. The stimulation indices (SI) were calculated according to the formula:

SI= $E_{540} - E_{630}$ (stimulated cells) / $E_{540} - E_{630}$ (unstimulated cells)

Proliferative responses were measured separately for lymphocytes isolated from each mouse per group.

2.4. Number of CD4+ and CD8+ T cells

Lymphocytes from the spleens and depleted of erythrocytes were resuspended in PBS (pH 7.2) at a final concentration of 1x 10^6 cells /ml. Monoclonal antibodies rat anti-mouse CD4 fluorescein isothiocyanate-conjugated and rat anti-mouse CD8 phycoerythrin-conjugated monoclonal antibodies (BD Biosciences PharMingen, Belgium) were used at the concentration of 0.4 μg/10^6 cells at 4°C for 30 min. After washing in PBS three times, cells were analyzed by the FACScan flow cytometer (Becton Dickinson Biosciences, Germany) and CellQuest software. Cells from each mouse per group were analyzed individually. The final numbers of both cell populations were calculated as proportion from the total isolated lymphocytes per spleen/mouse.

2.5. Concentration of IFN-γ and IL-5 in serum

The capture ELISA was employed to determine the concentration of cytokines IFN-γ and IL-5 in serum according to the method [22]. IFN-γ and IL-5 were used as marker cytokines for the Th1 and Th2 responses, respectively. Cytokine-specific monoclonal antibodies were used, for IFN-γ detection: pure anti-mouse IFN-γ (R4-6A2) and biotin anti-mouse IFN-γ (XMG1.2); for IL-5 detection: pure anti-mouse IL-5 (TRFK5) and biotin anti-mouse IL-5 (TRF4) (all BD Biosciences PharMingen, Belgium). Results were expressed at pg/ml using murine recombinant IFN-γ and IL-5 (BD Biosciences PharMingen, Belgium) as standards. The detection limit of the assay for the both cytokines was 40 pg/ml.

2.6. Superoxide anion assay

Production of superoxide anion (O_2^-) by peritoneal macrophages was detected as superoxide dismutase (SOD) – reduction of ferricytochrome C with and without stimulation with phorbol myristate acetate (PMA) [23]. Cells were obtained by peritoneal lavage and after washing in PBS were diluted at concentration of 1 x 10^6 cells/ml in RPMI 1640 (Sigma-Aldrich, Germany).

Cell suspension (1 ml/well) was added to 24-well plate (Falcon, France) and incubated at 37 °C in 5 % CO_2 and 85 % humidity for 2 h. Nonadherent cells were removed by washing with ice-cold Earls Balanced Salt Solution (EBSS) (pH 7.2). The reaction was carried out in 0.3 ml/well of 160 μM ferricytochrome C (Sigma-Aldrich, Germany) in EBSS. In control, the reaction was immediately blocked by 300 μg SOD/10 μl in EBSS. The stimulation of cells was induced by 10 μl of PMA in ethanol. Cells were incubated at 37 °C in 5 % CO_2 and 85 % humidity for 2 h. Supernatant from wells was centrifuged at 170 x *g* for 3 min at 4 °C. The optical density (OD) of supernatant was measured at 550 nm in a 96-well plate reader (Multiscan Plus, Labsystems, Finland). Bradford protein microassay was used to determine cell-protein concentration in each well with standard reagent and bovine serum albumin as the protein standard (BioRad, UK). The OD was read at 595 nm. The resulting value was used to calculate nmol of O_2^- produced according to the formula: nmol O_2^- = $(OD_{\text{blocked by SOD}} - OD_{\text{without SOD}} /6.3) \times 100$ and determinated for 1 mg of cell proteins.

2.7. Statistical evaluation

Statistical differences were assessed using Kruskal-Wallis ANOVA and post hoc Tukey's HSD test (a value of $p<0.05$ was considered significant) in the program Statistica 6.0 (Stat Soft, Tulsa, USA) statistical package.

3. Muramyltripeptide

Muramylpeptides – components of bacterial cellular wall are classified as biological immunomodulators. Muramylpeptides primarily activate macrophages to a high production of oxygen radicals and a secretion of inflammatory cytokines, which activate neutrophils, T and B lymphocytes [24]. Muramyldipeptide (MDP) is the smallest bacterial structure with immunopotent activity. The positive effect of MDP on the host immune response was also observed in several parasitic infections [25–27]. Muramyltripeptide phosphatidylethanolamine (MTP-PE) is a lipofilic derivate of MDP. Liposome-encapsulated MTP-PE has an enhanced effect on macrophages to secrete pro-inflammatory cytokines, which results in increasing of cytotoxicity of these cells [28–30].

Affinity of liposomized forms of MTP-PE to the reticuloendotelial system, in particular to macrophages located in the liver and the spleen [30, 31], could be useful in therapy of alveolar echinococcosis, by which the parasite cysts primarily develop in the liver. The biological effect of MTP-PE takes place in Kuppfer cells in the liver (macrophage's equivalent) [32]. Macrophages activated by liposomized MTP-PE stimulate Th1 subpopulation of lymphocytes and proinflammatory mediators via cytokine secretion [28, 29, 33, 34]. T lymphocytes therefore constitute an active component of immune reactions after immunomodulation with muramylpeptides.

The effect of muramyltripeptide phosphatidylethanolamine incorporated into multilamellar liposomes (L-MTP-PE) on immune response of intermediate host infected with *E. multilocularis* was examined.

3.1. Experimental design

Experiments were carried out on male BALB/c mice (n=150) weighing 20–25 g. Mice were randomly divided into five groups as follows:

Group 1 – uninfected and untreated (control)

Group 2 – infected intraperitoneally with 5000 *E. multilocularis* protoscoleces/mouse on Day 0 and no treatment

Group 3 – *E. multilocularis* infected (as Group 2) and treated with liposomized muramyltripeptide phosphatidylethanolamine (L-MTP-PE) (Ciba-Geigy, Switzerland) intravenously (i.v.) twice a week at the dose of 1 mg/kg of body weight (b.w.) starting at weeks 5 and 6 post infection (p.i.)

Group 4 – *E. multilocularis* infected (as Group 2) and treated with albendazole (ABZ) (Sigma, Germany) per os (p.o.) twice a week at the dose of 10 mg/kg of b.w. starting at week 5 up to week 10 p.i.

Group 5 – *E. multilocularis* infected (as Group 2) and treated with combination of L-MTP-PE and ABZ as above.

Samples of blood, spleen, and peritoneal macrophages were obtained at the following weeks: 0 (prior infection), 2, 4, 8, 10, 12, 14, 18, 22, and 26 p.i. from all groups (3 mice per experimental day).

4. Results and discussion

In our experiment, the *E. multilocularis* infection induced an inhibition of the proliferative activity of T and B lymphocytes almost in the course of the whole experiment (Figures 4, 5).

However, the application of L-MTP-PE to infected mice had a positive stimulatory effect on T and B lymphocytes, especially in combination of L-MTP-PE+ABZ, where proliferative activity of lymphocytes was increased for a long time, from week 8 p.i. (2 weeks after the end of the therapy) till week 14 p.i. (lasted almost 2 months). Muramylpeptides belongs to the polyclonal activators of B lymphocytes, inducing a high proliferation and production of polyclonal antibodies. Muramyldipeptide activates B cells particularly during a late phase of their differentiation because the specific receptors for MDP are expressed on B cell surface at a definitive stage of their maturation [35].

T lymphocytes play a major role in the control of immune response in intermediate host organism infected with *E. multilocularis* [36]. In alveolar echinococcosis CD4+ T cells represent the main T subpopulation, being abundant in the first phase of the periparasitic granuloma formation and later these cells are replaced by CD8+ T cells [17]. A long-term stimulation of CD4+ T cell subpopulation after the immunotherapy could participate in antiparasite defence (to form the periparasitic granuloma) and increase its efficacy. Both L-MTP-PE alone and

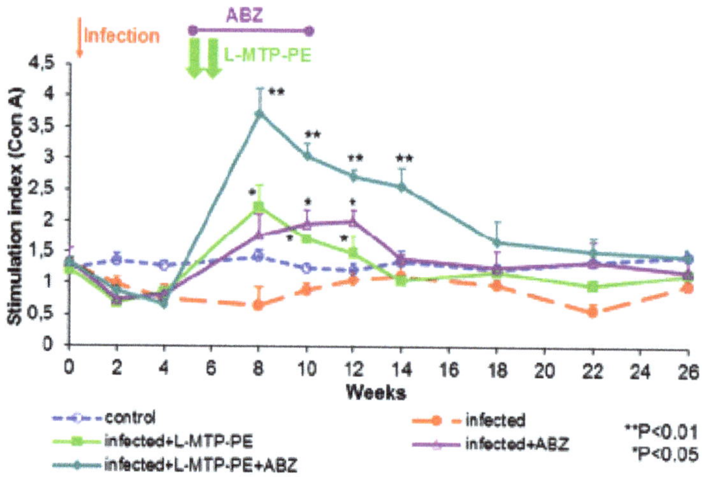

Figure 4. Proliferative activity of T lymphocytes in *E. multilocularis* infected mice after therapy L-MTP-PE+ABZ. *(p<0.05); **(p<0.01) statistically significant from infected mice.

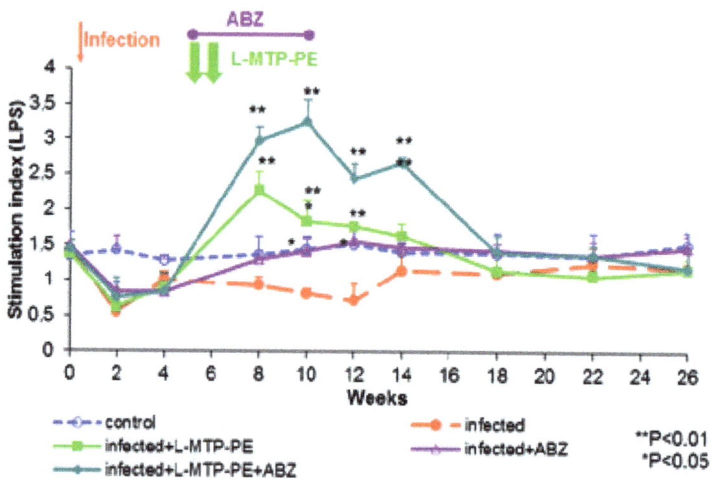

Figure 5. Proliferative activity of B lymphocytes in *E. multilocularis* infected mice after therapy L-MTP-PE+ABZ. *(p<0.05); **(p<0.01) statistically significant from infected mice.

combination of L-MTP-PE+ABZ increased the presence of CD4+ T cells in the spleen of infected mice within 6 weeks after the immunotherapy (Figure 6).

Previous experimental studies have manifested that *E. multilocularis* infection can lead to an expansion of CD8+ T cell clones [18, 37, 38]. In our study (Figure 7), the CD8+ T cells occurrence was higher for a short time in mice after therapy with L-MTP-PE than in infected and non-treated mice. Combined therapy L-MTP-PE+ABZ induced high values of CD8+ T cells, which remained increased till the end of the experiment. Splenic suppressive CD8+ T cells in alveolar

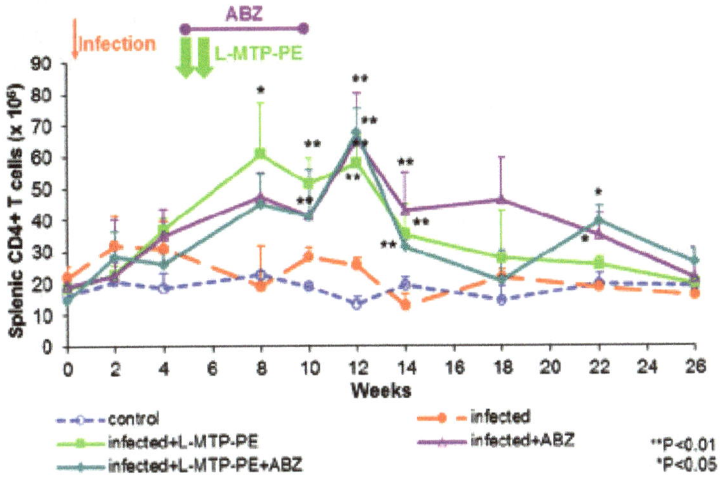

Figure 6. Number of splenic CD4 T cells in *E. multilocularis* infected mice after therapy L-MTP-PE+ABZ. *($p<0.05$); **($p<0.01$) statistically significant from infected mice.

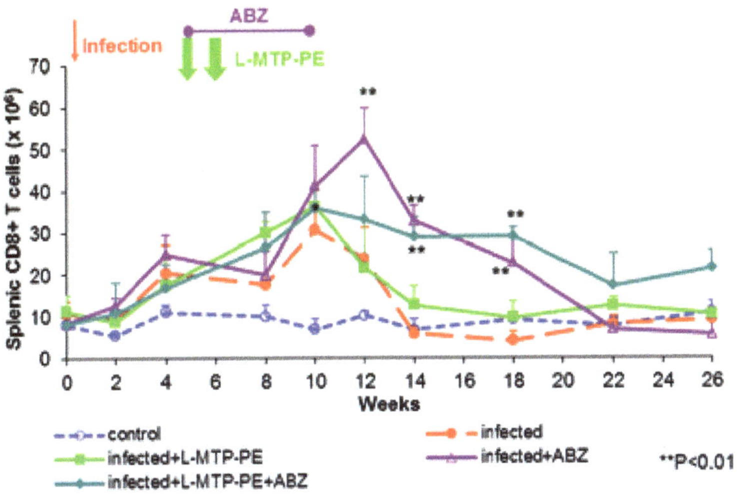

Figure 7. Number of splenic CD8 T cells in *E. multilocularis* infected mice after therapy L-MTP-PE+ABZ. **($p<0.01$) statistically significant from infected mice.

echinococcosis have a key role in modulation of immunosuppression and ensure the parasite survival in a host [20, 38]. Results in our experiment do not differentiate between cytotoxic and suppressor subtypes of CD8+ T cells and which one of them dominates. In alveolar echinococcosis, the CD8+ T splenocytes consist mostly of T suppressors with a low density of the CD8 antigen [37]. In our experiment, the immunotherapy suppressed the proliferation of *E. multilocularis* cysts and therefore we suppose L-MTP-PE could increase the occurrence of cytotoxic CD8+ T cells. Immunomodulator L-MTP-PE has also stopped a decrease of the CD4/

CD8 ratio and the CD4/CD8 index was stabilized over 2.00. This reflects that CD4+ T lymphocytes were in the majority despite the increased values of CD8+ T lymphocytes. CD4+ T cells together with macrophages and IFN-γ actively participate in parasite's destruction [39].

In many parasitic infections, the clinical outcome of the disease is associated with Th1 or Th2 cell activation. *E. multilocularis* metacestode is able to direct a host immune response to a less efficient, "tolerant" Th2 profile [20, 40]. In [34, 41] it was found that liposomized immunomodulators induce a development of splenic Th1 lymphocyte subpopulation. The dominance of Th1 response is important in defensive reactions of a host infected with *E. multilocularis*. IFN-γ is an important activator of macrophages and affects their energetic system [21]. In our study (Figure 8), the level of IFN-γ peaked after L-MTP-PE+ABZ therapy from weeks 8 to 18 p.i. (i.e., almost 3 months), which outlines an important credit of common administration of immunomodulators and anthelmintic drugs for therapy of alveolar echinococcosis. The protective effect of combined therapy L-MTP-PE+ABZ was the most evident during the time with IFN-γ stimulation (lasting 3 months after the therapy), manifesting in breaking of parasite's development (Figure 11).

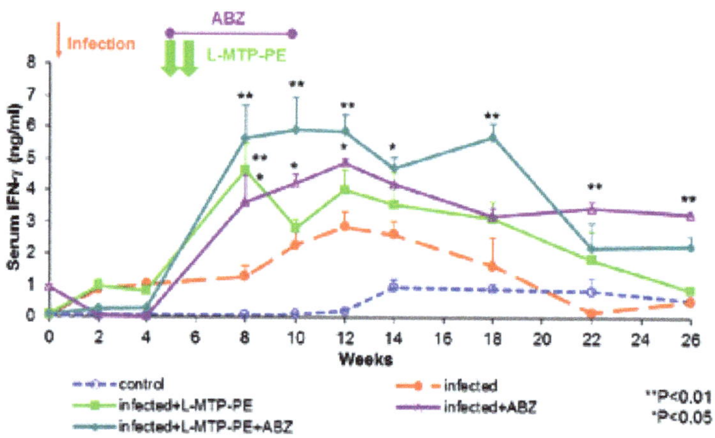

Figure 8. Serum IFN-γ in *E. multilocularis*-infected mice after therapy L-MTP-PE+ABZ. *(p<0.05); **(p<0.01) statistically significant from infected mice.

Liposomized MTP-PE suppressed the Th2 response, associated with a progressive development of larval cysts in *E. multilocularis* infection. In our experiment, the Th2 response was suppressed in mice treated with L-MTP-PE; we recorded almost twofold reduction of IL-5 production (Figure 9) during the whole experiment. We observed a total IL-5 cytokine suppression in mice treated with combined therapy L-MTP-PE+ABZ. The cytokine IL-5 is related to eosinophilia, IgE production, and may induce allergic reactions of the disease [19, 42, 43]. The therapeutic regime of L-MTP-PE in our experiment was timed on the first stage of the *E. multilocularis* infection, which is characterized by secretion of Th1 cytokines IL-2 and IFN-γ [20]. In this early phase of the infection, Th2 response has not been activated in substantial extent. Th2 response decreases a synthesis of proinflammatory Th1 cytokine IFN-γ by antagonistic IL-10 secretion and by inhibited IL-12 production in macrophages [44, 45]. Therefore, there is a higher possibility of an activation of protective Th1 response by immunomodulator before the stage when an expansive metacestode growth takes place (approx. from week 8 p.i.).

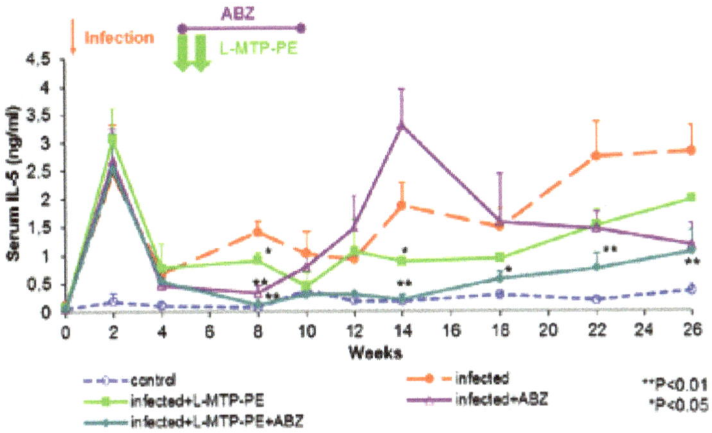

Figure 9. Serum IL-5 in *E. multilocularis* infected mice after therapy L-MTP-PE+ABZ. *(p<0.05); **(p<0.01) statistically significant from infected mice.

Macrophages participate in the destruction of the parasite through synthesis of O_2^- and other free radicals and, together with T cells, control the parasite development [39]. In our experiment (Figure 10), therapy L-MTP-PE stimulated O_2^- generation in infected mice from weeks 8 to 12 p.i. (i.e. for 1 month). The combination of L-MTP-PE+ABZ significantly increased the superoxide production from weeks 8 to 18 p.i. (almost for 3 months).

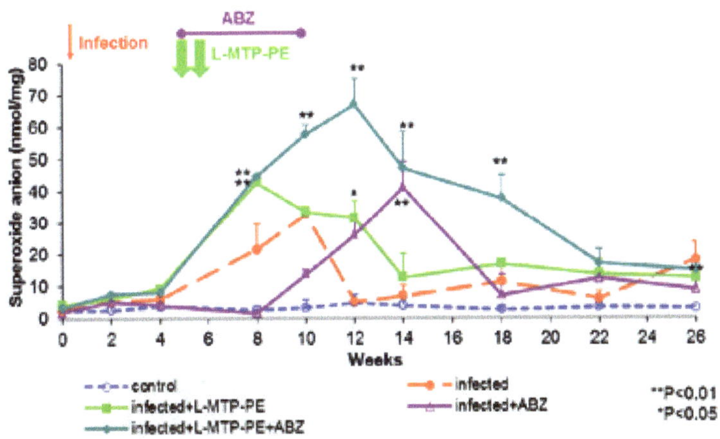

Figure 10. Macrophage's activity in *E. multilocularis* infected mice after therapy L-MTP-PE+ABZ. *(p<0.05); **(p<0.01) statistically significant from infected mice.

It documents a long-term and strong activation of macrophage's metabolism accompanied with a huge release of other biologically effective substances. In parallel, the proliferative activity of B cells was also increased, which could be related to macrophages' stimulation induced by B cell secrets [46]. Positive effect of L-MTP-PE on macrophages had been confirmed in immunosuppressed mice [25], in which the immunomodulator induced a macrophages restoration. An induction of cytotoxicity of liver macrophages against tumor cells after stimulation with L-MTP-PE was observed [28]. In addition, an increased tumoricidal activity of Kupffer cells in mice after application of L-MTP-PE was recorded [47]. Their results were later corroborated in the work [48], which described an activation of Kupffer cells with an increased production of superoxide anion and subsequent reduction of micrometastases in rats after MTP-PE therapy.

Macrophages' stimulation *in situ* is selectively influenced by a way of application of liposomized immunomodulator, and also by other biological substances. In [49], L-MTP-PE administered alone stimulated peritoneal macrophages with less effect than after coincubation of macrophages with L-MTP-PE and IFN-γ together, which doubled their cytotoxic activity. The synergetic and potentiating effect of IFN-γ in the immunomodulatory acting was also verified on macrophages infected with *Listeria monocytogenes* [50], in mice infected with *Klebsiella pneumoniae* [34]. These data confirmed an important role of T cells in immune activation of the host organism after the immunomodulator administration.

Potentiation of effector components of the immunity after the immunomodulation and anthelmintic therapy of *E. multilocularis* infected mice in our experiment resulted in a restriction of the parasite development and reduced larval cysts in a host organism (Figure 11). The immunomodulator L-MTP-PE administered alone slowed down *E. multilocularis* proliferation till week 14 p.i. and combination of L-MTP-PE+ABZ reduced the parasite development till week 22 p.i. (i.e., 3 months after the end of the experiment). A similar synergism of liposomized MDP and antiparasitic drug Glucantime was observed in visceral leishmaniasis [51].

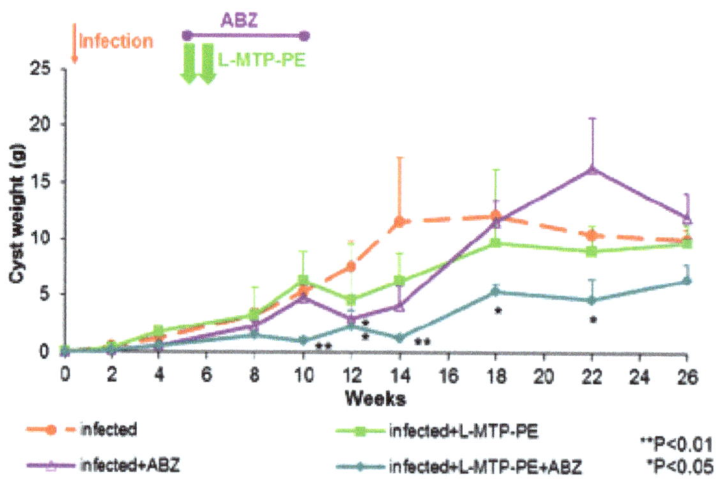

Figure 11. Cyst's weight in *E. multilocularis* infected mice after therapy L-MTP-PE+ABZ. *(p<0.05); **(p<0.01) statistically significant from infected mice.

In conclusion, our results show the possibility to increase antiparasitic efficacy of ABZ in *E. multilocularis* infection with L-MTP-PE, which properly stimulates the host immune response. Combined therapy L-MTP-PE+ABZ positively increased CD4+ T cells numbers and cytokine production that regulate the host immune response. The immunotherapy suppressed the Th2 response and *vice versa* activated the Th1 response with a restrictive impact on the parasite development. The immunomodulator L-MTP-PE stimulated macrophages' metabolism to produce reactive oxygen substances and together with IFN-γ increased an antiparasitic efficacy of albendazole.

5. Glucan and zinc

Glucans are β-(1,3)-D polymers of glucose occuring naturally as the basic component of the cell walls of bacteria, fungi, and yeast [52–54]. Glucans activate mainly nonspecific stimulation of the immune system [22], particularly proliferation and functional activity of phagocytic cells (macrophages, NK cells) as the part of innate immunity [55, 56], but also have an influence on specific immunity – increase of the T-lymphocyte activity and production of circulating antibodies [57–59]. The immunostimulative effect of glucan could be increased by its combination with the other components – immunoglobulin G, zinc, or vitamin C [60, 61]. Zinc interacts with cytokines and proteases and indirectly influences the immune system [62]. Its immunostimulative effect on T lymphocytes, macrophages has been known [63–65] and so zinc could potentiate the immunostimulative effect of the glucan during therapy of alveolar echinococcosis. Also living *Echinococcus* needs zinc for growth and its reproduction [66]. An obvious association between serum zinc concentration and disease severity in patients with alveolar echinococcosis was confirmed in [67]. Decreased zinc concentration in progressive cases may be a consequence of enhanced immune activation and also consumption of zinc by the growing parasite. Zinc deficiency in the host may thus contribute to the observed immunosupression in alveolar echinococcosis.

The role of glucan immunomodulator (GI, soluble β-(1,3)-D glucan) and/or glucan immunomodulator supplemented with zinc (GIZn) in stimulation of a host defence mechanism against *E. multilocularis* infection and the immunomodulator's effect on albendazole antiparasitic efficacy was observed.

5.1. Experimental design

Experiments were carried out on male BALB/c mice (n=220) weighing 20–25 g. Mice were divided randomly into five groups as folows:

Group 1 – uninfected and untreated (control)

Group 2 – infected intraperitoneally with 5000 *E. multilocularis* protoscoleces/mouse on Day 0 and no treatment

Group 3 – *E. multilocularis* infected (as Group 2) and treated with albendazole (ABZ) (Sigma, Germany) per os (p.o.) twice a week at the dose of 10 mg/kg of b.w. starting at week 5 up to week 10 p.i.

Group 4 – *E. multilocularis* infected (as Group 2) and treated with ABZ (as above) and glucan immunomodulator (GI) (Dimenzia, Slovak Republic) twice a week at the dose of 5 mg/kg b.w. at weeks 5 and 6 p.i.

Group 5 – *E. multilocularis* infected (as Group 2) and treated with ABZ (as above) with glucan supplied with zinc (GIZn) (Mevac, Slovak Republic) twice a week at the dose of 5 mg/kg b.w. at weeks 5 and 6 p.i.

Samples of blood, spleen, and peritoneal macrophages were obtained at the following weeks: 0 (prior infection), 2, 4, 6, 8, 10, 12, 14, 18, 22, and 26 p.i. from all groups (four mice per experimental day).

6. Results and discussion

The *Echinococcus multilocularis* infection in our experiment inhibited the proliferative activity of T and B lymphocytes within 26 weeks of the experiment (Figures 12, 13), with the minimum at weeks 2 and 4 p.i., that is, in the early stage of infection, during the time important for the parasite establishment. These data correlate to results of other authors [17, 68] and it could be caused by immunosuppressive factors released by protoscoleces of *E. multilocularis*. The T cell proliferation (Figure 12) was stimulated in infected mice with GI+ABZ therapy from week 6 to 10 p.i., at the beginning of the progressive larval growth in infected mice without treatment. The GI stimulatory activity was prolonged for 4 weeks by zinc supplementation in GIZn immunomodulator. This confirms an important role for zinc in immune response, specifically lymphocyte proliferation induced by mitogens. T-cell division, maturation, and differentiation require an adequate zinc content [65, 69]. Even after ABZ therapy, the proliferative activity of T lymphocytes was increased during drug's administration, from week 6 to 12 p.i., similarly to another works [68, 70]. The modulatory effect of albendazole could be derived from the fact that a drug induces direct morphological and structural changes of parasite cysts walls and protoscoleces [71], which lead to the revealing of normally unexposed structural antigens, which are presented to T lymphocytes. It results in inducing a Th2 response (chronic antigen stimulation) or a Th1 response (small parasitic lesions or reduced antigen output/recognition) [72]. The positive synergistic effect of anthelmintic ABZ and immunomodultor GIZn resulted in a prolonged increased T cell proliferation for 8 weeks after the end of drug's administration.

Immunomodulators GI and GIZn did not induce such stimulative effect on B cell proliferation (Figure 13); they restored a suppressed proliferative activity of B cells only for a short time. The similar restoring effect of glucan was observed in other parasitic infections with *Ascaris suum* or *Toxocara canis* [60, 73–75]. The weaker influence of GIZn on B cells could be explained by the fact that severe zinc deficiency impairment of B cell function is rarely seen [76, 77] and also the humoral response of patients with progressive alveolar echinococcosis was not affected by zinc deficiency [67]. Both combined therapies GI+ABZ and GIZn+ABZ reinforced

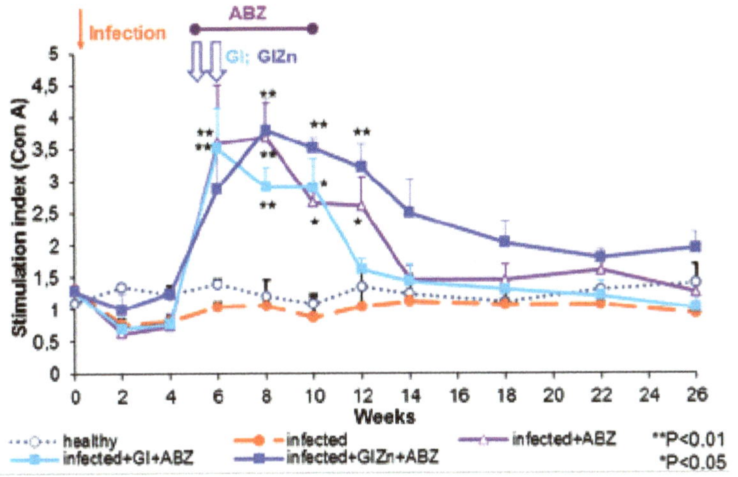

Figure 12. Proliferative activity of T lymphocytes in *E. multilocularis* infected mice after immunotherapy with GI or GIZn. *(p<0.05); **(p<0.01) statistically significant from infected mice.

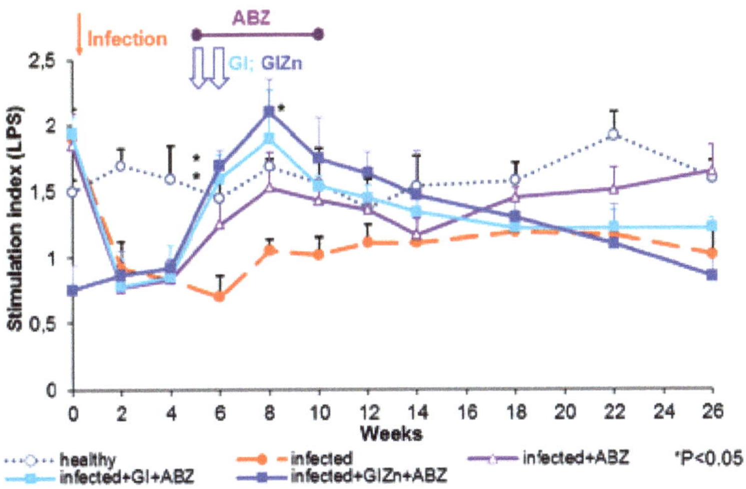

Figure 13. Proliferative activity of B lymphocytes in *E. multilocularis* infected mice after immunotherapy with GI or GIZn. *(p<0.05) statistically significant from infected mice.

a stimulatory activity of ABZ on B cell subpopulation from week 6 to 14 p.i., during the intensive cyst's growth in infected mice without treatment. The functional activity of T lymphocytes in cellular response to *E. multilocularis* infection is associated with two subpopulations of CD4+ and CD8+ T cells. A time-dependent supression of T cell proliferative response was observed in [78], and authors also recorded *in vitro* CD4 T cells' decrease and *vice versa* CD8 T cells' increase in splenocytes after activation with *E. multilocularis* protoscoleces.

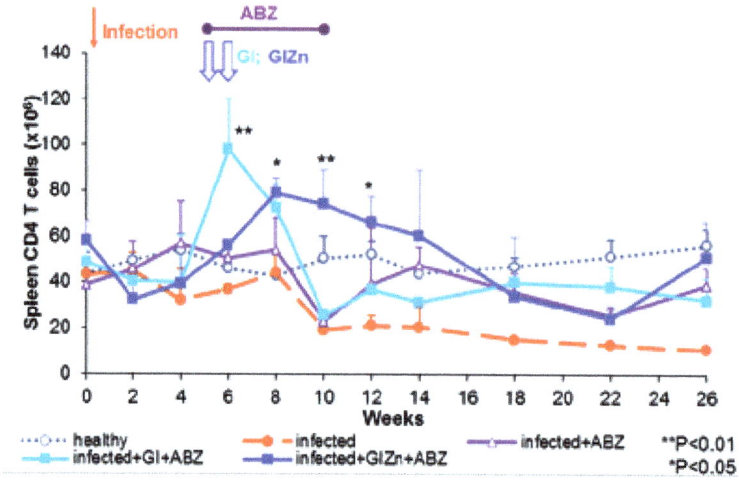

Figure 14. Number of splenic CD4 T cells in *E. multilocularis* infected mice after immunotherapy with GI or GIZn. *(p<0.05); **(p<0.01) statistically significant from infected mice.

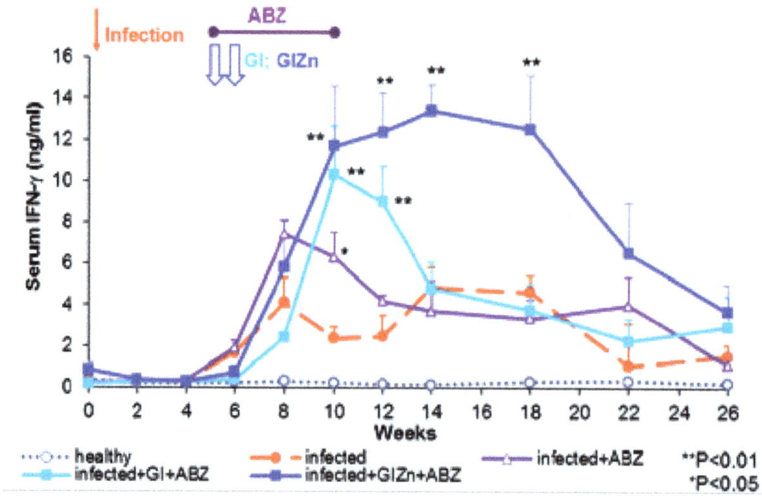

Figure 15. Serum IFN-γ in *E. multilocularis* infected mice after immunotherapy with GI or GIZn. *(p<0.05); **(p<0.01) statistically significant from infected mice.

CD4 T cells represent the main T subpopulation in the first phase of alveolar echinococcosis in granuloma formation around the parasite [17, 79]. In our experiment (Figure 14), the presence of CD4 T cells was stimulated from weeks 6 to 8 p.i. in the spleen of mice infected and treated with GI+ABZ. Supplementation of glucan with zinc could contributed to prolong an increase in the CD4 T cell subpopulation in mice treated with GIZn+ABZ from week 6 to 14 p.i. It has been known that zinc deficiency reduces the production of IL-4 cytokine acting

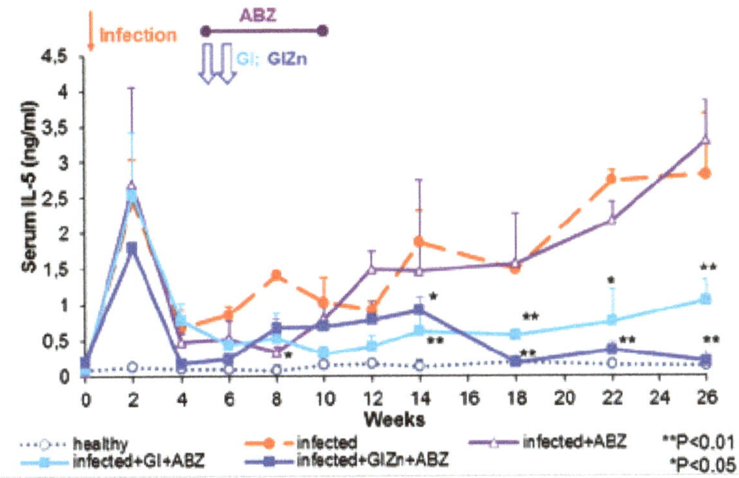

Figure 16. Serum IL-5 in *E. multilocularis* infected mice after immunotherapy with GI or GIZn. *(p<0.05); **(p<0.01) statistically significant from infected mice.

as a growth factor for helper CD4 T cells [80]. The long-term stimulation of CD4 T cells after GIZn+ABZ therapy could increase antiparasite defence. Periparasitic granuloma in regressive alveolar echinococosis is composed of great numbers of CD4 T lymphocytes, macrophages, and myofibroblasts [81]. In patients with progressive disease, the CD8 T lymphocytes are dominant [82]. In our experiment, *E. multilocularis* infection did not induce serious changes in T cells. The CD8 T lymphocytes were not influenced by immunotherapy, except for a light growth in the CD8 T cell numbers at weeks 12 and 14 p.i. in mice infected and treated with GIZn+ABZ, which could be helpful in the development of immunosuppression of the host.

The Th1 and Th2 cytokine balance regulates the immune response to *E. multilocularis* [19]. The possible effect of the immunotherapy on the Th1/Th2 balance was evaluated according to serum levels of cytokines IFN-γ and IL-5. GIZn+ABZ therapy stimulated the level of serum IFN-γ with the strongest and longest effect in mice with *E. multilocularis* infection from week 8 to 22 p.i. (Figure 15). This result documents the positive effect of GIZn immunomodulator on preferential Th1 stimulation. Immunomodulators GI and GIZn decreased the serum level of IL-5 from week 6 p.i. (Figure 16). The strong Th2 downregulative effect of both glucan immunomodultors stopped the rise of IL-5 (recorded in mice infected and without the treatment) from week 14 p.i till the end of the experiment.

IFN-γ is widely recognized as a major priming signal for macrophages' activation, which have a key role in effector phase of immune response to *E. multilocularis.* Macrophages provide for the protoscoleces destruction by reactive oxygen metabolites production (superoxide anion, hydrogenperoxide) [20]. The activation of peritoneal macrophages in the course of therapy was evaluated by generation and release of superoxide anion (O_2^-). Although the most increase in IFN-γ serum level in our experiment was found after GIZn therapy, GI had the strongest impact on O_2^- release (Figure 17). Both GI+ABZ and GIZn+ABZ therapies resulted in the huge generation of O_2^- from week 12 to 18 p.i., but with lower values in mice treated with GIZn+ABZ.

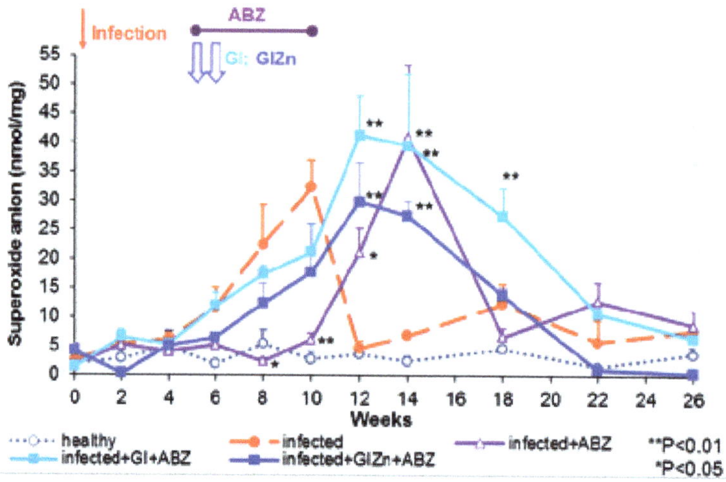

Figure 17. Macrophages' activity in *E. multilocularis* infected mice after immunotherapy with GI or GIZn. *($p<0.05$); **($p<0.01$) statistically significant from infected mice.

A notable finding in the treatment efficacy was that GI's presence in GI+ABZ therapy partly inhibited the parasitostatic effect of ABZ (Figure 18).

It could be explained by GI's stimulatory effect on fibrosis in periparasitic granuloma, which could inhibit anthelmintic drug from penetrating to parasite vesicle. The glucan's profibrotic activity in metacestode infection *Mesocestoides corti* was found in [83], where glucan therapy stimulated mononuclear-phagocytic cells in the liver followed by increased fibrotic process around parasite's larvae. In our experiment, GIZn+ABZ therapy was evaluated as the most effective therapeutic approach to alveolar echinococcosis, because it stopped larval cyst's growth in the host till week 14 p.i. This coincides with the highest levels of IFN-γ in our experiment – the cytokine with an antifibrotic property [21]. Cytokine IFN-γ plays a key role in the regulation of collagen metabolism and might ameliorate liver fibrogenesis. Also in [84] it was documented that IFN-γ downregulated lysyl oxidase gene expression, an essential catalyst for the cross-linking of extracellular collagen and elastin.

In our experiment, the stimulation of IFN-γ production induced by GIZn could reduce the irreversible fibrosis in periparasitic granuloma and thus allow penetration of anthelmintics to larvocyst. IFN-γ has not only an antifibrotic property, but it is also engaged in Th1 immune reactions, which are protective against *E. multilocularis* and include fibrogenesis. A correlation of T cell immune response and hepatic fibrosis was found in [85]; serum IFN-γ levels were negatively correlated with serological markers of fibrosis. Another immunological component connected with fibrogenesis appear to be reactive oxygen metabolites produced by macrophages. Superoxide anion, hydrogenperoxide, and hydroxyl radical are important stimuli to colagen gene induction of hepatic stellate cells (HSC) [86]. Collagen synthesis and subsequent cross-linking of collagen by pyridinoline, leading to irreversible fibrosis in periparasitic granuloma, is a substantial component of the host immune reaction in forming a resistance against parasite growth [87]. Therefore, the stimulation of fibrotic process could be beneficial

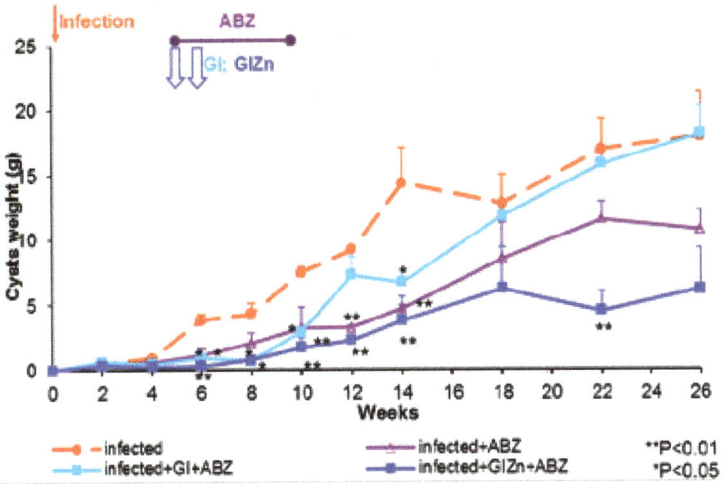

Figure 18. Cyst's weight in *E. multilocularis* infected mice after immunotherapy with GI or GIZn. *(p<0.05); **(p<0.01) statistically significant from infected mice.

for the host. On the contrary, overproduction of fibrous tissue may be harmful for host, as fibrosis results in many complications of alveolar echinococcosis in patients: vasculary and biliary obstructions in the liver [88]. In our experiment, the greatest inducer of O_2^- generation in peritoneal macrophages (connected with hepatic fibrosis) was GI. On the other hand, GI supplemented with zinc induced a short-time and a weaker production of this metabolite.

Zinc plays an important role as cofactor of enzymes involved in collagen synthesis [89] and zinc supplemention has favorable inhibitive effects on hepatic fibrosis [90, 91]. This fact can explain better the antiparasitic efficacy of treatment with GIZn and nearly twofold higher efficacy of GIZn+ABZ therapy in comparison with ABZ treatment (Figure 18).

According to host's immunosuppression and zinc deficiency in patients with alveolar echinococcosis [67], the combination of immunomodulator GIZn and anthelmintic drug ABZ achieved the most effective control of the parasite infection. The parasitostatic effect of therapy GIZn+ABZ lasted for the longest time; also after the end of the therapy it reached the greatest reduction of *E. multilocularis* cysts in the host. Zinc supplemention of glucan immunomodulator improved its immunostimulatory effects on cellular immunity, which activated Th1 response and significantly stimulated IFN-γ cytokine synthesis. We suppose zinc positively downregulated the liver fibrosis induced by glucan, because GIZn immunomodulator suppressed the generation of superoxide – an activator of hepatic stella cells involved in the fibrotic process.

7. Transfer factor

The dialysable leucocyte extract, a product of the immune system, is known as transfer factor (TF). Transfer factors are low molecular weight dialysable products extracted from immune cells which transmit the ability to express delayed-type hypersensitivity and cell-mediated immunity from sensitized donors to nonimmune recipients [92]. TF increases macrophage activation and IL-1, IL-2, and IFN-γ production *in vitro* and enhances leucocyte chemotaxis and natural killer function [93, 94]. The TF preparates activated the proliferation of splenocytes from animals with hypothyroidism [95] and stimulated hemopoiesis [96]. Transfer factor stimulated antigen-specific cell-mediated response in patients with various infections, and so administration of transfer factor has been recommended for patients with selective deficits in cell-mediated immunity such as refractory neoplasms and chronic infections [94]. Administration of dialysable leucocyte extract has been shown to be free of hypersensitivity, long-lasting side effects or complications, except for transitory hyperpyrexia.

Nonspecific transfer factor (TF) from the blood leukocytes of immunized swine was studied as an appropriate candidate for immunotherapy, supplementing conventional ABZ treatment of alveolar echinococcosis.

7.1. Experimental design

Experiments were carried out on male BALB/c mice (n=165) weighing 20–25 g. Mice were randomly divided into five groups as follows:

Group 1 – uninfected and untreated (control)

Group 2 – infected intraperitoneally with 5000 *E. multilocularis* protoscoleces/mouse on Day 0 and no treatment

Group 3 – *E. multilocularis* infected (as Group 2) and treated with transfer factor (TF) (Imunor, ImunomedicA, Czech Republic) per os (p.o.) twice a week at the dose of 200 μg/kg of body weight (b.w.) starting at week 5 up to week 10 p.i.

Group 4 – *E. multilocularis* infected (as Group 2) and treated with albendazole (ABZ) (Sigma, Germany) per os (p.o.) twice a week at the dose of 10 mg/kg of b.w. starting at week 5 up to week 10 p.i.

Group 5 – *E. multilocularis* infected (as Group 2) and treated with combination of TF and ABZ as above

Samples of blood, spleen, and peritoneal macrophages were obtained at the following weeks: 0 (prior infection), 2, 4, 6, 8, 10, 12, 14, 18, 22, and 26 p.i. from all groups (3 mice per experimental day).

8. Results and discussion

Transfer factors (TFs) are proteins that transfer specific cellular immunity from an immune donor to a nonimmune recipient and possess a number of nonspecific activities, such as the ability to increase the numbers of immunocompetent cells, to stimulate phagocytosis, to induce the production of interferons and interleukins, to stimulate hemopoiesis, etc. TF includes a lot of molecules, acting as antigens (MW cca 5 kDa), or acting as immunomodulators (less than 3.5 kDa) [97]. Transfer factors are very efficient in diseases in which cellular immunity plays an important role in protection and control of the disease, for example, viral, bacterial, and parasite infections, as well as immunodeficiencies and some types of cancer [98].

The host cellular immunity plays a principal role in the control of the *E. multilocularis* proliferation, which was documented by experiments, in which mouse strains not developing cellular immune response do not control metacestode growth, while mice deficient in humoral immunity control parasite growth up to a certain level [99]. Furthermore, T-cell immunity significantly contributes to the control of alveolar echinococcosis in human patients, demonstrated by the rapid fatal outcome of the infection in an immunodeficient patient coinfected with human immunodeficiency virus (HIV) [100]. Upon restoration of CD4-immunocomptence in another AIDS-patient coinfected with *E. multilocularis*, the course of disease was positively influenced again [101].

In our work, both the therapy with TF or combination of TF+ABZ abolished a suppressory impact of *E. multilocularis* infection on T- and B-cell proliferation (Figures 19, 20) and the therapeutic stimulatory effect was recorded up to week 14 p.i., that is, one month after the end of the therapy. Immunomodulating activity of TF on lymphocyte functional status was also recorded by [95], who detected an increased proliferation of splenocytes from rats with hypothyroidism induced by TF. A significant stimulative effect of TF on T- and B-cell populations was also confirmed in experimental ascariasis in pigs [63].

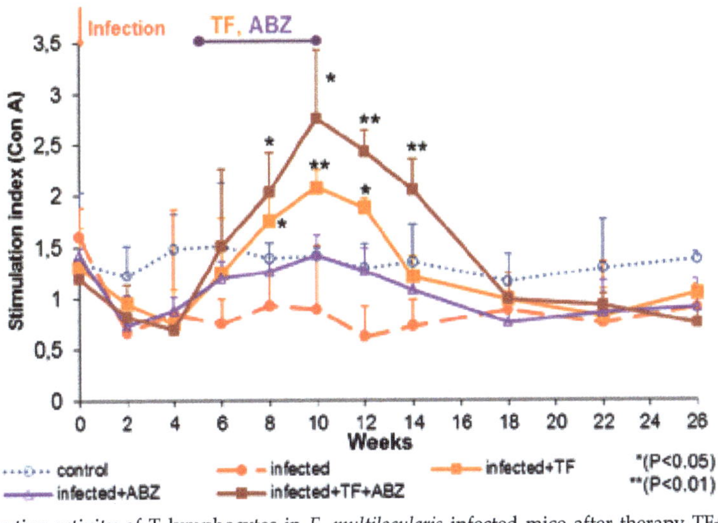

Figure 19. Proliferative activity of T lymphocytes in *E. multilocularis* infected mice after therapy TF+ABZ. *(p<0.05); **(p<0.01) statistically significant from infected mice.

T lymphocytes play a key role in the control of immune response in alveolar echinococcosis [18, 36]. In our study, the administration of TF alone or in combination of TF+ABZ caused the increase in numbers of CD4+ T cells in the spleen of infected mice up to week 14 p.i. (Figure 21). Patients with active alveolar echinococcosis showed increased numbers of CD8+ T lymphocytes [20] and also our results documented an increase in this subpopulation after *E.*

multilocularis infection from weeks 4 to 8 p.i., that is, during the massive proliferation of larval cysts. The CD8+ T cells were not markedly influenced with TF immunomodulator, because all therapeutic approaches inhibited the CD8+ T cell numbers during drug administration, from weeks 6 to 10 p.i., but with no effect after the end of therapies. The splenic CD8+ T subpopulation in alveolar echinococcosis are mostly T suppressor cells [78]. Therefore, we deduce that TF therapy stopped the development of host immunosuppression only for a short time, during the drug administration. The increase in CD4+ T lymphocytes induced by TF was also observed in viral infection (herpes zoster) and CD8+ T lymphocytes showed less decrease [102], similar to our results.

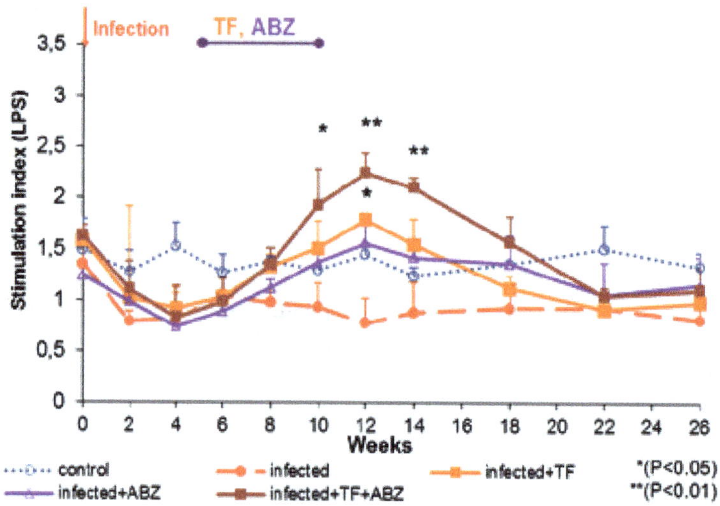

Figure 20. Proliferative activity of B lymphocytes in *E. multilocularis* infected mice after therapy TF+ABZ. *(p<0.05); **(p<0.01) statistically significant from infected mice.

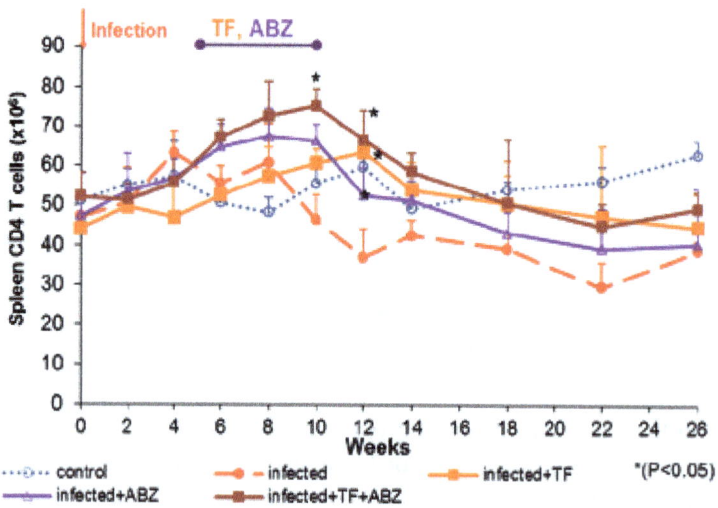

Figure 21. Number of splenic CD4 T cells in *E. multilocularis* infected mice after therapy TF+ABZ. *(p<0.05) statistically significant from infected mice.

Active alveolar echinococcosis is related to Th2 response – dominance of IL-5 and IL-10 and week production of IFN-γ [20]. The superiority of Th1 response plays a key role in the host defence reactions against *E. multilocularis*. TF therapy selectively affects cytokine production in response to antigen stimulation, particularly by secreting IFN-γ [93]. In our experiment, the results of cytokine proteins detected by capture ELISA may not correlate with the levels of bioactive cytokine protein. ELISA may utilize anticytokine antibodies that cannot discriminate between the precursor (inactive) and mature (bioactive) forms of a cytokine protein. Moreover, an ELISA may detect partially degraded cytokine proteins, which have retained their immunoreactive properties but may have lost their bioactivity [103, 104]. But capture ELISA is a helpful indicator of cytokine presence, although it does not reflect the biological potency of the detected cytokines.

The concentration of serum IFN-γ in mice infected with *E. multilocularis* and treated with TF or both TF+ABZ (Figure 22) was increased during therapy and also for one month after therapy (from weeks 6 to 14 p.i.). The stimulative effect of TF on Th1 response, particularly together with drug TF+ABZ, was observed in IFN-γ production *in vitro* [105], where high release of this cytokine from splenocytes was found till the end of the experiment. Similar results were achieved in mice with tuberculosis and treated with TF and antibiotics [98]. Th1-inducing effect of TF was also confirmed in antitumour immunotherapy [92]. The concentration of IL-5 in serum in mice infected with *E. multilocularis* and treated with TF or TF+ABZ in our work was suppressed till the end of the experiment. This is consistent with an inhibited production of IL-5 *in vitro* after immunotherapy with TF and TF+ABZ [105], which was significantly decreased two weeks after the end of the therapy. The intensive Th2 downregulative effect of TF was found by [93], who detected low splenocytes secretion of IL-10 and no IL-4. This cytokine IL-5 modulates eosinophilia, IgE production, and can enhance allergic reactions of the disease [20].

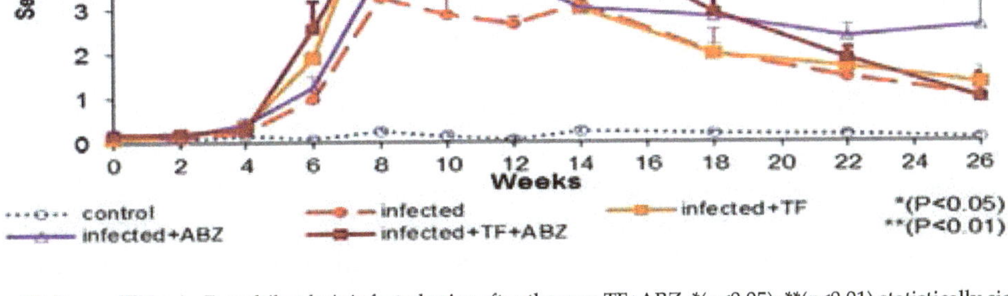

Figure 22. Serum IFN-γ in *E. multilocularis* infected mice after therapy TF+ABZ. *(p<0.05); **(p<0.01) statistically significant from infected mice.

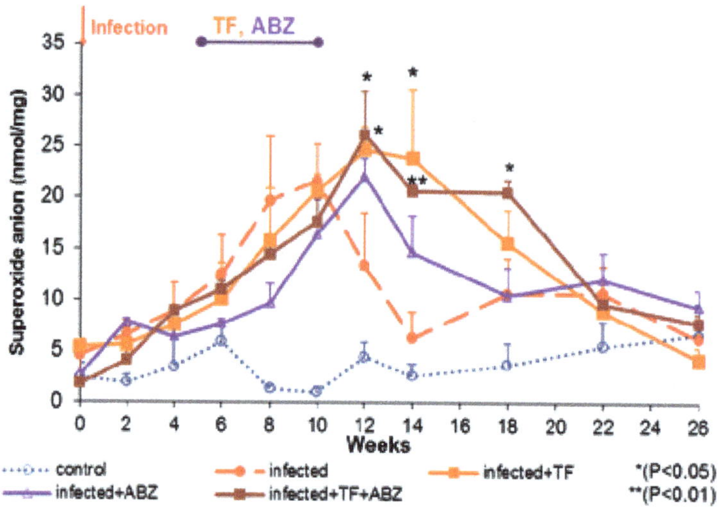

Figure 23. Macrophages' activity in *E. multilocularis* infected mice after therapy TF+ABZ. *(p<0.05); **(p<0.01) statistically significant from infected mice.

IFN-γ (that was stimulated after TF therapy) is an important activator of macrophages and affects their energetic system [21]. Immunotherapy with TF or TF+ABZ activated the respiratory burst in macrophages with high generation of O_2^- for a long time, from weeks 8 to 18 p.i. (Figure 23). This is documented by a long-term stimulation of macrophages' metabolic activity accompanied with a high production of also other biologically effective substances. At the same time, the proliferation of B cells and the IFN-γ level were increased. B cells release stimulation factors for macrophages after activation with antigens from destroyed *Echinococcus* protoscoleces [46] and cytokine IFN-γ markedly affects the macrophage energetic system. In our study, high concentrations of IFN-γ time-matched with intensive O_2^- production and slow parasite proliferation in infected mice treated with TF or TF+ABZ. Stimulative effect of TF on macrophages' metabolism had also been recorded by [106], who found the TF dialysis fraction (less than 3500 MW) activating the capacity of peritoneal macrophages to produce superoxide anion.

Activation of effector components of immune response after the immunotherapy of *E. multilocularis* infected mice in our experiment reduced the parasite growth and limited the development of larval cysts in the host (Figure 24). The immunomodulatory effect of TF suppressed the parasite proliferation till week 14 p.i. with the similar activity to anthelmintic drug albendazole and prolonged the parasite-reducing effect for one month, that is, till week 18 p.i. The TF-inhibiting effect on the parasite development was associated with the time of TF administration and a short time after it. The addition of TF to albendazole therapy resulted in a high antiparasitic effect with a significant cyst's reduction up to week 18 p.i. (2 months after the end of the therapy) in comparison to untreated group. Thereafter, the protective effect of anthelmintic therapy was lost.

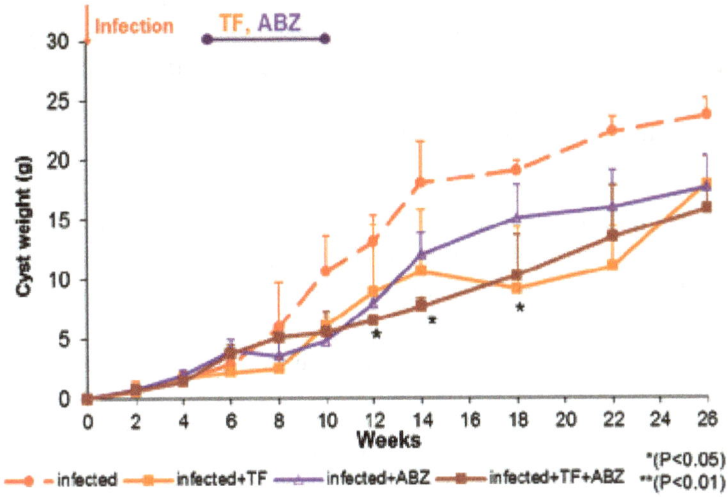

Figure 24. Cyst's weight in *E. multilocularis* infected mice after therapy TF+ABZ. *(p<0.05); **(p<0.01) statistically significant from infected mice.

In conclusion, the results of our study suggest that TF can have a positive effect on the host cellular immune response against the development of *E. multilocularis*. Nowadays, it is known that TF consists of a high quantity of low molecular weight proteins (> 200), and the exact chemical nature and molecular mechanisms of its action have not been defined yet. Low synthesis of IFN-γ induced by the *E. multilocularis* infection was restored with TF and exceeded the control concentration. The rise recorded in IFN-γ cytokine could be explained as a result of immunorestoration of CD4+ Th1 lymphocytes or due to the proliferation of another CD4 subpopulation. We think that regulation of immune homeostasis with TF therapy, which occurred between the CD4 cells and IFN-γ, played an important role in the immune response to *E. multilocularis* infection. Regulatory and effector mechanisms (CD4+ T cells, IFN-γ, and macrophages) which actively participate in the parasite destruction were stimulated with TF and supported antiparasitic effect of albendazole.

9. Conclusion

Our results suggest the possible way to increase ABZ antiparasitic efficacy in *E. multilocularis* infection by stimulation of the host immune response.

L-MTP-PE was recognized as a strong macrophage activator in mice infected with *E. multilocularis*. This immunomodulator stimulated the superoxide anion production for 3 months. The activity of macrophages was supported by dominant Th1 protective response – considered the highest serum IFN-γ level in that time. The antiparasitic effect of combined L-MTP-PE +ABZ therapy was manifested by marked reduction of cysts growth for 3 months after the end of treatment.

GIZn+ABZ has been shown to be the most effective immunomodulatory and antiparasitic treatment, the greatest reduction of metacestode growth was observed as early as 2 weeks from the beginning of this therapy, lasting till the end of experiment (for 4 months). The addition of zinc to immunomodulatory glucan substance has greatly contributed to the reduction of intensive fibrosis after glucan treatment, which attenuated the antiparasitic effect of ABZ alone.

TF could correct the immune balance disturbance after the *E. multilocularis* infection, which is responsible for lymphocyte suppressor activity. Inhibited IFN-γ production after the *E. multilocularis* infection was restored and increased with TF, which could result from a restoration of CD4+ Th1 lymphocytes. TF administration prolonged the parasitostatic effect of ABZ for 2 months. Restoration of suppressed host immune mechanisms that are important for restriction of parasite expansive growth seems to be a promising approach to *E. multilocularis* infection.

Immunomodulatory agents can be beneficial in the treatment of alveolar echinococcosis, where the developed Th1 immune response supports the improvement of the anthelmintic action of benzimidazoles. The type and development of the immune response are generally managed by the lymphocyte network and its immunoregulatory mechanism. Immunomodulators could regulate the immune disbalance after the *E. multilocularis* infection, which suppresses lymphocytes' and macrophages' activities. Restoring of this immunosuppresion may be one promising way to overcome this situation and to control chronic alveolar echinococcosis.

Acknowledgements

This study was supported by the Slovak VEGA agency, grants No. 2/0172/13 and No. 2/0081/15.

Author details

Emília Dvorožňáková*

Address all correspondence to: dvoroz@saske.sk

Institute of Parasitology, Slovak Academy of Sciences, Košice, Slovak Republic

References

[1] Wilson JF, Rausch RL, Wilson FR. Alveolar hydatid disease. Review of the surgical experience in 42 cases of active disease among Alaskan Eskimos. *Ann Surg* 1995;221(3) 315-323.

[2] Zhang W, McManus DP. Recent advances in the immunology and diagnosis of echinococcosis. *FEMS Immunol Med Microbiol* 2006;47(1) 24-41.

[3] Kern P. Medical treatment of echinococcosis under the guidance of Good Clinical Practice (GCP/ICH). *Parasitol Int* 2006;55(Suppl) S273-S282.

[4] Kinčeková J, Hrčková G, Bober J, Vrzgula A, Szabadošová V, Bohuš P, Zachar M. A rare case of alveolar echinococcosis in a 14-year-old child. *Helminthologia* 2008;45(1) 28-31.

[5] Reuter S, Jensen B, Buttenschoen K, Kratzer W, Kern P. Benzimidazoles in the treatment of alveolar echinococcosis: a comparative study and review of the literature. *J Antimicrob Chemo* 2000;46(3) 451-456.

[6] Venkatesan P. Albendazole. *J Antimicrob Chemo* 1998;41(2) 145-147.

[7] Capece BPS, Navarro M, Arcalis T, Castells G, Toribio L, Perez F, Carretero A, Ruberte J, Arboix M, Cristofol C. Albendazole sulphoxide enantiomers in pregnant rats embryo concentrations and developmental toxicity. *Vet J* 2003;165(3) 266-275.

[8] Ammann RW, Hirsbrunner R, Cotting J, Steiger U, Jacquier P, Eckert J. Recurrence rate after discontinuation of long-term mebendazole therapy in alveolar echinococcosis (preliminary results). *Am J Trop Med Hyg* 1990;43(5) 506-515.

[9] McManus DP, Zhang WB, Bartley PB. Echinoccosis. Lancet 2003; 362(9392) 1295-1304.

[10] Altintas Nuray, Orenay S, Reyhan E, Turk M, Asci M, Turel S, Yolasigmaz A, Altintas Nazmiye. Genotoxic effects of albendazole in patients medicated for cystic echinococcosis. *Helminthologia* 2007;44(2) 57-61.

[11] El-On J. Benzimidazole treatment of cystic echinococcosis. *Acta Tropica* 2003;85(2) 243-252.

[12] Gottstein B, Haag K, Walker M, Matsumoto J, Mejri A, Hemphill A. Molecular survival strategies of *Echinococcus multilocularis* in the murine host. *Parasitol Int* 2006;55(Suppl) S45-S49.

[13] [13]Vuitton DA, Zhang SL, Yang Y, Godot V, Beurton I, Mantion G, Bresson-Hadni S. Survival strategy of *Echinococcus multilocularis* in the human host. *Parasitol Int* 2006;55(Suppl) S51-S55.

[14] Gottstein B, Hemphill A. Immunopathology of echinococcosis. In: Freedman DO. (ed.) *Immunopathogenetic Aspects of Disease Induced by Helminth Parasites.* Book Series: *Chem Immunol,* 1997,66:177-208.

[15] Dixon JB. Echinococcosis. *Comp Immunol Microbiol Infect Dis* 1997;20(1) 87-94.

[16] Reimann J, Kaufmann SHE. Alternative antigen processing pathways in anti-effective immunity. *Curr Opin Immunol* 1997;9(4) 462-469.

[17] Emery I, Liance M, Deriaud E, Vuitton DA, Houin R, Leclerc C. Characterization of T-cell immune responses of *Echinococcus multilocularis*-infected C57BL/6J mice. *Paras Immunol* 1996;18(9) 463-472.

[18] Manfras BJ, Reuter S, Wendland T, Boehm BO, Kern P. Impeded Th1 CD4 memory T cell generation in chronic-persisting liver infection with *Echinococcus multilocularis*. *Int Immunol* 2004;16(1) 43-50.

[19] Sturm D, Menzel J, Gottstein B, Kern P. Interleukin-5 is the predominant cytokine produced by peripheral blood mononuclear cells in alveolar echinococcosis. *Infect Immun* 1995;63(5) 1688-1697.

[20] Vuitton DA. The ambiguous role of immunity in echinococcosis: protection of the host or of the parasite? *Acta Tropica* 2003;85(2) 119-132.

[21] Liance M, Ricard-Blum S, Emery I, Houin R, Vuitton DA. *Echinococcus multilocularis* infection in mice: in vivo treatment with a low dose of IFN-gamma decreases metacestode growth and liver fibrogenesis. *Parasite* 1998;5(3) 231-237.

[22] Šoltýs J, Quinn MT. Modulation of endotoxin- and enterotoxin-induced cytokine release by in vivo treatment with beta-(1,6)-branched beta-(1,3)-glucan. *Infect Immun* 1999;67(1) 244-252.

[23] Hrčková G, Velebný S. Effect of praziquantel and liposome-incorporated praziquantel on peritoneal macrophage activation in mice infected with *Mesocestoides corti* tetrathyridia (Cestoda). *Parasitology* 1997;114(5) 475-482.

[24] Pabst MJ, Beranova-Giorgianni S, Krueger JM. Effects of muramyl peptides on macrophages, monokines, and sleep. *Neuroimmunomodulation* 1999;6(4) 261-283.

[25] Adam A, Lederer E. Muramylpeptides as immunomodulators. *Atl Sci - Immunol* 1988;1(3-4) 205-214.

[26] Hui GS, Tam LQ, Chang SP, Case SE, Hashiro C, Siddiqui WA, Shiba T, Kusumoto S, Kotani S. Synthetic low-toxicity muramyl dipeptide and monophosphoryl lipid A replace Freund complete adjuvant in inducing growth-inhibitory antibodies to the *Plasmodium falciparum* major merozoite surface protein, gp195. *Infect Immun* 1991;59(5) 1585-1591.

[27] Dvorožňáková E, Borošková Z, Dubinský P, Tomašovičová O, Hříbalová V, Machnicka B. Immunomodulative effect of muramyldipeptide in mice with larval toxocarosis. *Parasitol Res* 1999;85(12) 1034-1040.

[28] Dieter P, Ambs P, Fityke E, Schwende H. Lipopolysaccharide and liposome-encapsulated MTP-PE-induced cytotoxicity and release of eicosanoids, tumor necrosis factor-alpha and nitric oxide in liver macrophages. In: Honn KV, Marnett LJ, Nigam S, et al. (eds.) *Eicosanoids And Other Bioactive Lipids in Cancer, Inflammation, and Radiation Injury 3* Book Series: *Adv Exper Med Biol* 1997;Vol407 485-490.

[29] Asano T, McWatters A, An T, Matsushima K, Kleinerman ES. Liposomal muramyl tripeptide up-regulates interleukin-1 alpha, interleukin-1 beta, tumor necrosis factor-alpha, interleukin-6 and interleukin-8 gene expression in human monocytes. *J Pharmacol Exper Therap* 1994;268(2) 1032-1039.

[30] Melissen PM, van Vianen W, Leenen PJ, Bakker-Woundenberg IA. Tissue distribution and cellular distribution of liposomes encapsulating muramyltripeptide phosphatidyl ethanolamide. Tissue and cellular distribution of LE-MTPPE. *Biotherapy* 1993;7(1) 71-78.

[31] Gay B, Cardot JM, Schnell C, van Hoogevest P, Gygax D. Comparative pharmacokinetics of free muramyl tripeptide phosphatidyl ethanolamine (MTP-PE) and liposomal MTP-PE. *J Pharmaceut Sci* 1993;82(10) 997-1001.

[32] Dieter P, Hempel U, Malessa B, Fitzke E, Tran-Thi TA, MacLouf J, Creminon C, Kanaoka Y, Urade Y. Lipopolysaccharide- and liposome-encapsulated MTP-PE-induced formation of eicosanoids, nitric oxide and tumor necrosis factor-alpha in macrophages. In: Honn KV, Marnett LJ, Nigam S, et al. (eds.) *Eicosanoids And Other Bioactive Lipids in Cancer, Inflammation, and Radiation Injury* 4 Book Series: *Ad Exper Med Biol* 1999;Vol469 443-448.

[33] Hsieh CS, Macatonia SE, Tripp CS, Wolf SF, O'Garra A, Murphy KM. Development of TH1 CD4+ T cells through IL-12 produced by *Listeria*-induced macrophages. *Science* 1993;260(5107) 547-549.

[34] ten Hagen TL, van Vianen W, Savelkoul HF, Heremans H, Buurman WA, Bakker-Woundenberg IA. Involvement of T cells in enhanced resistance to *Klebsiella pneumoniae* septicemia in mice treated with liposome-encapsulated muramyl tripeptide phosphatidylethanolamine or gamma interferon. *Infect Immun* 1998;66(5) 1962-1967.

[35] Souvannavong V, Brown S, Adam A. The synthetic immunomodulator muramyl dipeptide (MDP) can stimulate activated B cells. *Mole Immunol* 1988;25(4) 385-391.

[36] Graichen DAS, Gottstein B, Matsumoto J, Müller N, Zanotto PMA, Ayala FJ, Haag KL. 2007) Expression and diversity of *Echinococcus multilocularis* AgB genes in secondarily infected mice: evaluating the influence of T-cell immune selection on antigenic variation. *Gene* 2007;392(1-2) 98-105.

[37] Kizaki T, Kobayashi S, Ogasawara K, Day NK, Good RA, Onoe K. Immune suppression induced by protoscoleces of *Echinococcus multilocularis* in mice. Evidence for the presence of CD8dull suppressor cells in spleens of mice intraperitoneally infected with *E. multilocularis*. *J Immunol* 1991;147(5) 1659-1666.

[38] Gottstein B, Wunderlin E, Tanner I. *Echinococcus multilocularis*: parasite-specific humoral and cellular immune response subsets in mouse strains susceptible (AKR, C57B1/6J) or 'resistant' C57B1/10) to secondary alveolar echinococcosis. *Clin Exper Immunol* 1994;96(2) 245-252.

[39] Harraga S, Godot V, Bresson-Hadni S, Mantion G, Vuitton DA. Profile of cytokine production within the periparasitic granuloma in human alveolar echinococcosis. *Acta Tropica* 2003;85(2) 231-236.

[40] Hübner MP, Manfras BJ, Margos MC, Eiffler D, Hoffmann WH, Schulz-Key H, Kern P, Soboslay PT. *Echinococcus multilocularis* metacestodes modulate cellular cytokine and chemokine release by peripheral blood mononuclear cells in alveolar echinococcosis patients. *Clin Exper Immunol* 2006;145(2) 243-251.

[41] Sehra S, Chugh L, Gangal SV. Role of liposomes in selective proliferation of splenic lymphocytes. *Mole Cell Biochem* 1998;183(1-2) 133-139.

[42] Jenne L, Kilwinski J, Scheffold W, Kern P. IL-5 expressed by CD4+ lymphocytes from *Echinococcus multilocularis*-infected patients. *Clin Exper Immunol* 1997,109(1):90-97.

[43] Vuitton DA. Echinococcosis and allergy. *Clin Rev Aller Immunol* 2004;26(2) 93-104.

[44] Sher A, Fiorentino D, Caspar P, Pearce E, Mosmann T. Production of IL-10 by CD4+ T lymphocytes correlates with down-regulation of Th1 cytokine synthesis in helminth infection. *J Immunol* 1991;147(8) 2713-2716.

[45] Fiorentino D, Zlotnik A, Vieira P, Mosmann TR, Howard M, Moore KW, O'Garra A. IL-10 acts on the antigen-presenting cell to inhibit cytokine production by Th1 cells. *J Immunol* 1991;146(10) 3444-3451.

[46] Šoltýs J, Turčeková L, de Rycke PH. The effect *Echinococcus* hydatid cyst fluid and protoscoleces on mouse peritoneal macrophages and spleen lymphocytes. *Helminthologia* 1999;36(1) 25-30.

[47] Xu Z, Fidler IJ. The *in situ* activation of cytotoxic properties in murine Kupffer cells by the systemic administration of whole *Mycobacterium bovis* organisms or muramyl tripeptide. *Can Immunol Immunother* 1984;18(2) 118-122.

[48] Karpoff HM, Jarnagin W, Delman K, Fong Y. Regional muramyl tripeptide phosphatidylethanolamine administration enhances hepatic immune function and tumor surveillance. *Surgery* 2000;128(2) 213-218.

[49] Tanguay S, Bucana CD, Wilson MR, Fidler IJ, von Eschenbach AC, Killion JJ. *In vivo* modulation of macrophage tumoricidal activity by oral administration of the liposome-encapsulated macrophage activator CGP 19835A. *Canc Res* 1994;54(22) 5882-5888.

[50] Melissen PM, van Vianen W, Bidjai O, van Marion M, Bakker-Woundenberg IA. Free versus liposome-encapsulated muramyl tripeptide phosphatidylethanolamide (MTPPE) and interferon-γ (IFN-γ) in experimental infection with *Listeria* monocytogenes. *Biotherapy* 1993;6(2) 113-124.

[51] Adinolfi LE, Bonventre PF, Vanderpas M, Eppstein DA. Synergistic effect of glucantime and a liposome-encapsulated muramyl dipeptide analog in therapy of experimental visceral *Leishmaniasis*. *Infect Immun* 1985;48(2) 409-416.

[52] Morikawa K, Takeda R, Yamazaki M, Mizuno D. Induction of tumoricidal activity of polymorphonuclear leukocytes by a linear beta-1,3-D-glucan and other immunomodulators in murine cells. *Can Res* 1985;45(4) 1496-1501.

[53] Sakurai T, Suzuki I, Kinoshita A, Oikawa S, Masuda A, Ohsawa M, Yadomae T. Effect of intraperitoneally administered beta-1,3-glucan, SSG, obtained from *Sclerotinia sclerotiorum* IFO 9395 on the functions of murine alveolar macrophages. *Chem Pharmaceut Bull* (Tokyo) 1991;39(1) 214-217.

[54] Williams DL, Pretus HA, Mcnamee RB, Jones EL, Ensley HE, Browder IW, Di Luzio NR. Development, physicochemical characterization and preclinical efficacy evaluation of a water soluble glucan sulfate derived from *Saccharomyces cerevisiae*. *Immunopharmacology* 1991;22(3) 139-155.

[55] Větvička V, Thornton BP, Ross GD. Soluble beta-glucan polysaccharide binding to the lectin site of neutrophil or natural killer cell complement receptor type 3 (CD11b/CD18) generates a primed state of the receptor capable of mediating cytotoxicity of iC3b-opsonized target cells. *J Clin Invest* 1996;98(1) 50-61.

[56] Sakurai T; Kaise T; Yadomae T; Matsubara C. Different role of serum components and cytokines on alveolar macrophage activation by soluble fungal (1-->3)-beta-D-glucan. Eur J Pharmacol 1997;334(2-3) 255-263.

[57] Kidd PM. The use of mushroom glucans and proteoglycans in cancer treatment. Alt Med Rev 2000;5(1) 4-27.

[58] Gallin EK, Green SW, Patchen ML. Comparative effects of particulate and soluble glucan on macrophages of C3H/HeN and C3H/HeJ mice. *Int J Immunopharmacol* 1992;14(2) 173-183.

[59] Rasmussen LT, Seljelid R. Novel immunomodulators with pronounced *in vivo* effects caused by stimulation of cytokine release. *J Cell Biochem* 1991;46(1) 60-68.

[60] Šoltýs J, Borošková Z, Dubinský P, Tomašovičová O, Auer H, Aspock H. Effect of glucan immunomodulator on the immune response and larval burdens in mice with experimental toxocarosis. *Appl Parasitol* 1996;37(3) 161-167.

[61] Ditteová G, Velebný S, Hrčková G. Modulation of liver fibrosis and pathophysiological changes in mice infected with *Mesocestoides corti* (*M. vogae*) after administration of glucan and liposomized glucan in combination with vitamin C. *J Helminthol* 2003;77(3) 219-226.

[62] James K. Interactions between cytokines and alpha 2-macroglobulin. *Immunol Today* 1990;11(12) 163-166.

[63] Benková M, Borošková Z, Šoltýs J. Immunostimulatory effects of certain substances in experimental ascaridiasis in pigs. *Vet Med* (Prague) 1991;36(12) 717-724.

[64] Wellinghausen N, Kirchner H, Rink L. The immunobiology of zinc. *Immunol Today* 1997;18(11) 519-521.

[65] Rink L, Kirchner H. Zinc-altered immune function and cytokine production. *J Nutr* 2000;130(Suppl) S1407-S1411.

[66] Chowdhury N, Singh R. Distribution of zinc in parasitic helminths. *J Helminthol* 1989; 63(2) 149-152.

[67] Wellinghausen N, Jochle W, Reuter S, Flegel WA, Grunert A, Kern P. Zinc status in patients with alveolar echinococcosis is related to disease progression. *Paras Immunol* 1999;21(5) 237-241.

[68] Borošková Z, Dvorožňáková E, Ševčíková Z. Cellular immune reactions of mice with alveolar echinococcosis after albendazole therapy. *Helminthologia* 2003;40(4) 187-194.

[69] Baum MK, Shor-Posner G, Campa A. Zinc status in human immunodeficiency virus infection. *J Nutr* 2000;130(Suppl) S1421-S1423.

[70] Dvorožňáková E, Hrčková G, Borošková Z, Velebný S, Dubinský P. Effect of treatment with free and liposomized albendazole on selected immunological parameters and cyst growth in mice infected with *Echinococcus multilocularis*. *Parasitol Int* 2004;53(4) 315-325.

[71] Pérez-Serrano J, Denegri G, Casado N, Rodríguez-Caabeiro F. *In vivo* effect of oral albendazole and albendazole sulphoxide on development of secondary echinococcosis in mice. *Int J Parasitol* 1997;27(11) 1341-1345.

[72] Abbas AK, Murphy KM, Sher A. Functional diversity of helper T lymphocytes. *Nature* 1996;383, 787-793.

[73] Šoltýs J, Benková M, Borošková Z. Immunorestorative effect of glucan immunomodulator on guinea pigs with experimental ascariosis. *Vet Immunol Immunopathol* 1994;42(3-4) 379-388.

[74] Borošková Z, Dvorožňáková E, Dubinský P, Velebný S, Tomašovičová O, Machnická B. Effect of free and liposomised albendazole on the immune responses in healthy and *Toxocara canis* infected mice. *Vet Med* (Prague) 1998;43(10) 293-300.

[75] Dvorožňáková E, Akao A. 2000: Th1 and Th2 response after glucan immunomodulation in murine larval toxocarosis. Reports of Czech Parasitological Society, Prague, Czech Republic, 2000. S8:53.

[76] Bach JF. The multi-faceted zinc dependency of the immune system. *Immunol Today* 1981;2(11) 225-227.

[77] Crea A, Guérin V, Ortega F, Hartemann P. Zinc and the immune system. *Annales de Médecine Interne* 1990;141(5) 447-451.

[78] Kizaki T, Ishige M, Kobayashi S, Bingyan W, Kumagai M, Day NK, Good RA, Onoe K. Suppression of T-cell proliferation by CD8+ T cells induced in the presence of protoscoleces of *Echinococcus multilocularis in vitro. Infect Immun* 1993;61(2) 525-533.

[79] Bresson-Hadni S, Liance M, Meyer JP, Houin R, Bresson JL, Vuitton DA. Cellular immunity in experimental *Echinococcus multilocularis* infection. II. Sequential and comparative phenotypic study of the periparasitic mononuclear cells in resistant and sensitive mice. *Clin Exper Immunol* 1990;82(2) 378-383.

[80] Dowd PS, Kelleher J, Guillou PJ. T-lymphocyte subsets and interleukin-2 production in zinc-deficient rats. *Brit J Nutr* 1986;55(1) 59-69.

[81] Vuitton DA. New trends in the treatment of echinococcosis. *Helminthologia* 1999;36(3) 167-170.

[82] Gottstein B. Molecular and immunological diagnosis of echinococcosis. *Clin Microbiol Rev* 1992;5(3) 248-261.

[83] Hrčková G, Velebný S, Daxnerová Z, Solár P. Praziquantel and liposomized glucan-treatment modulated liver fibrogenesis and mastocytosis in mice infected with *Mesocestoides vogae* (*M. corti*, Cestoda) tetrathyridia. *Parasitology* 2006;132(4) 581-594.

[84] Song YL, Ford JW, Gordon D, Shanley CJ. Regulation of lysyl oxidase by interferon-gamma in rat aortic smooth muscle cells. *Arterioscler, Thromb Vasc Biol* 2000;20(4) 982-988.

[85] Tang JT, Fang JY, Gu WQ, Li EL. T cell immune response is correlated with fibrosis and inflammatory activity in hepatitis B cirrhotics. *World J Gastroenterol* 2006;12(19) 3015-3019.

[86] Casini A, Ceni E, Salzano R, Biondi P, Parola M, Galli A, Foschi M, Caligiuri A, Pinzani M, Surrenti C. Neutrophil-derived superoxide anion induces lipid peroxidation and stimulates collagen synthesis in human hepatic stellate cells: Role of nitric oxide. *Hepatology* 1997;25(2) 361-367.

[87] Guerret S, Vuitton DA, Liance M, Pater C, Carbillet JP. *Echinococcus multilocularis*: relationship between susceptibility/resistance and liver fibrogenesis in experimental mice. *Parasitol Res* 1998;84(8) 657-667.

[88] Miguet JP, Bresson-Hadni S, Vuitton DA. Echinococcosis of the liver. In: Mcintyre N, Benhamou JP, Bicher J, Rizetto M, Rodes J. (eds.) *Oxford Textbook of Clinical Hepatology*. Oxford University, Oxford, 1991; 721-730.

[89] Anttinen H, Ryhanen L, Puistola U, Arranto A, Oikarinen A. Decrease in liver collagen accumulation in carbon tetrachloride-injured and normal growing rats upon administration of zinc. *Gastroenterology* 1984;86(3) 532-539.

[90] Kojima-Yuasa A, Ohkita T, Yukami K, Ichikawa H, Takami N, Nakatani T, Opare Kennedy D, Nishiguchi S, Matsui-Yuasa I. Involvement of intracellular glutathione in zinc deficiency-induced activation of hepatic stellate cells. *Chemico-Biologic Interact* 2003; 146(1) 89-99.

[91] Kojima-Yuasa A, Umeda K, Ohkita T, Opare Kennedy D, Nishiguchi S, Matsui-Yuasa I. Role of reactive oxygen species in zinc deficiency-induced hepatic stellate cell activation. *Free Rad Biol Med* 2005;39(5) 631-640.

[92] Pineda B, Estrada-Parra S, Pedraza-Medina B, Rodriguez-Ropon A, Pérez R., Arrieta O. Interstitial transfer factor as adjuvant immunotherapy for experimental glioma. *J Exp Clin Can Res* 2005;24(4) 575-583.

[93] Alvarez-Thull L, Kirkpatrick Ch. Profiles of cytokine production in recipients of transfer factors. *Biotherapy* 1996;9(1-3) 55-59.

[94] Foschi FG, Marsigli L, Bernardi M, Salvi F, Mascalchi M, Gasbarrini G, Stefanini G. Acute multifocal cerebral white matter lesions during transfer factor therapy. *J Neurol Neurosurg Psychiat* 2000;68(1) 114-115.

[95] Holeva OH, Paster IP, Liubchenko TA, Paster IeU, Kholodna LS, Zamotaierva HA, Hrodzinskyi DM. The immune reactivity transfer factor as a modulator of lymphocyte functional activity in rats. *Fiziolohichnyĭ zhurnal* 2000;46(4) 58-65.

[96] Vacek A, Hofer M, Barnet K, Čech K, Pekárek J, Schneiderová H. Positive effects of dialyzable leukocyte extract (DLE) on recovery of mouse haemopoiesis suppressed by ionizing radiation and on proliferation of haemopoietic progenitor cells in vitro. *Int J Immunopharmacol* 2000;22(8) 623-634.

[97] Foschi FG, Marsigli L, Bernardi M, Salvi F, Mascalchi M, Gasbarrini G, Stefanini G. Acute multifocal cerebral white matter lesions during transfer factor therapy. *J Neurol Neurosurg Psychiat* 2000;68(1) 114-115.

[98] Kirkpatrick CH. Activities and characteristics of transfer factors. *Biotherapy* 1996;9(1-3) 13-16.

[99] Fabre RA, Pérez TM, Aguilar LD, Rangel MJ, Estrada-Garcia I, Hernández-Pando R, Estrada Parra S. Transfer factors as immunotherapy and supplement of chemotherapy in experimental pulmonary tuberculosis. *Clin Exp Immunol* 2004;136(2) 215-223.

[100] Dai WJ, Waldvogel A, Siles-Lucas M, Gottstein B. *Echinococcus multilocularis* proliferation in mice and respective parasite 14-3-3 gene expression is mainly controlled by an alpha beta(+) CD4(+) T-cell-mediated immune response. *Immunology* 2004;112(3) 481-488.

[101] Sailer M, Soelder B, Allerberger F, Zaknun D, Feichtinger H, Gottstein B. Alveolar echinococcosis of the liver in a six-year-old girl with acquired immunodeficiency syndrome. *J Pediat* 1997;130(2) 320-323.

[102] Zingg W, Renner-Schneiter EC, Pauli-Magnus C, Renner EL, vanOverbeck J, Schlapfer E, Weber M, Weber R, Opravil M, Gottstein B, Speck RF. Swiss HIV Cohort Study. Alveolar echinococcosis of the liver in an adult with human immunodeficiency virus type-1 infection. *Infection* 2004;32(5) 299-302.

[103] Estrada-Parra S, Nagaya A, Serrano E, Rodriguez O, Santamaria V, Ondarza R, Chavez R, Correa B. Comparative study of transfer factor and acyclovir in the treatment of herpes zoster. *Int J Immunopharmacol* 1998;20(10) 521-535.

[104] Mosmann TR, Fong TAT. Specific assays for cytokine production by T cells. *J Immunol Meth* 1989;116(2) 151-158.

[105] Carter LL, Swain SL. Single cell analyses of cytokine production. *Curr Opin Immunol* 1997;9(2) 177-182.

[106] Dvorožňáková E, Porubcová J, Ševčíková Z. Immune response of mice with alveolar echinococcosis to therapy with transfer factor, alone and in combination with albendazole. Parasitol Res 2009; 105(4):1067-1076.

[107] Karhumaki E, Marnela KM, Krohn K. Chromatographic and enzymatic effects on transfer factor-like activity from human leukocytes and porcine spleen dialysate. Int J Biochem 1988;20(10) 1067-1072.

12

Surgical Management of Hydatid Disease

Angeliki Vidoura, Mariana Parisidou,
Christina Chatedaki and Dimitris Zacharoulis

Management of hydatid disease carries a substantial risk of complications and recurrence. The ultimate goal of surgery is to kill the parasites, evacuate the cyst, remove the germinal layer, and obliterate the residual cavity all while preserving the healthy liver tissue. In endemic areas, a conservative approach is preferred. The open surgeries have a substantial risk of complications, such as bile leakage, parasite contamination, and presence of dead spaces, in which an abscess can form. These complications then have to be managed with more radical surgical approaches. The most commonly used surgical approaches are pericystectomy, partial pericystectomy, and even hepatic resection. With the right indications, subadventitial cystectomy has low postoperative complication, mortality, and recurrence. The condition of the cyst and the patient, the general status of the patient and the cyst size, location, and pathology are factors that indicate the optimal surgical approach.

Keywords: echinococcosis, hydatid disease surgical approach, pericystectomy, cystic hepatic echinococcosis, hepatic hydatid cyst, open surgical approach

1. Introduction

Hydatid disease is a global parasitic zoonosis, mostly found in the northern hemisphere, caused by the larval stages of the dog tapeworm *Echinococcus granulosus*. Humans become intermediate hosts through ingestion of the parasite eggs and are infected directly by contact with dogs or indirectly by contaminated food or dirt. The eggs then develop into larvae after crossing the intestinal wall and migrate to the liver, where they form cysts. The liver is the most frequent site for the cystic lesions seen in hydatid disease, followed by the lung and brain. Liver cysts, such as these usually remain asymptomatic and untreated for years until they compress their adjacent organs, form fistulas into them or even rupture into the abdomen. Complete elimination of the parasite with minimum morbidity and mortality is the goal of the surgical treatment. There are three treatment options (**Table 1**): surgery, medical therapy, and interventional procedures. Management of hydatid cysts in the liver typically involves an open surgical approach with meticulous operative site packing and employment of a variety of conservative and radical operative techniques. This chapter reviews the available surgical approaches used to treat cystic echinococcosis of the liver and summarizes the safety and effectiveness of surgical interventions [1].

Pharmaceutical: medical therapy	• Mebendazole • Albendazole • Praziquantel
Percutaneous	• PAIR technique (puncture, aspiration, injection, reaspiration) • Catheterization (percutaneous evacuation, modified catheterization, dilatable multifunction trocar)
Surgical treatment: open or laparoscopic	• Conservative: external drainage, omentoplasty, capitonnage • Radical: subadventitial pericystectomy, (partial) pericystectomy, hepatic resection

Table 1. Treatment options of echinococcal (hydatid) hepatic cysts.

2. Surgical treatment

To date, surgical management remains the treatment of choice for most cases of hydatid hepatic cysts. It is the only method that allows complete eradication of the parasite, treatment or prevention of complications, and evasion of relapse. Indications for surgical management are mentioned in **Table 2** [9].

In general, the physical condition of the patient and the characteristics of the hydatid cyst indicate the necessity of surgical treatment. In cases where surgical treatment is contraindicated, systematic monitoring in combination with drug therapy—with or without minimally invasive, nonsurgical techniques—is the recommended treatment approach (wait and watch). The goals of surgical treatment are mentioned in **Table 3**.

Indications	Contraindications
• Superficial cysts with a high rupture risk	• Multiple cysts
• Large cysts, containing multiple daughter cysts	• Inactive, difficult to access cysts
• Hepatobiliary communication	• Dead cysts
• Compression of neighboring organs (symptomatic)	• Inactive cysts that are partially or totally calcified
• Pus containing, infected echinococcal cyst	• Very small cysts
• Nonhepatic echinococcal cysts (lungs, kidneys, etc.)	• unsuitable patient's condition
• Cysts exerting pressure on adjacent vital organs	

Table 2. Indications for surgical treatment of hydatid echinococcal hepatic cysts.

• Obliteration of the cyst
• Prevention of intraoperative transfer of the parasites
• Treatment of the remaining hepatic parenchyma
• Identification and treatment of possible hepatobiliary communication

Table 3. The goals of surgical treatment of echinococcal (hydatid) hepatic cysts.

Surgical treatment is reserved for complicated cysts, for example, cysts that develop a biliary fistula or perforated cysts and cysts that contain daughter cysts. In addition, it is a treatment of choice for superficial cysts that are smaller than 10 cm or are at high risk of rupture and for patients not suitable for percutaneous treatment. Complete obliteration of the parasite, evacuation of the cyst cavity, elimination of the residual cavity, inactivation of the parasite, and removal of the germinal layer are the main goals of a surgical approach to treating hydatid disease. There are three treatment approaches, and they consist of a conservative or a radical open approach and a laparoscopic approach [6]. Regardless of the technique chosen to treat each patient, it must be noted that medical treatment with benzimidazole prior to any surgery must take place to achieve sterilization of the cyst content and prevent dissemination or anaphylaxis. The operating field must be scrupulously packed in all cases, along with the use of solutions that are capable of eradicating even the protoscolices of the parasite, within the content of the cyst [2]. Some of the scolicidal solutions used in surgical approaches are hypertonic saline, povidone iodine, hydrogen peroxide, iodine, formalin, silver nitrate, and albendazole. These scolicides can be used alone or in combination. Regarding cystic echinococcosis, deep, endoparenchimatic, or rear cysts, close to large vessels, containing multiple daughter cells or calcified cysts must be treated with open surgery. On the other hand, superficial cysts on the anterior side of the liver are more suitably treated with laparoscopic surgery [3].

Surgical options include radical and conservative surgeries. Recurrence and complication rates tend to be higher with conservative surgery as compared to those with radical surgery. The recurrences are usually relative to failure of complete removal of the endocysts and/or their dissemination during the surgery. As in all techniques, the choice of the patients that will be operated on laparoscopically or openly should be made considering the indications. Known advantages of minimally invasive methods, smaller incision, and shorter hospitalization time also take place here. Most common laparoscopic technique used is that of injection evacuation omentoplasty.

2.1. Conservative operations

In conservative procedures, only the parasitic cyst contents are removed, whereas the pericystic membrane is retained and the residual cavity is managed with different techniques such as omentoplasty, capitonnage, or external drainage. The cyst is exposed safely. The pericystic area and operating field are covered with pads soaked with scolicidal agent to prevent the spillage of parasites into the surrounding tissue and peritoneal cavity. The cyst is punctured and aspirated. Before instilling the scolicidal agent, as much fluid as possible is aspirated to prevent dilution of the scolicidal agent. Then, the scolicidal agent is instilled into the cyst cavity and left for approximately 5–15 minutes [4]. Then, the scolicidal agent is aspirated, and the cyst is unroofed. The cyst contents, such as the germinative membrane and daughter cysts, are evacuated. At this point, the cavity should be explored carefully for any gross communication with the biliary tract and for the presence of exogenous cysts embedded in the wall. The next step in conservative treatment is managing the residual cavity. This can be done using various methods such as external drainage, marsupialization, internal drainage, capitonnage, introflexion, and omentoplasty. The Mabit procedure consists of deroofing the cyst and extraction of the parasite with omentoplasty and external drainage of the cyst cavity. The Posadas procedure consists of deroofing of the cyst with capitonnage (the surgical closure of a cyst cavity by applying sutures so as to cause approximation of the opposition surfaces) of the cavity without drainage. During partial pericystectomy, a deeply situated part of cyst wall is left within the liver. Marsupialization is the surgical exteriorization of a cyst by resection of the anterior wall and suture of the cut edges of the remaining cyst to the adjacent edges of the skin, thereby establishing a pouch of what was formally an enclosed cyst. Conservative surgery is easy, safe, and rapid, but has high morbidity and recurrence rates.

2.2. Radical operations

Radical surgery refers to the removal of the cyst along with the pericystic membrane and parasitic contents; it may also include liver resection if indicated. Radical surgical approach aims toward the eradication or elimination of local relapse or complications due to false orbiting. Additionally, it radically deals with the residual cavity, especially in cysts with partial calcification of the wall and biliary communication. There are two methods: the open-cyst method and the closed-cyst method. Radical procedures include: subadventitial cystectomy, (partial) pericystectomy, and hepatic resection. The subadventitial pericystectomy technique is enabled by understanding the surrounding structure of the cyst. The pericyst consists of two layers of different histological origin. Closest to the liver parenchyma is located the subadventitial layer, which is formed by fibrosis and by compression of the Glisson's capsules and hepatic veins. Next up closest to the parasitic cyst is the exocyst layer, which is caused by granulomatous reaction. In between the exocyst and the adventitial layer, there can be found the pericyst and it is the space formed in the in-between that is ideal for smooth detachment [3]. This approach however is not suitable for patients with cysts near the vital vessels or bile ducts. During the pericystectomy procedure, the cyst is dissected along its boundary with healthy liver tissue, blood vessels, and small biliary structures passing through the plane between the normal liver tissue and cyst are clamped and divided. During a hepatic resection operation, the cyst along with the pericyst and in conjunction with normal hepatic parenchyma is removed. Hepatic resection takes longer time to perform and is associated with more blood loss but presents a low rate of cyst recurrence. Pericystectomy and partial pericystectomy are easy to perform and associated with minimal blood loss and operation time. The rate of recurrence of cysts is lower in subadventitial cystectomy and hepatic resection. Subadventitial cystectomy causes less damage to healthy liver tissue than hepatic resection. In any case, treatment aims to one great common goal, that is, the residual cavity must always be treated with excellent care. This is critical to prevent biliary leakage, biliary fistula, and abscess formation. It is in the hands of the surgeon to decide how to go about treating each case separately, depending on the location of the cyst and always aiming towards the safest and most effective method [3]. Radical surgical approaches are associated with a low risk of postoperative complications, fewer relapse cases, long postoperative hospitalization, and low mortality rates; they are all operations with a high difficulty level mostly suitable for highly specialized to the liver surgeons. Radical surgery is superior to conservative surgery with lower morbidity, mortality, and reoccurrence rates [10].

2.3. The use of radiofrequency energy in hydatid disease surgery

The use of radiofrequency under ultrasound guidance allows for very little blood loss and results in minimal coagulation on the liver parenchyma. Ultrasonography (US)-guided RF pericystectomy is recommended specifically for cases where the cyst is not located near the liver helium (**Figures 1** and **2**) [5].

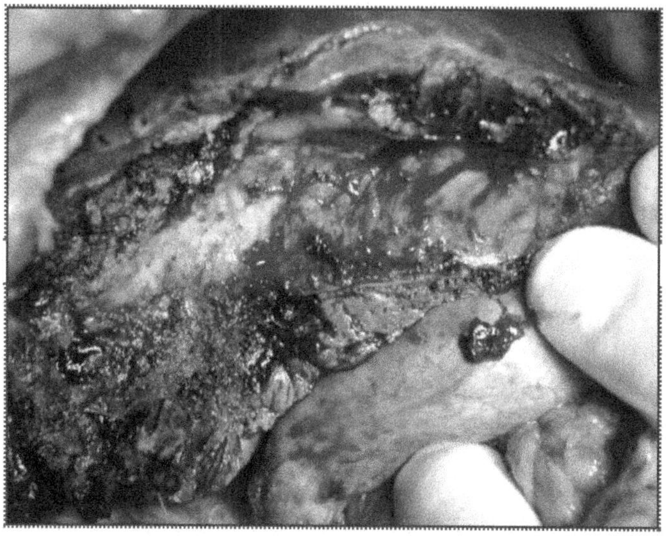

Figure 1. The liver parenchyma is shown with minimal coagulation and hemorrhage, after a radiofrequency assisted closed pericystectomy. (Image kindly supplied by Dr Zacharoulis) [5].

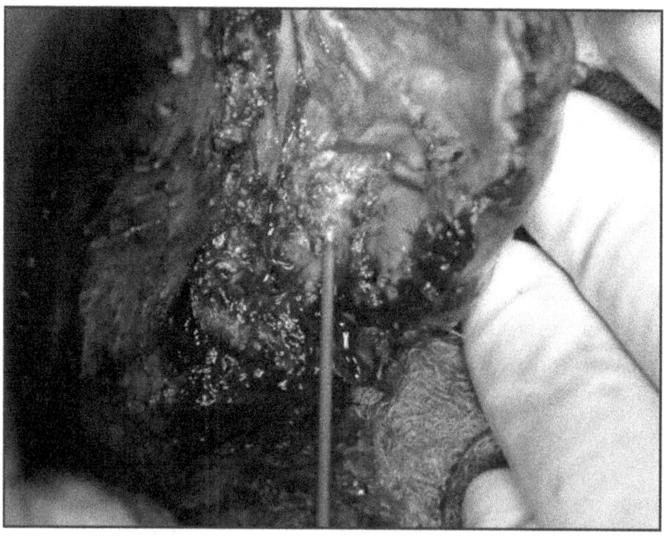

Figure 2. Radiofrequency assisted excision of the pericyst (open pericystectomy). (Image kindly supplied by Dr Zacharoulis) [5].

3. Complication

Potential major complications associated with the surgical treatment of hepatic hydatid cysts include secondary infection; obstructive jaundice due to pressure or rupture into the biliary tree, peritoneum, or an adjacent structure; anaphylaxis, postoperative hemorrhage, bile exudation from the residual cyst cavity, incisional fistula formation, cholangitis, wound infection, sepsis, incisional fistulae; pulmonary complications such as pneumonia and pulmonary embolization; complications of anesthesia; and death. Infection and biliary communication with the cyst (i.e., leakage or rupture with cholestasis) can occur before or after surgical interventions. In the case of intrabiliary rupture either during or after the completion of the operation, treatment can consist of a simple placement of a suture on the orifice, in cases with normal common bile duct caliber and no contamination. In the cases where the common bile duct has an abnormal caliber and the biliary tree is contaminated by cyst contents, firstly the leak must be thoroughly drained and decontaminated and t-tube drainage must be placed, moreover it might even be necessary for a choledochoduodenostomy procedure to be performed. Cases such as these can also be treated endoscopically by sphincterectomy and replacement of the nasobiliary catheter. Another complication or bile leakage which can be symptomatic or cause the formation of a high output biliary fistulae, this can also be managed endoscopically by performing sphincterectomy, nasobiliary drainage, or biliary stenting [7]. Surgical operations except from hepatic resections may leave behind a residual cavity that may easily be mistaken due to imaging techniques for a reoccurrence or any other condition. Recurrence, both local and as secondary echinococcosis, is associated with spillage during removal of the cyst, incomplete removal of the endocyst, and possibly the presence of unnoticed exophytic cyst development. Intraoperative US improves the quality of hepatic surgery [8].

4. Conclusion

In conclusion, hydatid disease remains to be a significant public health problem, and the main treatment goal should be parasite elimination, without recurrence and with minimal morbidity and mortality. Surgical techniques for the treatment of hepatic hydatid cysts range from hepatic resection to simple cyst evacuation and partial pericystectomy. These procedures eventually eradicate the entirety of the parasitic tissue, resulting in complete cure without recurrence. Even though surgical procedures are the golden therapeutic option, an optimal surgical technique is impossible to be decided on since each operation plan is specifically designed to each patient.

Author details

Angeliki Vidoura[1*], Mariana Parisidou[1], Christina Chatedaki[2] and Dimitris Zacharoulis[1]

*Address all correspondence to: angeliki.vid@gmail.com

1 University of Thessaly, Larissa, Greece

2 Department of Microbiology, University Hospital of Larissa, Larissa, Greece

References

[1] Mihmanli M, Idiz UO, Kaya C, Demir U, Bostanci O, Omeroglu S, Bozkurt E. Current status of diagnosis and treatment of hepatic. World Journal of Hepatology. 2016;**8**(28):1169-1181. DOI: 10.4254/wjh.v8.i28.1169

[2] Smego Jr RA, Sebanego P. Treatment options for hepatic cystic echinococcosis. International Journal of Infectious Diseases. 2005;**9**(2):69-76. DOI: 10.1016/j.ijid.2004.08.001

[3] Chen X, Chen X, Shao Y, Zhao J, Li H, Wen H. Clinical outcome and immune follow-up of different surgical approaches for human cyst hydatid disease in liver. The American Society of Tropical Medicine and Hygiene. 2014;**91**(4):801-805. DOI: 10.4269/ajtmh.14-0177

[4] Abdelraouf A, El-Aal AAA, Shoeib EY, Attia SS, Hanafy NA, Hassani M, Shoman S. Clinical and serological outcomes with different surgical approaches for human hepatic hydatidosis. Revista da Sociedade Brasileira de Medicina Tropical. 2015;**48**(5):587-593. DOI: 10.1590/0037-8682-0223-2015

[5] Zacharoulis D, Poultsidis A, Roundas C, Tepetes C. Liver hydatid disease: Radiofrequency-assisted pericystectomy. The Royal College of Surgeons of England. 2006; **88**:499-505. DOI: 10.1308/003588406X116864

[6] Rinaldi F, Brunetti E, Neumayr A, Maestri M, Goblirsch S, Tamarozzi F. Cystic echinococcosis of the liver: A primer for hepatologists. World Journal of Hepatology. 2014;**6**(5):293-305. DOI: 10.4254/wjh.v6.i5.293

[7] Sozuer E, Akyuz M, Akbulut S. Open surgery for hepatic hydatid disease. International Surgery. 2014;**99**(6):764-769. DOI: 10.9738/INTSURG-D-14-00069.1

[8] Graeter T, Ehing F, Oeztuerk S, Mason RA, Haenle MM, Kratzer W, Seufferlein T, Gruener B. Hepatobiliary complications of alveolar echinococcosis: A long-term follow-up study. World Journal of Gastroenterology. 2015;**21**(16):4925-4932. DOI: 10.3748/wjg.v21.i16.4925

[9] Pakala T, Molina M, Wu GY. Hepatic echinococcal cysts: A review. Journal of Clinical and Translational Hepatology. 2016;**4**(1):39-46. DOI: 10.14218/JCTH.2015.00036

[10] Baraket O, Moussa M, Ayed K, Kort B, Bouchoucha S. Predictive factors of morbidity after surgical treatment of hydatid cyst of the liver. Arab Journal of Gastroenterology. 2014;**15**(3-4):119-122. DOI: 10.1016/j.ajg.2014.05.004

13

Biliary Complications of Hepatic Hydatid Cyst Surgery and Prevention Methods

Can Konca and Deniz Balcı

Abstract

Cystic echinococcosis is still one of the main reasons for liver surgery especially in endemic areas. The most common complication of liver hydatid cyst is cystobiliary communication (CBC). Preoperative or intraoperative diagnosis of CBC is essential for the treatment, since it leads to postoperative bile leakage and fistula formation eventually without intervention. Predictive factors such as cyst size, history of jaundice, and degenerated cysts are described for preoperative evaluation. Further preoperative study can be performed for diagnosis in their presence. At the intraoperative phase, every effort should be performed for diagnosis. There are several methods for the investigation of CBC. When a CBC is found, it is also essential to evaluate the biliary system as well. By this way, postoperative complication rates can be lowered. Biliary leakage and fistula formation are the most common postoperative complication of liver hydatid surgery and they are the main reasons of morbidity and mortality. Their rates can be lowered by knowing how to interfere for the treatment. As a result, every effort should be made to detect and prevent these complications during the evaluation and management of cystic echinococcosis.

Keywords: hydatid cyst, hydatid surgery, bile leakage, bile fistula, biliary complication, prevention, echinococcus

1. Introduction

Cystic echinococcosis (CE) affects liver in approximately 70% of the cases and is still one of the main indications for liver surgery in endemic areas [1]. Reported CE-related mortality rates are between 0.5 and 4%, majority of which are mainly a consequence of the complications [1, 2].

In the past decades, surgery was the only treatment method for hepatic hydatid cysts [3]. With the advancements in medical and percutaneous therapy techniques, surgery is reserved mainly for the complicated hydatid cysts and cysts classified as CE2 or CE3B according to the World Health Organization Informal Working Group on Echinococcosis (WHO-IWGE) classification [1–4].

There are two modalities for surgery: radical and conservative approaches. Pericystectomy (**Figure 1**) and hepatectomy are examples for radical surgery, which aim a complete excision of the cyst and the pericyst [5]. They have lower complication (0–26%) and recurrence (0–3%) rates than the conservative methods [1, 6], but their usage is limited by the anatomic localization and multiplicity of the cysts, since especially in centrally located or bilobular disease, the extent of the surgery exceeds the purpose of the treatment of a benign disease. Also, hepatobiliary surgical expertise and longer operation time are needed for radical surgery, which can be a limitation in endemic regions. By contrast, conservative approaches such as partial pericystectomy (also known as unroofing) with drainage or omentoplasty (**Figure 2**) require less experience and shorter duration of operation. However, their complication and recurrence rates are higher [5]. Simply, they aim to remove the germinal and laminar membrane along with the cystic content and excise the pericystic membrane as much as possible without parenchymal dissection [5]. They have morbidity rates between 6 and 47% and recurrence rates between 4 and 25% [6].

Postoperative bile leakage and fistula formation are a result of cystobiliary communication (CBC) due to intrabiliary rupture (IBR) of the cyst, and this is most common complication of liver surgery for hydatid cyst [7]. Incidence of postoperative bile leakage is between 2.5 and 28.6%. When the postoperative bile leakage is drained externally and persists for more than 10 days, this is called biliary fistula. It is the major cause of morbidity and is encountered in 1–25% of the cases [6, 8]. In the absence of adequate internal or external drainage, bilioma, biliary abscesses, or biliary peritonitis may develop, which can lead to sepsis resulting in serious morbidity and even mortality. Postoperative biliary fistula is the major cause of prolonged hospitalization and complications requiring intervention after hydatid surgery. However, fistulas may close spontaneously in the first postoperative week. It can be classified as "low-flow fistula" if the daily drainage volume is less than 300 ml/day or "high-flow fistula" if more than 300 ml/day [8, 9]. If the fistula persists more than 3 weeks or is a high-flow fistula, then endoscopic or surgical intervention should be considered rather than a conservative approach [8, 10, 11].

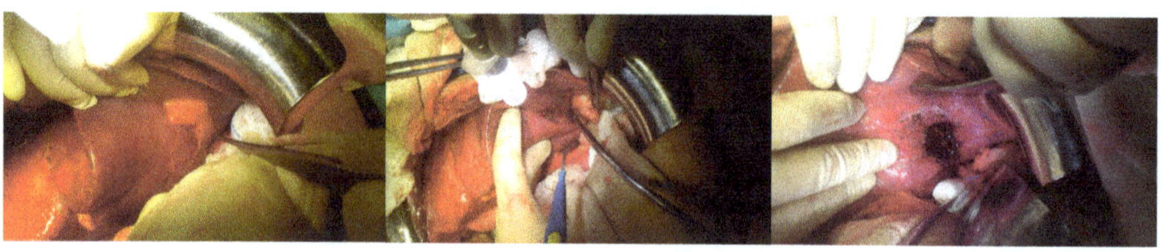

Figure 1. Pericystectomy procedure.

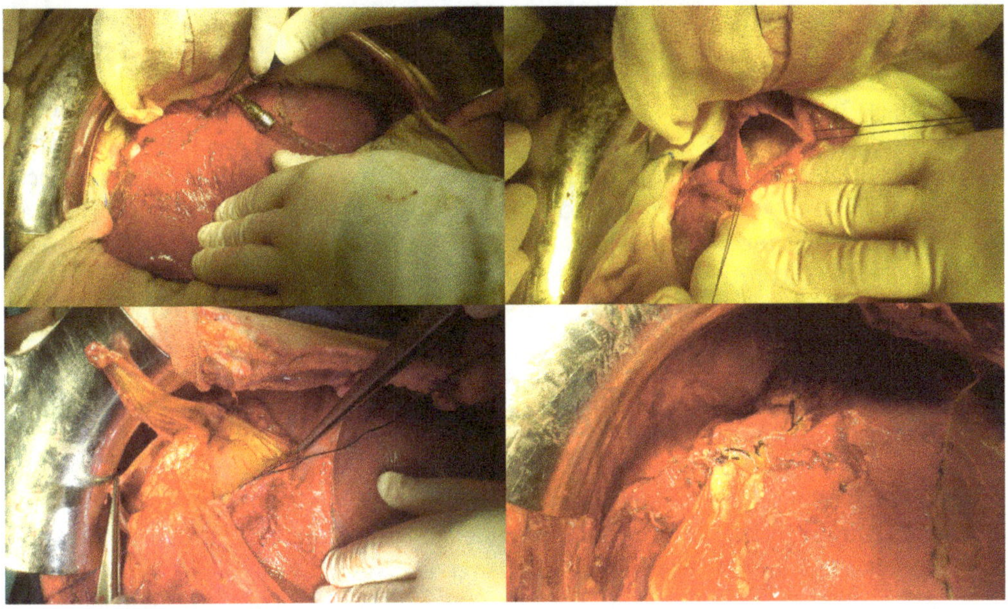

Figure 2. Partial pericystectomy with omentoplasty.

The most common complication of CE is a cystobiliary communication occurring in about 60% of the complicated patients [7]. Two theories have been proposed for pathogenesis: the first is progressive necrosis developing on the wall of biliary duct due to the compression of the hydatid cyst. Such necrosis may lead to a communication between the cyst and the biliary system. The second one suggests that small biliary radicals, which are trapped in the pericystic membrane, become atrophic due to the cystic pressure and rupture eventually [11]. Even though some studies stated communication rates up to 90% during the cysts evolution, the reported incidence of clinical CBC is only 13–37% [8, 11].

There are two types of CBC, **frank** (major, ≥5 mm) and **occult** (minor, <5 mm) CBC [6]. Frank CBC is a wide communication between the cyst and the biliary system. Since intracystic pressure is higher than the biliary pressure, frank CBC allows the cystic contents such as daughter cysts or membrane fragments to enter the biliary system and leads to clinical symptoms like **obstructive jaundice, cholangitis, cyst infection, or anaphylaxis**. Its incidence varies between 3 and 17% in liver hydatid cyst patients [6, 11]. If frank CBC is wider than 5 mm, cystic contents can be seen in the bile ducts during the preoperative evaluation in up to 65% of the patients [11]. Therefore, frank CBC can be diagnosed preoperatively, and treatment can be planned accordingly. By contrast, occult CBC is a smaller communication between the cyst and the biliary radicals. Its incidence varies between 10 and 37% of the patients with liver hydatid cyst [6, 12]. It is usually asymptomatic at the preoperative period, and thus, it is difficult to diagnose. So, careful intraoperative evaluation and postoperative follow-up are needed to overcome the consequences of this morbidity. It is reported that lower postoperative morbidity and bile leakage rates are achieved when the diagnosis is made in the pre- or intraoperative periods [11, 13].

2. Preoperative evaluation

Preoperative evaluation for CBC is essential for liver hydatid surgery, since diagnosis directly affects the treatment plan and the surgical outcome. Diagnosing a frank CBC is easy when a patient presents with symptoms of cholangitis and obstructive jaundice. However, occult CBC is usually asymptomatic and clinical suspicion is essential for its diagnosis. There are few studies investigating the predictive factors for CBC. While Akcan et al. reported that older age, larger cysts, and presence of multiple and bilobar cysts are associated with increased intrabiliary rupture rates, El Nakeeb et al. suggested that only the cyst size (>10 cm) is a significant predictor for CBC, regardless of the type [10, 14]. Because clinical presentation differs between frank and occult CBC, preoperative evaluation will be discussed separately.

2.1. Frank CBC evaluation

Frank CBC can be diagnosed preoperatively. In an unruptured cyst, the intracystic pressure is between 30 and 80 cm H_2O, while the normal intrabiliary pressure is 15 and 20 cm H_2O. When a frank CBC develops, intracystic materials like daughter cysts and membrane fragments, along with the hydatid fluid, enter the biliary ducts as a consequence of the pressure gradient toward the biliary system [8]. Hydatid material in the bile ducts leads to clinical symptoms. Obstructive jaundice can be seen in 57–100% and cholangitis in 20–37% of the patients. Without treatment, both may lead to sepsis and death, with mortality rates as high as 50% [12]. Acute pancreatitis, acute cholecystitis, and, as a late complication, biliary cirrhosis have also been reported [15–17].

In 30–74% of the cases, diagnosis can be made by ultrasonography (US) [11]. Irregular linear echogenic structures without acoustic shadowing in bile duct and a dilated biliary system are ultrasonographic findings in cases with intrabiliary-ruptured frank CBC [6]. The sensitivity of computed tomography (CT) for the diagnosis of frank CBC is 75% [11]. Hydatid materials in the bile ducts or a cystic wall defect due to a frank CBC can be seen via CT. In 75% of the cases, cyst wall discontinuity can be seen as a direct sign of CBC [18]. Magnetic resonance cholangiopancreatography (MRCP) is another alternative and more effective method for the preoperative diagnosis of the suspected cases [18]. For frank CBC diagnosis, MRCP has 92% sensitivity and 83% specificity [11].

There are some clinical predictors described for the presence of frank CBC (**Table 1**) [12]. In our review of 301 cases, our analysis also showed that a high preoperative alkaline phosphatase (ALP), history of cholangitis, and a larger cyst diameter (>10 cm) were significantly more common in patients who developed postoperative biliary fistula (PBF) [19].

Clinical predictors
History of jaundice
Central location of large cysts >10 cm
Presence of suggestive USG findings
Type IV (Gharbi classification) or CE4 (WHO-IWGE Classification) cyst on USG

Table 1. Clinical predictors of frank CBC.

In cases of clinical suspicion and presence of predictive factors, further studies can be planned such as MRCP or endoscopic retrograde cholangiopancreatography (ERCP). Because MRCP is a noninvasive test, it can be used as a primary method for the diagnosis. After confirmation of CBC diagnosis, ERCP can also be used for treatment [20].

ERCP can be used for both diagnostic and therapeutic purposes. It has 86–100% diagnostic sensitivity for frank CBC. It serves for (i) the treatment of acute conditions to defer for elective surgery, (ii) decreasing the postoperative complication rates and achieving shorter postoperative hospitalization time, and (iii) evacuation of biliary and cystic hydatid contents [20]. ERCP with endoscopic sphincterotomy (ES) is the first line of treatment for patients presenting with jaundice or findings of IBR [11]. In case of documented CBC, it helps with planning the elective surgery and prevention of intraoperative common bile duct exploration during the operation [10–12]. Additionally, lower postoperative biliary fistula rates were reported with preoperative ERCP with ES [11]. Performing ERCP with ES prior to surgery decreases the risk from 11.1 to 7.6% for postoperative biliary fistula [21]. It was also reported that 25% of the patients with frank CBC have been cured with ERCP without the need for further surgery [20]. In addition to ES, extraction with balloon or basket catheter, nasobiliary drainage, and biliary stenting can be used as therapeutic tools during ERCP [20].

2.2. Occult CBC evaluation

Occult CBC is hard to diagnose preoperatively since a small communication usually cannot be seen on radiologic studies [12, 22, 23]. Most of the cases are asymptomatic until surgery or postoperative period when it presents as bile leakage and fistula. The flow gradient of contents is toward the biliary system in an unruptured cyst. As a result, small biliary radicals are compressed with the pressure and remain silent until the gradient is reversed. The median intracystic pressure is around 25 mm Hg (range, 5–55 mm Hg) and there is a positive correlation between cyst size and pressure in viable cysts. Manometric studies indicate that the sphincter of Oddi pressure (basal 10 mmHg, peak 124 mmHg) is higher than the normal common bile duct pressure (10 mmHg). According to the LaPlace Law, the expansion of the cyst due to increased intracystic pressure results in an increased cyst diameter, which causes increased tension on the cyst wall containing the neighboring bile ducts. The pressure dynamics arising from higher intracystic pressures than the resting bile duct pressure may explain how the cyst communicates with the biliary system as the pericyst becomes thinner and thinner, eventually eroding into the bile ducts and leading to the development of an IBR [19]. During an operation with conservative approach, bile staining of the cystic content during first aspiration cannot be seen in most cases. Once the gradient is reversed with aspiration and evacuation of the cystic content, bile leakage begins [8]. So, the principal evaluation of occult CBC must be undertaken during surgery. Even with an attempt to control a detected BF intraoperatively, there might be a significant failure rate if that was used as the only method to control the cyst-biliary communication [19].

However, there are some clinical predictors described for the presence of occult CBC (**Table 2**) [8, 12]. Taking these predictors into consideration, a clinical suspicion can further lead to evaluation for an occult CBC. However, unlike frank CBC, diagnostic sensitivity of MRCP and ERCP is low [12]. In cases with high suspicion, preoperative ERCP with ES can be done to decrease the postoperative leakage rate and to determine the biliary anatomy [20]. Yet, this is not a standard therapeutic modality.

A diagnostic and therapeutic algorithm for preoperative evaluation of CBC can be seen in **Figure 3**.

History of nausea and vomiting
ALP level >144 U/L
gamma-glutamyltransferase (GGT) level >34.5 U/L
Total bilirubin level >0.8 mg/dL
Direct bilirubin level >0.4 mg/dL
Eosinophil rate >0.09
Cyst diameter >8.5 cm
Multilocular cysts (Gharbi type III)
Degenerate cysts (Gharbi type IV or WHO-IWGE CE4)

*The data in this table are derived from different studies having common and uncommon predictive parameters and among similar parameters, ones with the lowest cut-offs were selected to aim for the widest patient range [8, 12].

Table 2. Clinical predictors of occult CBC*.

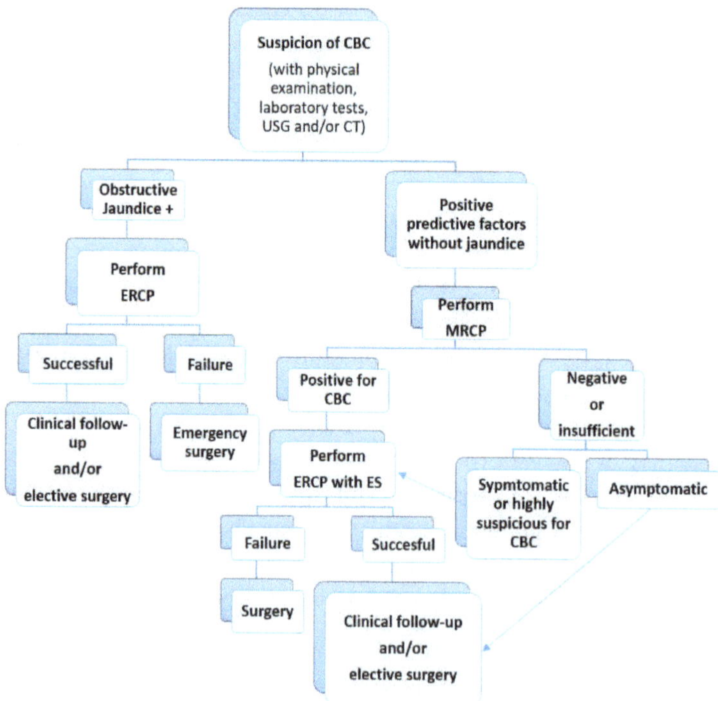

Figure 3. Diagnostic and therapeutic algorithm for preoperative evaluation of CBC.

3. Operative decision making

Radical surgical techniques should be undertaken whenever feasible because of their lower postoperative morbidity and recurrence rates [5, 8, 11]. In the last decade, major liver surgery became much more safer with very low morbidity and mortality rates. The decision making is usually complex with various factors interplaying different roles. Patient-related factors with general condition and comorbidities, liver parenchymal quality (steatosis, age, diabetes, etc.), and center expertise are leading factors. On the other hand, these factors, taken together, may pose a higher risk for a benign disease unless complicated [11]. As a result, conservative approaches are still the most common method applied, especially in the endemic regions [8]. Among all the conservative methods, partial cystectomy with omentoplasty has the lowest reported postoperative leakage rate [1, 24]. In our center, we favor anatomical liver resections whenever feasible, especially in patients with frank CBC.

4. Intraoperative evaluation

Frank CBC is usually easy to diagnose intraoperatively. The communication should be sutured whenever feasible. If it is diagnosed with MRCP or ERCP preoperatively, it is essential to understand the type and anatomical location of the communication of the duct with the cyst. If the frank communication is related with the primary or secondary biliary pedicules, suture closure of the communication could lead to biliary obstruction for distal branches [12]. In such cases, conversion to radical surgery, biliary drainage procedures like t-tube drainage or choledochoduodenostomy or postoperative ERCP and ES with or without biliary stenting/nasobiliary drainage should be considered [11]. In patients with frank CBC without preoperative evaluation, cholangiography or choledochoscopy can be performed before and after the evacuation of hydatid material in bile ducts. After that, placing a t-tube and closure over t-tube or decompression through cystic duct can be preferred [8, 11]. It is reported that when a communication is wider than 5 mm, hydatid material in biliary system can be seen in 65% of the cases [25]. For that reason, an intraoperative cholangiography via the communication, cystic duct, or common bile duct can be done in patients without preoperative ERCP [12].

Careful evaluation should be done to diagnose occult CBC. At the first aspiration of the hydatid cyst fluid, bile staining should be checked. If the fluid is positive for bile, a surgeon should avoid using scolicidal agents to prevent sclerosing cholangitis [2, 6, 11]. After evacuation of the hydatid material in the cyst cavity, careful inspection for bile leakage should be done inside the cavity. Using a coloring scolicidal agent like povidone iodine can be a handicap for this purpose [8]. On the other hand, using a non-coloring scolocidal agent like hypertonic saline or chlorhexidine may increase diagnostic accuracy. If a communication is found, it should be sutured [11].

Surgical telescopes with 2.5 × or 3.5 × magnification can enhance the quality of inspection. In cases of negative inspection for bile leakage, there are several methods for additional evaluation. The simplest method is filling the cavity with gauze [8]. In addition, manual clamping of the main bile duct can provoke bile staining through the communication by increasing intrabiliary pressure. When discovered, occult CBCs should also be sutured. Another method described especially for large and multilobar cysts, which can be at difficult locations for inspection, is using a videotelescope [26]. The rotation and magnification abilities of the videotelescope facilitate a more precise diagnosis, especially in multilobar and deep localized cavities. Endoscopic instruments can also be used for suturation of unreachable communications [26].

When bile staining is present but the communication cannot be localized, there are two options: external drainage from cavity can be performed and postoperative ERCP with ES can be scheduled or, as a more invasive option, methylene blue or air injection with or without intraoperative cholangiography can be performed [11, 12]. In such cases, cholangiography can be performed via cystic duct or main bile duct [12]. A cholecystectomy is needed to perform a transcystic cholangiography. If the patient has cholelithiasis or the gallbladder wall constitutes the cyst wall, then transcystic approach should be preferred. Otherwise, cholangiography through the main duct with a thin-needled syringe—like insulin syringe—should be done. Separately, or in addition to cholangiography, methylene blue or air injection through cholangiography access should be done for detecting the localization of the communication [11, 12, 27]. With methylene blue injection, covering of the cavity with gauze technique can be used for localization. If air injection is preferred, filling the cavity with saline should be done. Next, air bubbles in the cavity must be checked for the presence of a communication.

If a frank or occult CBC has been detected intraoperatively and the patient has not been evaluated preoperatively with MRCP or ERCP, cholangiography should be performed for the presence of hydatid material in the biliary system. In cases with hydatid material, choledochotomy should be done and after evacuation of the hydatid material, t-tube drainage should be performed for further access and evaluation. In cases of biliary stricture, choledochoduodenostomy may be preferred. Intraoperative ERCP can be a less invasive approach in available centers [14, 20].

In all cases that underwent conservative hydatid liver surgery, continuous suturation of pericystectomy line can be used to eliminate the risk of leakage from biliary radicals at pericystic wall and an external drainage catheter should be placed at the entrance or in the cavity to avoid the risk of uncontrolled postoperative biliary leakage and biliary peritonitis.

In some series, fibrin sealant usage to prevent postoperative biliary leakage is used, but controversial results have been reported. Therefore, efficacy of fibrin sealant is still questionable [5, 9].

5. Postoperative evaluation

A close follow-up should be done at the postoperative period for complications. In acute conditions, necessary interventions should be planned promptly. Emergency laparotomy is indicated if the patient has biliary peritonitis. Peritoneal irrigation, correction of leakage by suturation or more radical methods as needed and maintaining an adequate external drainage should be performed accordingly. If bile leakage persists after the operation, ERCP with ES and biliary stenting should be considered [20].

In cases of postoperative jaundice, first therapeutic modality should be ERCP with ES and evacuation of the hydatid contents within the bile ducts [20]. If ERCP fails, then bile duct exploration with t-tube drainage or choledochoduodenostomy should be considered.

Biliomas should be evaluated with percutaneous drainage first. When biliary leakage persists, then ERCP with ES should be scheduled [20].

The most common postoperative complication of hydatid liver surgery is bile leakage and fistula formation as mentioned before. In such cases, every effort should be made at the preoperative and intraoperative period to decrease its rates. When postoperative bile fistula is present, it is essential to determine the flow rate of fistula. In low-flow fistulas (flow rate of <300 ml/day), conservative follow-up for 3 weeks is appropriate since most of low-flow fistulas close spontaneously in this period [8, 9]. If the fistula persists after 3 weeks, then ERCP

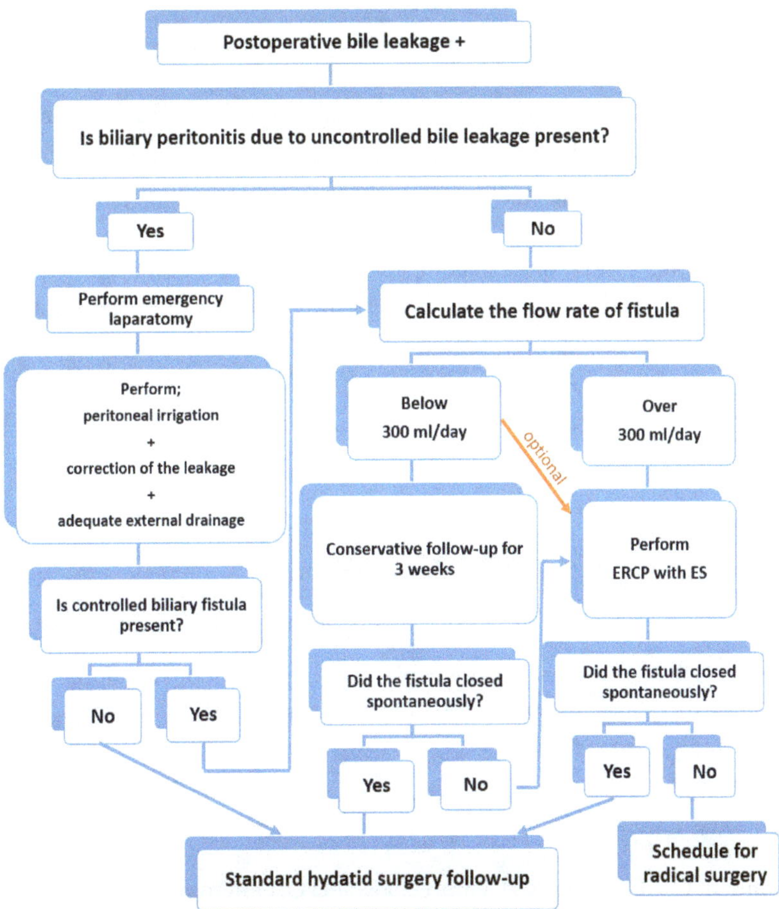

Figure 4. Therapeutic algorithm for postoperative bile leakage.

with ES should be planned [8, 10, 11]. In high-flow fistulas (>300 ml/day), spontaneous closure of the fistula is unlikely; thus, ERCP with ES should be performed without delay [8, 20]. The success rate of ERCP is very high (90%) [11]. Most of the fistulas close in the first week after ERCP [8]. Spontaneous closure of a fistula from a calcified cyst wall is usually unexpected [2]. In our series, PBF occurred in 46 (16%) patients, despite preoperative and operative efforts to prevent this complication. The fistula closed spontaneously in only 12 (26%) of the patients with PBF without further intervention, confirming that patients with PBF often have a complicated postoperative course, requiring multiple endoscopic and other interventional procedures with serious morbidity and mortality [19].

In a small group of patients in whom all interventions fail, as repeated ERCP and stenting, radical surgery could be an alternative for the correction of the leakage [6, 28]. A therapeutic algorithm for postoperative bile leakage evaluation is offered in **Figure 4**.

6. Conclusion

Hydatid liver surgery is still one of the main indications for liver surgery in endemic regions. It is hard to refer all patients to an experienced hepatobiliary surgery center due to high volume of disease in those regions. As a result, conservative methods are still preferred therapeutic modalities for many surgeons.

Cystobiliary communication is the most common complication of hydatid liver disease. Without appropriate evaluation and intervention, this will eventually lead to postoperative bile leakage and fistula formation, a major cause of morbidity and mortality. By that means, every effort should be made to detect and prevent these complications during the evaluation and management of cystic echinococcosis liver disease.

Author details

Can Konca[1] and Deniz Balcı[2*]

*Address all correspondence to: denizbalci1@yahoo.com

1 Department of General Surgery, Ankara University School of Medicine, Ankara, Turkey

2 Department of General Surgery and Transplantation Division of Hepatopancreatobiliary Surgery, Ankara University School of Medicine, Ankara, Turkey

References

[1] Mihmanli M, Idiz UO, Kaya C, Demir U, Bostanci O, Omeroglu S, Bozkurt E. Current status of diagnosis and treatment of hepatic echinococcosis. World Journal of Hepatology. 2016;8(28):1169-1181

[2] Brunetti E, Kern P, Vuitton DA, Writing Panel for the WHO-IWGE. Expert consensus for the diagnosis and treatment of cystic and alveolar echinococcosis in humans. Acta Tropica. 2010;**114**(1):1-16

[3] Junghanss T, da Silva AM, Horton J, Chiodini PL, Brunetti E. Clinical management of cystic echinococcosis: State of the art, problems, and perspectives. American Journal of Tropical Medicine and Hygiene. 2008;**79**(3):301-311

[4] Guidelines for treatment of cystic and alveolar echinococcosis in humans. WHO Informal Working Group on Echinococcosis. Bulletin of the World Health Organization. 1996;**74**(3):231-242

[5] Gomez IGC, Lopez-Andujar R, Belda Ibanez T, Ramia Angel JM Moya Herraiz A, Orbis Castellanos F, Pareja Ibars E, San Juan Rodriguez F. Review of the treatment of liver hydatid cysts. World Journal of Gastroenterology. 2015;**21**(1):124-131

[6] Sozuer E, Akyuz M, Akbulut S. Open surgery for hepatic hydatid disease. International Surgery. 2014;**99**(6):764-769

[7] Chautems R, Buhler LH, Gold B, Giostra E, Poletti P, Chilcott M, Morel P, Mentha G. Surgical management and long-term outcome of complicated liver hydatid cysts caused by *Echinococcus granulosus*. Surgery. 2005;**137**(3):312-316

[8] Demircan O, Baymus M, Seydaoglu G, Akinoglu A, Sakman G. Occult cystobiliary communication presenting as postoperative biliary leakage after hydatid liver surgery: Are there significant preoperative clinical predictors? Canadian Journal of Surgery. 2006;**49**(3):177-184

[9] Atahan K, Kupeli H, Deniz M, Gur S, Cokmez A, Tarcan E. Can occult cystobiliary fistulas in hepatic hydatid disease be predicted before surgery? International Journal of Medical Sciences. 2011;**8**(4):315-320

[10] El Nakeeb A, Salem A, El Sorogy M, Mahdy Y, Ellatif MA, Moneer A, Said R, El Ghawalby A, Ezzat H. Cystobiliary communication in hepatic hydatid cyst: Predictors and outcome. The Turkish Journal of Gastroenterology: The Official Journal of Turkish Society of Gastroenterology. 2017;**28**:125-130

[11] Ramia JM, Figueras J, De la Plaza R, Garcia-Parreno J. Cysto-biliary communication in liver hydatidosis. Langenbeck's Archives of Surgery. 2012;**397**(6):881-887

[12] Atli M, Kama NA, Yuksek YN, Doganay M, Gozalan U, Kologlu M, Daglar G. Intrabiliary rupture of a hepatic hydatid cyst: Associated clinical factors and proper management. Archives of Surgery. 2001;**136**(11):1249-1255

[13] Prousalidis J, Kosmidis C, Kapoutzis K, Fachantidis E, Harlaftis N, Aletras H. Intrabiliary rupture of hydatid cysts of the liver. The American Journal of Surgery. 2009;**197**(2):193-198

[14] Akcan A, Sozuer E, Akyildiz H, Ozturk A, Atalay A, Yilmaz Z. Predisposing factors and surgical outcome of complicated liver hydatid cysts. World Journal of Gastroenterology. 2010;**16**(24):3040-3048

[15] Kattan YB. Intrabiliary rupture of hydatid cyst of the liver. Annals of the Royal College of Surgeons of England. 1977;**59**(2):108-114

[16] Saez-Royuela F, Yuguero L, Lopez-Morante A, Perez-Alvarez JC, Martin-Lorente JL, Ojeda C. Acute pancreatitis caused by hydatid membranes in the biliary tract: Treatment with endoscopic sphincterotomy. Gastrointestinal Endoscopy. 1999;**49**(6):793-796

[17] Abou-Khalil S, Smith BM, MacLean JD, Poenaru D, Fried GM, Bret P, Barkun AN. Acute cholecystitis and cholangitis caused by *Echinococcus granulosus.* The American Journal of Gastroenterology. 1996;**91**(4):805-807

[18] Ormeci N, Kir M, Coban S, Emrehan Tuzun A, Ekiz F, Erdem H, Palabiyikoglu M, Dokmeci A. The usefulness of endoscopic retrograde cholangiopancreatography and (99m)Tc-labeled albumin macroaggregates in diagnosing hydatid disease fistulae. Digestive Diseases and Sciences. 2007;**52**(6):1410-1414

[19] Zeybek N, Dede H, Balci D, Coskun AK, Ozerhan IH, Peker S, Peker Y. Biliary fistula after treatment for hydatid disease of the liver: When to intervene. World Journal of Gastroenterology. 2013;**19**(3):355-361

[20] Dolay K, Akbulut S. Role of endoscopic retrograde cholangiopancreatography in the management of hepatic hydatid disease. World Journal of Gastroenterology. 2014;**20**(41): 15253-15261

[21] Galati G, Sterpetti AV, Caputo M, Adduci M, Lucandri G, Brozzetti S, Bolognese A, Cavallaro A. Endoscopic retrograde cholangiography for intrabiliary rupture of hydatid cyst. The American Journal of Surgery. 2006;**191**(2):206-210

[22] Ozaslan E, Bayraktar Y. Endoscopic therapy in the management of hepatobiliary hydatid disease. Journal of Clinical Gastroenterology. 2002;**35**(2):160-174

[23] Spiliadis C, Georgopoulos S, Dailianas A, Konstantinidis A, Rimikis M, Skandalis N. The use of ERCP in the study of patients with hepatic echinococcosis before and after surgical intervention. Gastrointestinal Endoscopy. 1996;**43**(6):575-579

[24] Mentes A, Yuzer Y, Ozbal O, Coker A, Ilter T, Musoglu A. Omentoplasty versus introflexion for hydatid liver cysts. Journal of the Royal College of Surgeons of Edinburgh. 1993;**38**(2):82-85

[25] Zaouche A, Haouet K, Jouini M, El Hachaichi A, Dziri C. Management of liver hydatid cysts with a large biliocystic fistula: Multicenter retrospective study. Tunisian Surgical Association. World Journal of Surgery. 2001;**25**(1):28-39

[26] Ozmen MM, Coskun F. New technique for finding the ruptured bile duct into the liver cysts: Scope in the cave technique. Surgical Laparoscopy, Endoscopy & Percutaneous Techniques. 2002;**12**(3):187-189

[27] Kayaalp C, Sengul N, Akoglu M. Importance of cyst content in hydatid liver surgery. Archives of Surgery. 2002;**137**(2):159-163

[28] Akcakaya A, Sahin M, Karakelleoglu A, Okan I. Endoscopic stenting for selected cases of biliary fistula after hepatic hydatid surgery. Surgical Endoscopy and Other Interventional Techniques. 2006;**20**(9):1415-1418

Permissions

All chapters in this book were first published by InTech Open; hereby published with permission under the Creative Commons Attribution License or equivalent. Every chapter published in this book has been scrutinized by our experts. Their significance has been extensively debated. The topics covered herein carry significant findings which will fuel the growth of the discipline. They may even be implemented as practical applications or may be referred to as a beginning point for another development.

The contributors of this book come from diverse backgrounds, making this book a truly international effort. This book will bring forth new frontiers with its revolutionizing research information and detailed analysis of the nascent developments around the world.

We would like to thank all the contributing authors for lending their expertise to make the book truly unique. They have played a crucial role in the development of this book. Without their invaluable contributions this book wouldn't have been possible. They have made vital efforts to compile up to date information on the varied aspects of this subject to make this book a valuable addition to the collection of many professionals and students.

This book was conceptualized with the vision of imparting up-to-date information and advanced data in this field. To ensure the same, a matchless editorial board was set up. Every individual on the board went through rigorous rounds of assessment to prove their worth. After which they invested a large part of their time researching and compiling the most relevant data for our readers.

The editorial board has been involved in producing this book since its inception. They have spent rigorous hours researching and exploring the diverse topics which have resulted in the successful publishing of this book. They have passed on their knowledge of decades through this book. To expedite this challenging task, the publisher supported the team at every step. A small team of assistant editors was also appointed to further simplify the editing procedure and attain best results for the readers.

Apart from the editorial board, the designing team has also invested a significant amount of their time in understanding the subject and creating the most relevant covers. They scrutinized every image to scout for the most suitable representation of the subject and create an appropriate cover for the book.

The publishing team has been an ardent support to the editorial, designing and production team. Their endless efforts to recruit the best for this project, has resulted in the accomplishment of this book. They are a veteran in the field of academics and their pool of knowledge is as vast as their experience in printing. Their expertise and guidance has proved useful at every step. Their uncompromising quality standards have made this book an exceptional effort. Their encouragement from time to time has been an inspiration for everyone.

The publisher and the editorial board hope that this book will prove to be a valuable piece of knowledge for researchers, students, practitioners and scholars across the globe.

List of Contributors

Myriam Oudni-M'rad and Selim M'rad
LP3M: Laboratory of Medical and Molecular Parasitology-Mycology, LR12ES08, Faculty of Pharmacy, University of Monastir, Monastir, Tunisia

Hamouda Babba
LP3M: Laboratory of Medical and Molecular Parasitology-Mycology, LR12ES08, Faculty of Pharmacy, University of Monastir, Monastir, Tunisia
Laboratory of Parasitology, teaching hospital F. Bourguiba, Monastir, Tunisia

Ana Flisser
Departamento de Microbiologia y Parasitologia, Facultad de Medicina, Universidad Nacional Autonoma de Mexico, DF, Mexico

Pablo Maravilla and Fernando Martinez-Hernandez
Departamento de Ecologia de Agentes Patogenos, Hospital General "Dr. Manuel Gea Gonzalez", Secretaria de Salud, DF, Mexico

Pilar Mata-Miranda
Coordinación Auxiliar de Investigación en Salud, Delegación Veracruz Norte, Xalapa, Veracruz, Mexico

Alfonso J. Rodriguez-Morales
Public Health and Infection Research Group, School of Medicine and School of Veterinary Medicine and Zootechnics, Faculty of Health Sciences, Universidad Tecnológica de Pereira, Pereira, Risaralda, Colombia
Committee on Zoonoses and Haemorrhagic Fevers, Asociación Colombiana de Infectología, Bogotá, DC, Colombia
Working Group on Zoonoses, International Society for Chemotherapy, Aberdeen, United Kingdom

Lauren Sofia Calvo-Betancourt
Fundación Cardiovascular de Colombia, Floridablanca, Santander, Colombia

Camila Alarcón-Olave
Universidad Autónoma de Bucaramanga, Bucaramanga, Santander, Colombia

Adrián Bolívar-Mejía
Clínica FOSCAL Internacional, Floridablanca, Santander, Colombia

Shukun Yang
Image Diagnosis Department, The First Peoples' Hospital of Yinchuan City, Ningxia Hui Autonomous Region (NHAR), P.R. China

Yumin Zhao
Human Pathological Department of Guiling Medical College, Guilin City, Guangxi Province, P.R. China

Don Peter McManus
Molecular Parasitology Laboratory, QIMR Berghofer Medical Research Institute, Brisbane, Australia

YuRong Yang
Human Pathology & Immunology Department, Ningxia Medical University, Yinchuan City, Ningxia Hui Autonomous Region (NHAR), P.R. China
Ningxia Medical University, Yinchuan, Ningxia Hui Autonomous Region, P.R. of China
Molecular Parasitology Laboratory, QIMR Berghofer Medical Research Institute, Brisbane, Australia

Antonio Di Cataldo, Stefano Puleo, Amy Giarrizzo, Martina Calabrini, Rosalia Latino, Rosanna Portale, Antonella Agodi, Martina Barchitta and Annalisa Quattrocchi
Department of Medical and Surgical Sciences, Advanced Technologies GF Ingrassia, University of Catania, Italy

Giuseppe Petrillo, Claudia Trombatore and Stefano Palmucci
Radiodiagnostic and Radiotherapy Unit, University Hospital Policlinico-Vittorio Emanuele, Catania, Italy

Nunzio Crimi and Silvia Fichera
Department of Respiratory Diseases and Allergology, University of Catania, Italy

Said Hilmani
Neurosurgical Department, Hassan II University, Casablanca, Morocco

Dilek Emlik, Kemal Ödev, Necdet Poyraz and Hasan Emin Kaya
Necmettin Erbakan University, Meram Medicine School, Department of Radiology, Meram, Konya, Turkey

Adel Spotin
Department of Parasitology and Mycology, Tabriz University of Medical Sciences, Tabriz, Iran

Santosh Kumar and Shivanshu Singh
Advanced Urology Center, Department of Urology, Postgraduate Institute of Medical Education and Research, Chandigarh, India

Emília Dvorožňáková
Institute of Parasitology, Slovak Academy of Sciences, Košice, Slovak Republic

Angeliki Vidoura, Dimitris Zacharoulis and Mariana Parisidou
University of Thessaly, Larissa, Greece

Christina Chatedaki
Department of Microbiology, University Hospital of Larissa, Larissa, Greece

Can Konca
Department of General Surgery, Ankara University School of Medicine, Ankara, Turkey

Deniz Balcı
Department of General Surgery and Transplantation Division of Hepatopancreatobiliary Surgery, Ankara University School of Medicine, Ankara, Turkey

Index

A

Albendazole, 25-27, 40-41, 57-58, 62-66, 70, 103, 115, 117, 156-158, 177, 187, 189, 193, 199-201, 206-207, 210-211, 213, 218-219, 223-224

Alopecia, 65-66, 103, 157-158, 188-189

Alveolar Echinococcosis, 4-5, 17, 47-50, 53-54, 61-62, 65-66, 68-70, 74, 84-87, 92-93, 102-103, 106-107, 109, 141-142, 163-164, 171, 174-177, 179-185, 187-189, 192-193, 196-197, 199-209, 212-221, 228, 239

Anaphylaxis, 64, 69-70, 102-103, 106-107, 157-158, 167-168, 224, 227, 231

Animal Husbandry, 16-17, 47-48

Antibiotics, 24-25, 189, 209

Antiparasitic Drug, 74, 198-199

B

Benzimidazole, 103, 106-107, 183, 188-189, 213, 224

Bile Leakage, 63-64, 222, 227, 229-231, 233, 235, 237-238

C

Cestodes, 21, 41, 46-48, 71-72, 74, 76, 109

Chest Pain, 7, 59-60, 80, 120

Cholecystectomy, 24-25, 236

Computed Tomography, 24-25, 60, 122, 133-136, 150, 155-156, 162-164, 174-175, 232

Coproantigens, 23, 32-33

Cystic Echinococcosis, 3-6, 9, 15-21, 23-25, 39-45, 47-48, 52-54, 58-60, 62, 65-66, 68-70, 72-75, 79-80, 82-84, 95, 102-107, 109, 114-115, 149, 163-164, 167-168, 172-175, 180-186, 213, 223-224, 228-229, 238-239

Cystic Lesions, 87, 91-93, 96-99, 113, 117-118, 127-128, 153-154, 222

Cytokines, 74, 77, 82, 87, 175, 183, 187-189, 191-193, 196-197, 199, 203, 209, 217

D

Daughter Cysts, 51-52, 63-64, 96-99, 111, 126, 128-134, 140, 150, 153-154, 157-158, 160, 162, 223-224, 231-232

Dyspnea, 59-60, 119-120

E

Echinococcus Granulosus, 4-5, 17-25, 39-45, 47-48, 53-54, 58, 70, 74, 83-85, 88-89, 91-93, 102-103, 105, 118, 141-142, 150, 166, 171-173, 180-185, 222, 239-240

Echinococcus Ortleppi, 23, 26-27, 38-39

Endemic Areas, 3-5, 52, 56, 81, 92-93, 95, 104-105, 119-120, 123-124, 143-144, 172-173, 222, 229

Eosinophilia, 61-62, 114-115, 153-154, 196-197, 209

Epidemiological Survey, 23

Epidemiology, 1, 3, 5-7, 14-15, 18-19, 26-27, 41, 66, 68, 72, 83, 85, 92-93, 110-111, 138, 146, 172-173, 180-181, 184-186

F

Fibrosis, 79-80, 188-189, 204-205, 212-213, 217, 219, 225

G

Genitourinary Echinococcosis, 150-152, 162

Genitourinary Tract, 150-152, 154

Genotype, 4-9, 11, 13-17, 19, 24-25, 32-33, 38-41, 95, 105, 143-144, 148, 181

Germinal Layer, 26-27, 63-64, 78-79, 150-152, 160, 162, 222, 224

Glucan, 187, 189, 199-205, 212-215, 217-219

Gravid Proglottid, 75, 140

H

Helminthic Disease, 24-25, 96-97

Hemagglutination, 120, 153-154

Hemoptysis, 7, 59-60, 119-120

Hepatic Parenchyma, 224-225

Hepatitis, 110-111, 188-189, 219

Hepatomegaly, 24-25, 59-60, 174-175

Hydatid Cysts, 6-7, 13-15, 20-21, 23, 29-31, 33, 39, 42-43, 47-50, 56, 58, 72-73, 94-95, 97-99, 101, 103, 107-111, 113, 115-122, 127-128, 130-137, 151-154, 157-158, 160, 162-164, 166, 169, 181, 223, 227, 230, 239-240

Hydatid Disease, 19-21, 41-43, 46-48, 54, 67-72, 85, 88, 91-97, 99-101, 104-111, 117-120, 123-124, 127-128, 130, 133-137, 150-152, 157-158, 163-169, 178-183, 185, 212-213, 222, 224, 226-228, 239-240

Hydatidosis, 3-9, 16-17, 19, 21, 43, 52-54, 56, 69-70, 92-93, 98-99, 102-103, 107, 117-118, 127-128, 130, 134, 136, 152, 156, 164-166, 171, 174-175, 186, 228, 239

Hydaturia, 151-152

Hypertension, 97, 100-101, 106-107, 110-111, 116-117, 152

I

Iliac Fossa, 160-162

Immune Response, 79, 81, 96-97, 106-107, 175-177, 183, 187-189, 192-193, 196-197, 199-201, 203-205, 207, 210-213, 215, 217, 219-221

Immunoelectrophoresis, 120

Immunotherapy, 74, 82, 88, 187, 190-191, 193-195, 199, 201-207, 209-211, 220-221

Intermediate Host, 48, 50-52, 56, 71-72, 75, 78-79, 81, 86, 110-111, 118, 143-144, 176-177, 187-189, 192-193

Intestinal Tapeworm, 23, 48

K

Kidneys, 29, 58, 150-152, 223

L

Laparoscopic Surgery, 25-27, 63-64, 161-162, 224

Larval Stage, 4-5, 24-25, 31, 56, 187

Leukopenia, 61-62, 157-158

Light Microscopy, 26-27, 49-50

Liver, 3-9, 12-13, 23, 25-27, 29, 31, 33, 40-43, 46, 48-52, 57-66, 68-73, 127-128, 130, 136-137, 150-152, 156, 166-169, 172-177, 181-183, 188-193, 198-199, 204-205, 214-215, 217, 219-226, 228-232, 235-240

Livestock, 5, 9, 12-15, 20-21, 23-25, 28-29, 31-33, 35, 47-48, 58, 71-72, 75, 79, 81, 93, 109, 145-146, 149, 172-173

Lungs, 3-7, 13, 33, 48-52, 58, 60, 75, 80, 91-97, 100-101, 110-111, 118, 120-122, 135-136, 172-175, 223

M

Macrophages, 187-189, 191-193, 196-201, 203-207, 210-217

Magnetic Resonance Imaging, 60, 80, 154, 174-175

Malaise, 24-27, 60, 151-152

Malnutrition, 77, 174-175

Mebendazole, 64-66, 103, 107, 213, 223

Mediastinum, 95, 100-101, 120, 122, 128, 131-134, 137, 169

Medical Therapy, 64, 150-152, 156-158, 160, 162, 223

Metacestode, 4-5, 48-50, 58, 68, 74, 76-77, 79, 139-140, 187-191, 196-197, 204-205, 207, 212-213

Muramyltripeptide, 187, 192-193, 215

N

Necropsy, 14-15, 26-27, 33

O

Omentoplasty, 223-225, 230-231, 235, 240

P

Parasite, 5-9, 12-13, 19-21, 26-27, 29, 31-33, 37, 40-41, 48-50, 59-62, 68, 75-82, 85-88, 92-99, 102-103, 105, 109-111, 115, 119-120, 123-124, 138, 151-154, 171-177, 183-185, 188-193, 195-205, 207, 210-215, 220-225, 227

Parasitic Zoonosis, 46-48, 92-93, 222

Parasitism, 74-76, 81, 85

Pathogenesis, 119-120, 173, 231

Pathophysiology, 79, 110-111

Pelvicalyceal System, 153-154, 157-158

Pericystic Membrane, 224-225, 230

Pleural Cavity, 99, 119-120, 130

Povidone Iodine, 157-158, 161-162, 224, 235

Praziquantel, 32-33, 63-66, 69-70, 81, 103, 156, 177, 188-189, 214-215, 219, 223

Protoscolices, 26-27, 51-52, 62-64, 78-79, 224

R

Radiography, 118, 120, 122, 124-126, 135-136

S

Scolicidal Agent, 25, 157-160, 162, 224, 235

Streptomycin, 189, 191

Surgical Excision, 151-152, 156, 161-162

Surgical Incidence, 4-5, 7, 19

Symptomatology, 29, 59-60, 152

T

Taeniidae, 17, 41, 47-48, 83, 109, 143-144, 148-149, 185

Thoracic Wall, 119-120, 131-132

U

Ultrasonography, 23, 60-62, 69-70, 73, 150, 162, 226, 232

Ultrasound, 8-9, 23, 28-29, 60, 62, 64, 68, 80, 91, 101, 110-111, 118, 130, 135-136, 141-142, 153-154, 157-158, 164, 166, 174-175, 181, 226

Z

Zoonotic Infection, 91, 171

www.ingramcontent.com/pod-product-compliance
Lightning Source LLC
LaVergne TN
LVHW062232200926
848484LV00006B/1520
9798887403618